- Prevent Alzheimer's disease the simple way •
- Dissolve fibrocystic tumors naturally •
- Beat psoriasis in three days! •

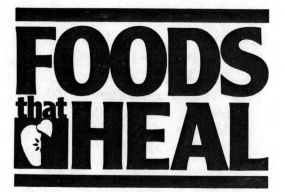

by
MAUREEN SALAMAN
and
JAMES F. SCHEER

M.K.S., Inc.

Published by
M.K.S., Inc.
1259 El Camino Real, Suite 1500
Menlo Park, CA 94025
Telephone: (415) 854-9355
FAX: (415) 854-9292

Printed by
BookCrafters

Last Printing July, 1994

Recipes and Cover Photo by
Jack Hanley

■ ISBN: 0-913087-025
Library of Congress Card No. 89-051450

DEDICATION

This book is dedicated to those valiant warriors — members, staff and board members of the National Health Federation — whose steadfast sacrifice has preserved these truths and to Jan Crouch, who inspired me to chronicle them.

IN GRATITUDE

The deepest gratitude a heart can feel goes to those who have helped me to know God better — these God-anointed messengers: Connie and Ronn Haus, Shirley and Kenny Foreman, Kenny Foreman, Jr., Steuart McBirnie, Dwight and Zonelle Thompson, Carla and Dick Bernal, and Mike Murdock.

INTRODUCTION

Let me introduce the book you are about to meet. "Foods That Heal" is different from any nutrition book you have ever read. It focuses on natural foods to help you stay well, keep well or to regain wellness.

What's so different about that?

Only that I have researched all over the world in person and on paper for the latest studies—many of them double-blind—on natural, God-given foods that contribute to prevention and healing. Some are based on folk medicine and plainly labeled as such.

When a single food will not suffice, I turn to a vitamin or mineral—or a combination of nutrients—which university research shows alleviates a particular physical condition. Then I list natural foods which contain the highest amounts of these nutrients.

Conspicuously absent are shellfish. Although oysters are the richest of all foods in zinc—160 mg for a helping of less than four ounces—they are omitted for a very good reason.

Shellfish can be hazardous to your health, because they nourish themselves with sewer-water loaded with industrial pollutants, bacteria and viruses. Outbreaks of gastroenteritis, infectious hepatitis, meningitis, polio, strep throat and typhoid fever have been traced to shellfish. Some authorities refer to the lobster as the cockroach of the sea. (I will offer this explanation again under the category of Acne, because it is the first ailment with which I deal.)

After the listings of nutrient-rich foods in most of the book's sections are specially crafted recipes utilizing them. Recipes are the creation of the celebrated gourmet cook Jack L. Hanley, my associate.

A distinctive aspect of the Hanley recipes is that, for the most part, they feature raw or lightly cooked natural foods. This is intentional, because cooking rearranges atoms and molecules and denatures protein. Non-cooked foods, for the most part, match our digestive tract better for maximum absorption. And greater absorption is the name of the game.

I stress natural, whole foods—not man-made foods such as margarine, egg substitutes, fractionated grain cereals, refined sugar and baked goods made from white flour and refined sugar.

Man-made, imitation foods are fine for imitation people. God-given, real foods are made for real people. I do not favor processed foods — canned and packaged — because they have lost too many needed nutrients, and they are embalmed with additives to give them greater shelf life — or shelf death — however you want to look at it.

Further, they have many hidden ingredients which can bring on food sensitivities and allergies. Illness is your body's typical response to man-made foods.

Cooperate with your body, and it will cooperate with you, making your visits to the doctor and hospital fewer and farther between. And, believe me, that is a distinct advantage. Norman Cousins has a great way of characterizing the institution of the hospital:

"...A hospital is no place for a person who is seriously ill."

Or anybody else, Norman.

Not long ago, somebody told us that he had seen statistics that patients' hospital stays were becoming shorter and shorter.

That's easy to believe. Patients will do anything to get away from that food.

Recently, I saw a survey in a reputable journal to the effect that patients who enter hospitals are usually malnourished and are even more malnourished when they leave, thanks to establishment dieticians.

Hospital food is a joke to everybody but those who have to consume it. Hospital dieticians should be sentenced to eat their own food.

Don't get me wrong. I am not against hospitals. They have to exist, but so do people. I love doctors. Some of my best friends are medical doctors — alternative practitioners.

The author does not intend for this book to substitute for or replace the doctor. As a matter of fact, over and over again, it advises readers to get needed medical care. However, it is a sad fact of life that most orthodox doctors are not as yet food-minded, despite the publication in leading medical journals of papers on preventive and therapeutic values of crucifer vegetables, beta carotene, fiber and various vitamins and minerals.

Can you imagine your phriendly phamily physician scribbling a prescription for one head of cabbage and a medium-size carrot before bedtime? Neither can I. Medicine and drug-oriented doctors are hardly the ones to offer the service of a Foods That Heal for the benefit of mankind.

That's why I did it. I enjoyed writing it for you. I hope you will enjoy reading it.

Maureen Salaman

TABLE OF CONTENTS

IN FRIENDSHIP

My life's most precious treasures, those who have been a pearl of great price, are my true friends. After this book goes to press, I'm sure I'll recall how remiss I've been in not listing many more, the "unforgettables" that I managed to forget. However, there will be other books.

Meanwhile, my thanks go out to the following for being my friends, for being a part of me and my life, and for being with me to share laughter and tears:

Gene Arceri, Karl Rolfes, Margaret Lesher, Dr. Steuart McBirnie, Dee & Glen Simmons, Anne Regel (Jim Regel, too); Jack L. Hanley, Jim Scheer, Peggy Boyd, Thelma Miller, Ruth McAnich, Lee Gruhn, Al and Lili Battista, Fran Sanchez, Jeanette Kennedy, Dr. Gary Gordon, Mary Harper, Holly and Dr. Jonathan Wright, Linda and Bob Lowinbrowski, Dan Ray, George Briggs, Harold Stueve, Paul Virgin, Dennis Itami, Ron Wright, Charley Fox, Larry Lindwall, Bob Bonk, Debra Fraser, Kathy and John Fitzpatrick, Vonda Haus, Kenny Foreman, Jr., Kurt Foreman, Dr. John Trowbridge, Dr. Bob Cathcart, Dr. Paul Lynn, Dr. Ted Rozema, Jack Ritchason, N.D., Dr. Donald Whitaker, David Capps, Pat Britt, Nancy Ostrander, Ron and Sue Gawthorne, Roger Wilbanks, Dan Nidess, Chuck and Taina Broes, Beverly and Dave Jaime, Lorraine and Jim Dennis, Janice Hartman, Dennis Deluca, Gina Foster, Dr. Doug Brody, William Holloway, Veronica and Fred Niero and Dr. Ernesto Contreras and family.

PLEASE NOTE

The purpose of this book is to offer the latest health and nutrition information based on worldwide research. This is not given or intended as medical advice. In fact, in many, if not most sections, you are referred to a medical doctor. A constant and clear differentiation is made between data gathered by scientists through experiments and study and information based on folklore.

ACKNOWLEDGEMENTS

In any comprehensive work of this kind, many years go into gathering material. Some of it was derived from in-person talks with eminent researchers throughout the world, from attending national and international conferences on biochemistry and nutrition, from interviewing leading authorities on my weekly television program, from gathering material for articles and editorials as a health magazine editor for 20 years and for my book, "Nutrition: The Cancer Answer," from attending and presiding over national and regional National Health Federation meetings, where speakers presented information at the forefront of health research.

Some of it was acquired by my collaborator, Jim Scheer, from authorities whom he interviewed as a health magazine editor and writer and from research studies in many journals, as well as from books.

My thanks go to everybody who contributed information: Gary Gordon, M.D., Jonathan Wright, M.D., Dr. Steuart McBirnie, Edward R. Pinckney, M.D. and his wife Cathey; William Campbell Douglass, M.D., Stephen Langer, M.D., Robert Cartright, M.D., Richard Kunin, M.D., John Trowbridge, M.D., William Crook, M.D., Stephen Gyland, M.D., James Braly, M.D., James Julian, M.D., Richard Casdorph, M.D., Paul Lynn, M.D. and from George and Evon Shutt, who helped bring world attention to the late Broda O. Barnes, M.D., Ph.D, and his pioneering studies of the thyroid gland.

To Jack L. Hanley for having an instinct for essentials. To my secretary, Jayne (Reaction) Sousa, who helps to bring order out of chaos. To Anita Smith whose sweet countenance brightens my life; and to Alesia Stevenson, who has mastered the strange world of computers in my behalf.

Special thanks go to Peggy Boyd for her excellent suggestion that symptoms of ailments be included in write-ups of physical disorders. We have done this.

Special thanks to Bill and Linda Goin who have been the instrument of God's harvest in my life. And, to Carolina Hanley, whose sharp proofreading structured the text.

My thanks also go to the hundreds of researchers who performed the experiments and studies that are the bedrock of this book—some mentioned in references and others who remain anonymous. In the latter instance, their discoveries speak for themselves in the pages that follow.

FOREWORD

My latest book, "Dr. Atkins' Medical Revolution" documents my metamorphosis from drug-oriented training into natural healing modalities.

At one time, medicine was my God. Now God is my medicine.

This places me in an ideal position to evaluate Foods That Heal, a fresh, innovative, exhaustively researched book, whose greatest strength is offering gentle, natural healing systems that follow God's laws.

Contrast this approach with that of money-motivated, mainstream, 20th century medicine, closely allied with the multi-billion dollar drug industry. Only man-made, never-before-existing drugs can be patented, so they, alone, can be profitable. Consequently foods are of little interest to practitioners of medicine. You can't patent them.

Nutritionists Maureen Salaman and James F. Scheer offer you an alternative, the best possible healing choice, utilizing novel and tasty recipes created by Jack Hanley from whole, nutrient-rich, natural foods.

It is simple concepts such as this that confound the wise, that are often considered revolutionary. Only a few years ago—before the breakthrough with the crucifer vegetables and bioflavonoids—the idea that foods could prevent or control to a significant degree all the major diseases, caused by both over and under-consumption, was considered Utopian by many, and absurd by some.

However, in reality, the regimes detailed in this book do that very thing.

Regardless of ivory-tower, armchair logic and deductive reasoning of medical academicians, the empirical approach, as demonstrated here, goes straight to the bottom line. Does it work? It if works, it must be worth considering. Foods That Heal works.

Skeptics will question themselves, "Can these foods actually effect healing? Really, now, isn't that a little too much? Some will protest and ask, "Isn't healing reserved for doctors and their medications?"

Orthodox doctors would like to think so.

The more certain the questioner is about his or her objections, the more certain it is that he or she is a product of the 20th century's propaganda mind-set.

We have all been propagandized to consider healing as the product of medicines and doctors, to respect medicine as a science which deals with what is proved beyond a doubt, something one can deduce through an understanding of the mechanics which explain it and agreed-upon by the scientific community.

From this perspective, the advice to use something simply because it works, is, at best, wishful thinking and, at the worst, quackery. Yet the medical minds which demand double-blind studies from others rarely realize that certain procedures they hold dear — heart bypass surgery as one instance — was never double-blind tested and yet is generally accepted.

Foods That Heal offers quintessential examples of natural, low-risk, empirically-demonstrated approaches to health preservation and enhancement. As such, it will probably seem entirely proper to most of us to devour these writings in hope of devouring foods described that promise to maintain or restore health.

One of the rare qualities of this book is that it not only instructs but entertains in the process, offering charming insights and an intimacy and warmth and color never before found in a nutrition book. It is an easy book to pick up, but hard to put down. The writer presents difficult concepts in over-the-backyard-fence language.

Encores are hard for most best-selling authors to earn, but apparently not for these outstanding nutritionists, who are at the top of their game.

There is little doubt that those who page through the book out of curiosity about their own physical dilemmas will be unable to avoid reading the rest of this fascinating, richly textured, good-humored work.

Full of vitality and emotional intensity, this book is likely to be rated one of the most useful books on natural healing published in this century.

Many features set it apart from the plethora of pedestrian and ordinary books on nutrition and healing—particularly its documentating the most effective type of healing—natural healing—because it comes to us from the Creator.

The authors then substantiate their faith with many credible controlled studies, with clinical scientific research and, in many instances, double blind experiments.

This gentle way of preventing and healing may help you live longer and more happily to make longer living more worthwhile, because the book's methods follow the instruction which Hippocrates, the father of medicine, offered to would-be doctors training under him:

"First, do no harm."

A superbly savvy work, Foods That Heal will not only keep you turning pages to the end, it is destined to become a cherished family bible of natural healing for the millions.

The Salaman-Scheer team—along with Hanley—have crafted a book that will live on through the ages of natural healing literature. And those who read it should live on and on in a state of well-being and health beyond their most extravagant expectations.

Robert Atkins, M.D.

CHAPTER 1

Acne

The most touching letter I have ever received came from a middle-aged woman in response to an article I wrote for a national magazine, Effects of Zinc on Acne, based on an interview with Robert Cathcart, M.D., who had made a dazzling record of healing acne patients with the mineral zinc.[1]

This woman wrote:

"I had been embarrassed with acne vulgaris—pits and pustules—since late in my childhood. Doctors comforted me with, 'When you go through puberty, your acne will disappear.'

"It didn't. And the agonizing years of low self-esteem dragged by. Then doctors said, " 'Don't worry. It will go away when you have a child.' It didn't. Now at age 42—after many thousands of dollars spent on doctors, I began to hear, 'Don't worry. It will soon go away.' It didn't.

"Then I just happened to read your interview article with Dr. Cathcart and followed his advice about taking zinc supplements. Within weeks, I began to notice a difference. Every day I could see an improvement. Within three months, my skin has become acne-free and smooth. My pores are like satin.

"For the first time since I was a child, I am liberated from self-consciousness and embarrassment. My self-esteem is coming back. I'm beginning to feel like a person. And I owe it all to your article. Bless you and thank you for your service to mankind."

What It Is And What Causes It

Acne vulgaris, common to adolescents and young adults, is an inflammation of the skin's sebaceous glands, which secrete a greasy substance called sebum. These glands on the face, neck, back and chest become plugged with sebum and infected and turn into pustules.

Doctors warn patients not to squeeze the pustules, because this can disfigure the face, leaving the skin scarred and pitted.

An ailment which leaves emotional as well as physical scars, acne can be caused by many factors: (1) a diet heavy in junk foods; (2) a diet deficient in zinc and/or vitamin A; (3) too little hydrochloric acid in the stomach, and, therefore, the inability to absorb critical nutrients properly — and (4) food sensitivities and allergies, particularly to milk.

On the positive side, most nutrition-oriented doctors recommend a diet high in fresh vegetables with some fresh fruit with high quality protein such as fish, poultry, meat and eggs.

Dr. Cathcart's Therapy

This is a quick summary of what Dr. Cathcart told me:

While practicing in Incline Village, Nevada, he began using zinc on 27 acne patients, following the regimen of a doctor named Michaelson, of Sweden's Upsala University Hospital:

"I used 50 milligrams of elemental zinc three times a day with meals. Dr. Michaelson used 45 mg, so I started a little bit higher. It became apparent after I was into this a while that some people require more zinc than that to get maximum effect.

"People who would take 50 mg with each meal did not always get the desired result, but if they increased to 100 and maybe 150 mg with each meal, they would get much better results," he explained.

His statistics showed that within 12 weeks, the zinc group of patients improved by 87 percent. Dr. Cathcart used dosages from 50 mg to 150 mg three times daily. He cautioned people not to go on the zinc regime without being supervised by a nutrition-oriented medical doctor.

The Case Of The Absent Acne

I was privileged to see the Cathcart regimen work right under my eyes. It was snow season at glorious Lake Tahoe. I was having my boots fitted for longer skis, and almost gasped when I saw the neck of the young man doing the job: a mass of unsightly and angry red pustules. A scraggly, long beard tried in vain to cover skin eruptions that looked like boils pressing against one another, competing for space.

Concerned, I asked what he was doing for his acne.

"Nothing now. I've seen every dermatologist in creation with nothing to show for it."

I told him about the Cathcart therapy and gave him Dr. Cathcart's name and address.

"Sounds great!" he replied. "I'll try anything."

"It's not that bad — 50 milligrams of zinc after each meal."

A year later I was back in Tahoe during snow season. My skiing had improved, so I returned to the same place to be fitted for longer skis. As I was about to sit down, a young man approached me. He let out a howl of joy.

"You're the lady who advised me about my acne last year!" "I want to hug you to death."

He almost did.

I hardly had an instant to observe his clean-skinned ruddy, beardless face, because he gave me a loving and powerful hug that would have made Leo Buscaglia envious.

Naturally, I was bubbling over with joy for him and thankful that superb nutrition had preserved my ribs.

When he released me, and I could breathe again. I studied his face. It was hard to believe that he had ever had acne. His complexion was perfect!

Foods That Heal

All right. It was zinc tablets that brought about the young man's deliverance from acne, but can foods do the same?

Yes, foods with a high zinc content.

But can a person get as much as 150 milligrams (mg) a day from foods alone?

Yes. The diet may be a bit monotonous, but it can be done, because I know people who have done it.

And cleared up their acne?

Yes. They ate quite a bit of herring, wheat germ, sesame seeds, liver, soybeans, sunflower seeds, egg yolk and lamb.

(As mentioned earlier, certain seafoods—oysters, crab, clams—are rich in nutrients, but some authorities refer to them as the garbage collectors of the sea, full of pollutants. Therefore, such seafood—not saltwater fish, which are okay—has been omitted from lists of foods with the highest content of vitamins and minerals.)

Oysters are the richest foods in zinc—160 mg per a less than a four ounce serving. However, I am starting the list with herring, whose zinc content is the next highest: 110 mg per less than a four ounce serving.

Some individuals prefer to take zinc supplements and eat foods with a high content of this mineral as a nutritional base. Following are foods richest in zinc in milligrams for less than a four ounce portion:

Herring, 110; wheat germ, 14; sesame seeds, 10; torula yeast, 9.9; blackstrap molasses, 8.3; maple syrup, 7.5; liver, 7.0; soybeans, 6.7; sunflower seeds, 6.6; egg yolk, 5.5; lamb, 5.4; chicken, 4.8; regular molasses, 4.6; brewer's yeast, 3.9; oats, 3.7; bone meal, 3.6; rye, 3.4; whole wheat, 3.2; corn, 3.1; coconut and beef, 3.0; beets, turkey and walnuts, 2.8; barley, 2.7; beans and avocados, 2.4; peas, 2.3; bleu cheese, 2.2; eggs, 2.1; and buckwheat, 2.0.

Fried Smoked Herring

8 smoked herrings
Pepper
1 cup olive oil
Cornmeal

Wash herring and soak in cold water for 24 hours, changing water twice. Rinse and dry. Sprinkle with pepper and roll in cornmeal. Fry in shallow oil (⅛ to ¼ inch) in skillet for approximately 12 to 15 minutes, or until brown and crisp, turning twice. Makes 4 servings.

Gene's Tangerine Chicken Salad

3 cups cooked chicken, diced
6 tangerines, peeled,
  separated into segments, seeded
½ cup slivered toasted almonds
½ cup celery, chopped
½ cup green pepper, chopped
⅓ cup home-made mayonnaise
  (not salad dressing)
⅓ cup dairy sour cream (raw certified)
2 tablespoons candied ginger,
  finely chopped
Salad greens

In large bowl, combine chicken, tangerine segments, almonds, celery and green pepper. Thoroughly combine mayonnaise, sour cream and ginger. Pour over salad. Toss lightly to mix well. Chill at least one hour before serving on crisp salad greens. Serves 5 to 6.

Home-Made Mayonnaise

1 egg
½ teaspoon sea salt
¼ teaspoon cayenne pepper
2 tablespoons honey

4 teaspoons apple cider vinegar
7 teaspoons lemon juice
1¼ cups safflower oil

Put all ingredients into a blender, except the safflower oil. When well blended, slowly add safflower oil. Soon the mixture will become thickened. If you desire more sweetness, add honey.

CHAPTER 2

Alcohol
How To Shatter
The Glass Prison

As a person who has never touched a drop of alcohol—wrong, I once had my tennis elbow rubbed with some—I have spent many years studying it.

Is alcohol as bad for you as the biochemists say?

See what you think, based on the surprising new data pouring out of the labs, relative to alcohol and the brain, the heart, and the body's vitamins and minerals?

Anyone who has studied anatomy, will remember that various organs are preserved in alcohol. Does this mean that brains of alcoholics are well preserved by the intoxicants they drink? No way. Their brains deteriorate much faster than those of non-drinkers.[1]

This is the finding of psychologists Aaron Noenberg, a Baltimore private practitioner, Gerald Goldstein, of the University of Pittsburgh School of Medicine and Horace Page, of Kent State University. These researchers tested 40 Veterans Administration patients in their 30s, 40s, 50s and 60s with 40 non-alcoholics matched for age, intelligence, formal education, and social and economic status.

Frightening Facts

Measuring a range of functions—eye and hand coordination and spatial ability, among others—revealed a sharp contrast in the groups. Brains of long-time alcoholics seemed to have aged 10 years. Performance of alcoholics in the 40 to 50 age groups were comparable with those of non-alcoholics in their 50s and 60s.[2]

Deterioration takes very little time to happen. Even alcoholics in their 30s who had done heavy drinking for just 10 years showed poorer brain performance than non-alcoholics in the same age group. In whatever age bracket, alcoholism exacts a severe penalty in this highly competitive world.[3]

Obviously heavy drinking over a long period will damage brains and the body, as well, including the liver. Now, however, researchers have found that even an occasional heavy drinking bout can bring on strokes and brain hermorrhages — even in young people.[4]

Explanation Of Unexplained Strokes

Unexplained strokes and cerebral hemorrhages in young adults—happening more and more—have been explained by a team of investigating physiologists at the State University of New York's Downstate Medical Center in Brooklyn.[5]

Such medical occurrences usually happen within 24 hours after a heavy drinking period. Sometimes less than an ounce of alcohol causes spasms of the arterioles, branches of arteries a little larger than capillaries, and a cut-off of oxygen—a condition called hypoxia. It is like what happens in a stroke.[6]

Investigation by the team also reveals why alcohol eventually invites blackouts, brain damage and hallucinations, among other psychiatric problems.

Initially, a reduced amount of oxygen produces an exaggerated feeling of well-being, fuzzy-mindedness and then talkativeness. Next, along with additional alcohol, come more marked spasms of brain arterioles, somewhat impaired vision, slurred speech, unsteadiness and staggering. Beyond this stage comes coma, stupor and what seem to be strokes.[7]

Arterioles constrict and choke off oxygen, damaging brain cells or complexes of them—temporarily or permanently. A stroke takes place when the damage covers a sufficiently large area. Blood blockages due to a series of spasms then cause blood pressure to rise.[8]

With a frequent and high intake of alcohol, arteriole walls weaken and, under extreme pressure, rupture. This research explains why chronic alcoholics on a binge experience a high rate of strokes, more high blood pressure and sudden death.[9]

Brains of chronic alcoholics after death are not usable by medical students for dissection. The cells have lost structure and have turned into mush.[10]

Attack On The Liver

A leading cause of cirrhosis of the liver is over-use of alcohol. Cirrhosis means the forming of scar tissue. Scar tissue replaces liver cells, reducing circulation and causing the liver to malfunction. Although cirrhosis can't be cured, its progress can usually be halted by cutting out alcohol and adding protein and B-complex to the diet.

The liver's capacity for handling large amounts of alcohol—pure carbohydrate—is limited. The remaining alcohol attacks and kills liver cells, depositing fat throughout the organ. The next step is cirrhosis, which must be stopped early or it will take over the entire liver, shut off its many functions and kill the person.

Much research indicates that proper diet and certain added nutrients can discourage the craving for alcohol. Non-alcoholics given a diet extremely high in raw foods immediately and spontaneously avoided alcohol and tobacco.[11] Thirty-two patients with high blood pressure followed a diet averaging 62 percent raw foods for six and a half months. Four out of five of those who smoked and drank abstained from both spontaneously.[12]

Chronic alcoholics given a nutritious diet, plus a multi-vitamin supplement, managed far better to stay away from alcohol than controls.[13]

How To Reduce Cravings For Alcohol

Test results with rats were similar to those with human beings. Placed on a junk food diet—particularly when given coffee, too—rats increased their alcohol intake.[14] Animals made deficient in vitamin B-complex, preferred alcohol to water.[15]

A sixteen week rat experiment at Loma Linda University School of Public Health underscores the fact that a high carbohydrate junk food diet encourages the tendency to drink more alcohol.[16]

Rats placed on a junk food diet drank a weekly average of what would be a quart of 100 proof whiskey a day for a man. Rats on the same diet but with the addition of vitamin-mineral supplements drank in a week the equivalent of what would be one-third of a quart of 100 proof whiskey a day for a man. The last group of rats, fed a balanced human diet, drank in a week what would be one-seventh of a quart of whiskey per day for a man.[17]

Now here's a staggering fact. (No play on words intended). In a previous study, 20 percent of rats on a high carbohydrate diet failed to develop a taste for alcohol. Then sugar was added to the alcohol, and these rats suddenly became the heaviest alcohol users of all, drinking in a week the equivalent of what would be a 1.4 quarts a day for a man.[18]

Another nutrient supplement, L-Glutamine, may decrease the craving for alcohol, as it did in animals, indicates noted biochemist Dr. Roger Williams, who participated in the experiment.[19]

In an experimental, single-blind crossover study, nine of 10 test subjects—in addition to friends and relatives—said that glutamine lessened their urge to drink, diminished anxiety and improved their quality of sleep. This is one-half a teaspoon daily in divided doses, taken particularly when the person craves alcohol.[20]

Reducing The Harm Of Alcohol

Until an alcoholic can break the habit, something can be done to help protect him or her from the worst damage. Any spouse of a hard drinker or parent of a child who drinks should know that all the toxic damage from alcoholism is not necessarily directly caused by the alcohol, but often by nutritional deficiencies brought on by it.

So many nutrients are lacking in so many alcoholics that it's best for them to start from a base of the 62 percent raw foods diet — mainly vegetables—and then supplement. So says Jonathan Wright, M.D., of Kent, Washington.[21]

Based on a careful survey of medical literature on alcoholism, Melvyn R. Werbach, M.D., assistant clinical professor, School of Medicine, UCLA, writes in Nutritional Influences on Illness (Third Line Press, Inc.) that the following nutrients may guard the liver from damage by alcohol: vitamins A, C, and E and magnesium, selenium and zinc. Then he adds accessory nutrients: L-carnitine, catechin (a naturally occurring flavonoid, gamma-linoleic acid, glutathione, and pantethine.[22]

Some authorities think alcohol can bring on reactive hypoglycemia. (See Section on hypoglycemia.) This disorder can trigger drinking more alcohol. Numerous small meals can often correct hypoglycemia.

Other nutrients which may be lacking in the alcoholic are vitamins B-1, B-2, B-6 and B-12, Evening Primrose oil, calcium, mixed freeform amino acids and glutathione.

These are good guidelines to follow. However, inasmuch as nutritional deficiencies of alcoholics—even of hard drinkers who aren't necessarily alcoholics—may be acute, I recommend that they or loved ones see an alternative physician or a nutrition-oriented medical specialist in alcohol-addiction for an appropriate regime and guidance.

Anita's Field Salad

5 ounces watercress

2 avocados, sliced

5 ounces fresh spinach

½ cup pistachio nuts

Italian salad dressing

Rinse, drain and tear spinach. Chill in bowl or plastic bag. Arrange avocado slices with nuts on spinach in salad bowl. Serves 6 to 8.

Organic Vegetable Dish

2 cups carrots, grated

2 cups celery or lettuce, chopped

½ cup cabbage, shredded

Sea salt and mixed herbs as desired

¼ cup raw cashews,
   ground and lightly toasted

1 teaspoon onion, minced

2 teaspoons lemon juice

1 tablespoon wheat germ

Mix all ingredients together and chill.

Harold's Exotic Lamb

1 tablespoon olive oil

1 pound boneless lean lamb shoulder,
   cut into 1½ inch cubes

1 medium onion, chopped

2 cups beef broth

½ teaspoon cinnamon

¼ teaspoon kelp

¼ teaspoon pepper

¼ teaspoon ginger, ground

2 medium apples, peeled and diced

2 sweet potatoes, cooked

6 prunes, pitted and cut in half

4 lemon slices

3 tablespoons honey

Heat oil in 12 inch skillet over low heat. Add lamb and onion and brown well on all sides, stirring occasionally. Pour off any drippings. Add broth, cinnamon, salt, pepper and ginger. Heat to boil. Reduce heat, cover and simmer for 1 hour and 15 minutes. Add apples, sweet potatoes, prunes, lemon and honey. Cook, uncovered, 10 minutes longer, or until apples are tender (stirring occasionally). Makes 4 servings.

CHAPTER 3

Allergies
(Food and Additives)

"The man with a thousand faces." That was the Hollywood publicity label applied some years ago to an actor who played a vast range of characters convincingly.

Like this performer, allergies have many faces—or symptoms—many more than we may think. We tend to recognize only the more obvious faces of food sensitivities or allergies—a rash, an itch, a runny nose, sniffles, sneezing and a headache. So, often, we don't even know that we are allergic.

Of course, certain symptoms of allergy can represent any number of ailments, but here's a list given me by alternative doctors:

Abnormal hunger, anxiety, arthritis, belching, bloating, blurred vision, chest congestion, crying jags, depression, dermatitis, diarrhea, difficulty in concentrating and remembering, dizziness, earache, ear infection, eczema, faintness, fatigue, flatulence, hives, hyperactivity, increased pulse rate, irritability, learning disabilities, mental slowness, muscle aches, nausea, pains, persistent and frequent need to urinate, post-nasal drip, sleeplessness, stomach distress and cramps, swelling ankles, feet and hands, vaginal discharge, vomiting, watery eyes and weakness.

How To Discover Culprit Foods

Foods are not the only environmental allergens, by any means, but they appear to affect more individuals than any other category of allergens.

Cathey Pinckney and Edward R. Pinckney, M.D., authors of the most complete and helpful book on medical tests, The Patient's Guide To Medical Tests (Facts on File) have told me that conventional tests for food allergies are not very accurate, that the food elimination diet is just as legitimate and as much a medical test as the others.

Clinical ecologists have created two tests which may help in discovering specific food allergens: the Coca Pulse Test and the Rotary Diversified Diet of the late Dr. Herbert Rinkel.

The late Dr. Arthur Coca, an eminent immunologist and founder-editor of the Journal of Immunology, discovered that foods to which a patient is sensitive or allergic rev up the heartbeat considerably. If the patient's heartbeat soars after he or she eats a certain food—say, 20 or more beats per minute above normal—that food is suspect. Here's how to take the test.

Find the area on the underside of the wrist where you can sense the pulse of blood pumped by your heart. Then, just count your pulse for six seconds and multiply by ten to find out your resting pulse.

First, take a pulse reading in bed, upon wakening in the morning. Repeat it right before eating. Eat just one food at a time, and take the test thirty minutes later and then sixty minutes later.

Food allergens can make heartbeat skyrocket from 72 to 92 or even as high as 180. One or more of the symptoms mentioned could follow within minutes or hours. Once a food turns out to be an allergen, just omit it. Results are not always straight-forward. Sometimes it takes 14 to 16 hours for a marked reaction to a food—at a time when you may no longer be keeping score.

Something More Accurate

A more accurate test is Rinkel's Rotary Diversified Diet which works in this way. Again, you eat only one food at a time. Then you avoid it for four days before eating it again. At this point, if you're sensitive or allergic to it, you will sense a heightened flare-up.

Repeat the process with other foods—suspected and unsuspected—until you develop a broad range of tolerable foods. According to the Rinkel theory, it is unwise to repeat even unsuspected foods more than every five days, because, by repetition, you could develop new sensitivities or allergies.

Rinkel explains that foods individuals enjoy eating often are foods to which they are sensitive. They tend to develop an addiction to them, similar to habituation to alcohol, cigarettes or coffee.

Then, if they miss a meal including these foods, they sense withdrawal symptoms. However, to minimize the withdrawal reaction, they unconsciously hunger for and eat the habituating food. As time goes by, they repeatedly eat the allergenic food before observable symptoms appear. Rinkel refers to this process as "masking".

Another Health Hazard

James Braly, M.D., who heads Optimum Health Laboratory in Encino, California, makes the process of testing foods easier by narrowing down the list to the following, which are suspect foods for most patients: beef, chocolate, eggs, citrus fruits, coffee, corn, malt, milk, nuts, pork, potatoes, soybeans, spices, tomatoes, wheat and yeast.[1]

Eating the same ten or twenty foods incessantly leads to reinforcing old food sensitivities and allergies and creating new ones, he states.

Braly warns against eating foods which have many ingredients, such as commercial bread, catsup or salad dressing. Hidden ingredients in canned and packaged foods can undo a non-allergenic diet. Several doctor friends have recommended eating little or no processed food. I rarely, if ever, eat processed packaged foods — not intentionally.

Incomplete Digestion

Dr. Braly mentions another cause of food allergies: a secretion of insufficient hydrochloric acid and digestive enzymes in the stomach, a slowdown which occurs in persons in their forties, fifties, sixties or beyond.

Poor digestion means that some over-large protein molecules reach the intestines, escape through the walls and end up in the bloodstream, where they cause allergies. Braly calls this condition "leaky gut syndrome".[2]

The gut becomes porous to undigested, large protein molecules for two major reasons: consuming of additives in processed foods—there are some 3,000 additives, states Braly — and following a nutrient-deficient diet. Inflammation and under-nutrition father the leaky gut syndrome. Numerous nutrient shortages contribute to this condition — mainly vitamin A and zinc.

There is evidence that certain vitamins block the release of histamine, the chemical substance that causes the misery of an allergic reaction, and that others may lessen sensitivity to monosodium glutamate (MSG) an artificial flavor-enhancer. Vitamins C[3] and E[4] have been shown to lower histamine in the blood and the following have been discovered to reduce sensitivity to MSG: vitamin B-6 and C.[5]

Watercress is an old folk remedy for the obvious symptoms of allergy: sneezing, a stuffy head and watering eyes. When I feel allergic, I eat a few handfuls of watercress.

Lactobacillus acidophilus, friendly organisms found in yogurt, may be helpful to children with food allergies, reveals one study.[6] Every child participating in a study was found deficient in this organism and related ones. (Let me issue a warning. Yogurt is fast becoming a junk food, loaded with sugars and syrups and fillers and additives such as potato starch. It is best to use pure yogurt sweetened with fruit.)

So the following nutrients may be able to help us battle allergies successfully: vitamins A, B-6, C, E and the mineral zinc.

Supplements and foods richest in vitamin A in International Units per less than a four ounce measure are: cod liver oil, 200,000; sheep liver, 45,000; cow liver, 44,000; calf's liver, 22,000; dandelion greens, 14,000; carrots, 11,000; yams, 9,000; kale, 8,900; parsley and turnip greens, 8,500; spinach, 8,100; collard greens and chard, 6,500; watercress, 5,000; red peppers, 4,400; squash, 4,000; egg yolk and cantaloupe, 3,400; endive, 3,300; persimmons and apricots, 2,700; broccoli, 2,500; pimentos, 2,300; swordfish, 2,100; whitefish, 2 ,000; romaine, 1,900; mangoes, 1,800; papayas, 1,700; nectarines and pumpkin 1, 600; peaches and cheeses, 1,300; eggs, 1,200; cherries, lettuce and cream, 1,000 and tomatoes and asparagus, 900.

Supplements and foods highest in vitamin B-6 in milligrams per units of less than four ounces are: brewer's yeast, 4; brown rice, 3.6; whole wheat, 2.9; royal jelly, 2.4; soybeans, 2.0; rye, 1.8; lentils, 1.7; sunflower seeds and hazelnuts, 1.1; alfalfa, 1.00; salmon, 0.98; wheat germ, 0.92; tuna, 0.90 bran, 0.85; walnuts, 0.73; peas and liver, 0.67; avocados, 0.60; beans, 0.57; cashews, peanuts, turkey, oats, chicken and beef, 0.40; halibut, 0.34 and lamb and banana, 0.32.

Here are supplements and foods with the largest amounts of vitamin C in milligrams per units of less than four ounces: rose hips, 3,000; acerola cherries, 1,100; guavas, 240; black currants, 200; parsley, 170; green peppers, 11 0; watercress, 80; chives, 70; strawberries, 57; persimmons, 52; spinach, 51; oranges, 50; cabbage, 47; grapefruit, 38; papaya, 37; elderberries and kumquats, 36; dandelion greens and lemons, 35; cantaloupe, 33; green onions, 32; limes, 31; mangoes, 27; loganberries, 24; tangerines and tomatoes, 23; squash, 22 and romaine lettuce and raspberries.

The richest sources of vitamin E in International Units in portions of less than four ounces are: wheat germ, 160; safflower nuts, 35; sunflower seeds, 31; wheat, 30; sesame oil, 26; walnuts, 22; corn oil and hazelnuts, 21; soy oil and peanut oil, 16; almonds, 15; olive oil, 14; cabbage, 7.8; brazil nuts and peanuts, 6.5; cod liver oil, 5.4; cashews, 5.1; soy lecithin, 4.8; spinach, 2.9; asparagus, 2.5; broccoli, 2.0; butter, 1.9; parsley, 1.8; oats, barley and corn, 1.7 and avocados and pecans, 1.5.

Foods and supplements with the highest amounts of zinc in milligrams per units of less than four ounces are: herring, 110; wheat germ, 14; sesame seeds, 10; torula yeast, 9.9; blackstrap molasses, 8.3; maple syrup, 7.5; liver, 7.0; soybeans, 6.7; sunflower seeds, 6.6; egg yolk, 5.5; lamb, 5.4; chicken, 4.8; regular molasses, 4.6; brewer's yeast, 3.9; oats, 3.7; bone meal, 3.6; rye, 3.4; wheat, 3.2; corn, 3.1; coconut and beef, 3.0; beets, turkey and walnuts, 2 .8; barley, 2.7; beans and avocados, 2.4; peas, 2.3; bleu cheese, 2.2; buckwheat, 2.0; mangoes, 1.9 and millet, brown rice and almonds, 1.5.

Broiled White Fish With Lemon Butter Sauce

2 lbs. White Fish Fillets	1 T. Parsley, Chopped
¼ c. Butter, Melted	2 t. Sea Salt
¼ c. Lemon Juice	Dash Pepper
2 T. Onion, Minced	6 Lemon Wedges for Garnish
1 T. Honey	

Preheat broiler. Place filets, skin-side down, in broiler pan. In small bowl, combine remaining ingredients, except lemon wedges. Broil filets 10 minutes until fish flakes easily when tested with a fork, generously basting filets with butter mixture. Serve with lemon wedges. Makes 6 to 8 servings.

Watercress Bean Sprout Salad

Watercress and any of the sprouts rich in Vitamin B-complex; alfalfa, bamboo, garbanzo, mung, wheat berry sprouts: Combine bean sprouts, green onion, celery and water chestnuts. Mix with sesame salad dressing and serve on a bed of watercress.

Sesame Salad Dressing

½ c. ground sesame seeds   Juice of ½ lemon
1 c. water, approximately   ½ garlic clove
1 t. kelp

Place seeds and 1 cup water in blender and blend until smooth. Add remaining ingredients and blend until smooth, adding more water if necessary to give correct consistency.

CHAPTER 4

Alzheimer's Disease (Refer To Memory Loss)

Long suspected for the crime against mind and body called Alzheimer's disease, the mineral aluminum so far has escaped being accused.

Always at the scene of the crime, at the site of tangled nerve fibers in the brain of the Alzheimer's disease victim, aluminum seems guilty due to circumstantial evidence. Yet, with typical scientific caution, authorities on this disease, say, "We can't be sure. Is aluminum the cause or is it a side effect of the disease process?"

While the evidence is being weighed, my alternative doctors' brain trust tells me, "Don't wait for an indictment. Just keep aluminum out of your life, your body and brain."

Sounds like a good idea, everything considered. About 15 years ago, a research team led by Dr. D. Crapper, at the University of Toronto, performed autopsies on Alzheimer's disease patients and, in each instance, found aluminum accumulated in localized brain areas and incredible tangles of nerve fibers, neurofibrils, tiny nerve conductors inside brain cells.[1]

Brain autopsies of numerous patients without Alzheimer's disease symptoms revealed neither aluminum nor neurofibril tangles.

Certain Diagnosis Is Difficult

It has been far from easy for doctors to offer a sure diagnosis for this disease for two reasons: it resembles other conditions of mental deterioration, as indicated in the section on Memory Loss, and, until recently, a certain diagnosis could be obtained only after death through autopsy. However, now, the brain can be studied in detail with nuclear magnetic resonance (known as NMR), which, unlike X-ray, is said to be harmless.

The initial symptoms of this disorder are so common they are likely to be overlooked, like inability to recall at once someone's address or a friend or neighbor's name.

Then the forgetfulness worsens, and the person, at first, fails to remember something such as where the tickets are for the baseball game and, then, even worse, forgets the location of the stadium. Or he or she writes a letter to someone. Then, later that day, does it all over again.

Added to a steadily deteriorating memory and impaired judgement come changes in personality and temperament: anxiety, nervousness, depression, irritability and temper flareups.

Next, the Alzheimer's disease victim has difficulty thinking and speaking, but this inability is not nearly as cruel to the dignity as the inability to control bladder or bowel and having to be diapered like a baby. The condition continues worsening until death seems merciful. This usually happens over a span of four to eight years.

Alzheimer's disease patients characteristically also experience porous, weakening, easily-fractured bones and painful arthritis.

Is Aluminum A Shining Killer?

Intent on learning the latest, I attended an international conference on Alzheimer's Disease several years ago in Zurich, Switzerland.

Authorities said that Alzheimer's disease victims are short of a neurotransmitter called acetylcholine. Neurotransmitters are chemicals at the ends of brain nerve cells which make message transmission possible.

Several papers read from the platform revealed that the nutrient choline, derived from lecithin, stimulates production of acetylcholine and improves Alzheimer's patients' short term memory and their general condition. The taking of acetylcholine itself also has proved helpful.

I was keenly disappointed that a subject of such obvious importance as aluminum was hardly mentioned. A researcher in one of the display booths told about experiments in which he had injected aluminum into the brains of lab animals and had observed the same kind of nerve fiber tangles that were found in Dr. Crapper's Alzheimer's disease autopsies. Large photographic blowups of nerve fiber tangles made an indelible impression on me.

Later I learned that another scientist had performed a similar experiment on rabbits with the same result: aluminum deposits and nerve fiber tangles in the brain.

More Strong Evidence

Other evidence is even stronger that aluminum may be a major contributor to Alzheimer's disease. Finger-pointing at aluminum began some years ago in clinics for dialysis treatments. Where aluminum content of the water used in treatments was high, dementia was high. Where it was low, dementia was low.[2]

Autopsies of dementia patients revealed brain concentrations of aluminum and the same devastation of nerve fibrils. When dementia patients were treated with drugs which lowered blood concentration of aluminum, they showed rapid improvement.

My friend Richard Casdorph, M.D., of Long Beach, California, informed a convention of the National Health Federation that his patients in the early or mid-stages of Alzheimer's disease had made marked improvement when aluminum was removed from them by means of chelation treatment with a chemical called EDTA.

Elevated blood levels of aluminum were found in many of 400 psychiatric patients experiencing senile episodes and memory loss, reports the Brain Bio Center in Princeton, New Jersey.[3]

Although aluminum can be reduced in the blood with supplements of zinc, magnesium and manganese, this doesn't mean it can be extracted from brain cells. So, prevention is still the best cure.

How Aluminum Does Its Damage

Now how can aluminum possibly invade the human body and stay there? After all, it has been believed for years that little, if any, aluminum could enter the body through the digestive tract. And this mineral certainly couldn't make it through the blood-brain barrier! This is why many doctors have felt safe in prescribing antacids, aluminum compounds. This is why so many makers of patent medicines felt it was all right to include liberal amounts of aluminum in their formulations.

All right, then, how does aluminum manage to do the impossible? A small but significant amount is absorbed through the intestines. And aluminum slips through the blood-brain barrier quite easily, because its ions are so tiny, less than half the size of those in minerals essential to the body—calcium, magnesium, potassium and sodium.[4]

Now, experiments performed at the University of Virginia in Charlottesville, show exactly how aluminum commits its brain sabotage.[5]

Researchers Timothy L. MacDonald, W. Griffith Humphreys and R. Bruce Martin say that aluminum works its crime against microtubules, which support cell structure. These tubules form filaments called spindles, without which cell division can't take place, and influence other structures and functions in nerve cells and other cells, as well.

Microtubules are always active, being assembled and disassembled, using a raw material called tubulin, made up of amino acids and magnesium. The researchers discovered that Good Guy magnesium and Bad Guy aluminum compete to be used for making tubulin.

What astonished them is that aluminum has a big advantage over magnesium. It is incorporated into tubulin 10 times faster than magnesium, making for weaker and more collapsible cell structures.

Another Alzheimer Mystery Solved

And, about those tangled neurofibrils, Alzheimer's disease authorities have been mystified as to how they destroy memory. Now a research team headed by Bradley T. Hymen, at the University of Iowa (Iowa City), has discovered that the tangled nerve fibers near aluminum deposits are concentrated in layers of cells that relay nerve impulses into and out of ⁺he brain's memory center.[6]

At one time, it was thought that the damage was in the hippocampus area, where memories are assembled. The University of Iowa researchers found that this was not so. However, the area surrounding the hippocampus showed significant nerve tangle damage.

Hymen indicates that the tangles cut off the input and output from the hippocampus, so that memory is not really lost. It is disconnected.

Why No Official Warning?

An accumulation of damning evidence mounds up against aluminum, which assails us in dozens of commonly used medicines and foods. It seems that an official public warning would be issued by the Food and Drug Administration, the Centers for Disease Control or the American Medical Association in view of an estimated 1.5 and 3 million Alzheimer's disease victims, more in the making and those with dialysis dementia. Yet there is only a loud silence from them.

Isn't there enough evidence against aluminum for the FDA, CDC or the AMA to issue a warning? Now that the truth is revealed, could they be afraid of public condemnation, a congressional investigation or lawsuits for their long silence? Or are they protecting the tender skin of manufacturers of products who might be sued as some cigarette makers have been in instances of lung cancer? Are they also fearful of making the public lose confidence in the implicated products and causing a plummeting of sales? Could it be that dollars are more important to them than your health and mine?

This leaves the ball in my court. And, right here and now, I want to list as many Trojan Horse products as I know which may threaten you by stealthily implanting aluminum in the body and mind: most acne medications and antacids — health food stores carry brands which are aluminum-free—anti-diarrhea products, anti-perspirants and deodorants, many cosmetics, douches, feminine hygiene products, some hemorrhoid preparations, lipstick, skin creams and lotions and tooth-paste.

Among the foods and food-related products containing various forms of aluminum are breads and pastries, most baking powders, baking powder biscuits, cheese, cheese sauces, pickles, many salad dressings, table salt, white flour, fruit juices stored in aluminum containers, water from most municipal sources and aluminum foil.

In a warning article, Barbara Bassett, the former Editor & Publisher of the health-nutrition magazine *Bestways*, points out that while natural cheese may contain one-half milligram to almost three milligrams of aluminum per a certain unit, processed cheese has up to 144 milligrams of aluminum in the same portion.[7]

That makes me shudder. How about you? Aluminum, among other additives, is one of many reasons why I recommend against eating any processed food.

Barbara also warns against using aluminum pots and pans, which impart small amounts of aluminum to foods. Fluoride in much municipal water increases the amount of aluminum leached from cookware and absorbed in foods cooked in it.

Self-Protection: Your Best Bet

Now that it is clear that we are on our own in safeguarding ourselves and loved ones from Alzheimer's disease (or from its worst ravages) the obvious measure to take is avoiding the intake of aluminum.

Dr. Stephen Davies, founding chairman of the British Society for Nutritional Medicine, and Dr. Alan Stewart, in their book, *Nutritional Medicine* (Pan Books), offer a special way of blocking absorption of aluminum from food: through supplements such as vitamin C (1,000 mg daily), calcium and magnesium. They feel that this regime may even reduce accumulated aluminum.[8]

Their recommendation is based on studies which lead them to believe that aluminum is involved in Alzheimer's disease as well as in a small percentage of non-specific joint disorders, and in childhood hyperactivity.

Another possible way to get rid of accumulated aluminum is through chelation, as mentioned earlier relative to Richard Casdorph, M.D.

Still another method of coping with Alzheimer's disease — successful in some experiments — is taking supplements. The B vitamin choline is converted to the brain neurotransmitter acetylcholine, a chemical contact between nerve cells. On this basis, alternative doctors often suggest that their patients take extra choline, acetylcholine or lecithin, the richest source of choline. Lecithin comes mainly from soybeans and eggs.

In a six-month London study, half of a group of Alzheimer's disease patients fed large doses of lecithin improved in certain mental functions as well as in the ability to care for themselves.[9]

An eminent authority on the biochemistry of the brain, Richard Wurtman, M.D., of Massachusetts Institute of Technology, has discovered that the amount of the neurotransmitter made from choline (derived from lecithin) is reduced by up to 90 percent in Alzheimer's disease patients, making for memory loss.[10]

A study by Dr. Raymond Levy, a brain researcher at the University of London, discloses that choline therapy accounted for continuing behavioral improvement of eight of 24 Alzheimer's disease patients.[11]

Improving patients averaged 79 years of age. Non-improving patients averaged 69 years of age. Apparently choline therapy is most effective for individuals who develop Alzheimer's disease late in life and in patients who have a milder form.

Declining ability of Alzheimer's disease patients to synthesize the neurotransmitter acetylcholine accounts for progression of this disorder, rather than the lack of lecithin or choline raw materials, states Dr. Neil R. Sims, an Alzheimer's disease project researcher at the Burke Rehabilitation Center in White Plains, New York.[12]

Maybe this is why lecithin is more effective in coping with Alzheimer's disease symptoms in the ailment's earliest stages, before the acetylcholine-making capability is slowed down.

Drs. Pierre Etienne, of Quebec, and Janice Christie, of Edinborough, have reported healing results in treating Alzheimer's disease patients with large amounts of lecithin.[13] The daily amount was not stated in the source I saw.

However, Dr. Brian L.G. Morgan, in his book *Nutrition Prescription* (Crown Publishers, p.27) lists his strategy against Alzheimer's disease as one to two grams of choline a day or 30 grams of lecithin. He recommends lecithin that is 100 percent phosphatidylcholine.

An arresting study by Judith Marquis in the Department of Pharmacology at Boston University offers significant information that may help to understand Alzheimer's Disease or even to prevent or moderate it.[10]

Aluminum appears to interrupt the metabolism of acetylcholine, a key brain neurotransmitter, she says. And being adequately nourished with calcium seems to limit the accumulation of aluminum in the brain.

Let's look at food and supplement sources said to block absorption of aluminum—vitamin C and the minerals calcium and magnesium—and at the nutrients claimed to stop the progression of Alzheimer's disease.

Richest supplements and food sources of vitamin C in milligrams per less than four ounce units are: rose hips, 3,000; acerola cherries, 1,100;

guavas, 240; black currants, 200; parsley, 170; green peppers, 110; watercress, 80; chives, 70; strawberries, 57; persimmons, 52; spinach, 51; oranges, 50; cabbage, 47; grapefruit, 38; papaya, 37; elderberries and kumquats, 36; dandelion greens and lemons, 35; cantaloupe, 33; green onions, 32; limes, 31; mangoes, 27; loganberries, 24; tangerines and tomatoes, 23; squash 22; raspberries and romaine lettuce, 17 and pineapple, 17.

Best food and supplement sources of calcium in milligrams per less than four ounce units are: sesame seeds, 1,200; kelp, 1,100; cheeses, 700; brewer's yeast, 420; sardines and carob, 350; regular molasses, 290; caviar, 280; soybeans and almonds, 230; torula yeast, 220; parsley, 200; brazil nuts, 190; watercress, salmon and chickpeas, 150; egg yolk, beans, pistachios, lentils and kale, 130; sunflower seeds and cow's milk, 120; buckwheat, 110; maple syrup, cream and chard, 100; walnuts, 99; spinach, 93; endive, 81; pecans, 73; wheat germ, 72; peas, 70; peanuts, 69 and eggs, 54.

Here are the supplements and foods which rate highest in magnesium content in milligrams in units of less than four ounces: kelp, 740; blackstrap molasses, 410; sunflower seeds, 350; wheat germ, 320; almonds, 270; soybeans, 240; brazil nuts, 220; bone meal, 170; pistachios and soy lecithin, 160; hazelnuts, 150; pecans and oats, 140; brown rice, 120; regular molasses, 81; chard, 65, spinach, 57; barley, 55; coconut, 44; salmon, 40; corn, 38; avocados, 37; bananas, 31; cheese, 30; tuna, 29 and potatoes and cashews, 27.

Richest supplements and food sources of choline in milligrams per less than a four ounce unit are: soy lecithin, milligrams per less than a four ounce unit are: soy lecithin, 2,900; egg yolk, 1,700; chickpeas, 780; lentils, 710; split peas, 700; brown rice, 650; liver, 550; caviar, 540; eggs, 500; wheat germ, 400; soybeans and green beans, 340; green peas, 270; cabbage and torula yeast, 250; spinach, peanuts and brewer's yeast, 240; sunflower seeds, 220; blackstrap molasses, 150; alfalfa, bran and barley, 140; asparagus, 130 and lamb and potatoes, 110.

Sweet And Sour Lentil Stew

⅓ c. raw brown rice
1 c. uncooked lentils
1 onion, chopped
3 carrots, chopped
1 green bell pepper, chopped
1 c. fresh tomatoes, chopped
2 T. liquid garlic
1 garlic clove, crushed
2 T. olive oil

1 bay leaf
2 T. kelp
1 t. basil
1 T. tamari soy sauce
1 T. lemon juice
1 T. molasses
½ T. vinegar
2 lbs. flank steak,
  cut in 1 inch squares

Put lentils, rice and water in large pot and bring to a boil. Reduce heat, cover and simmer for 30 minutes. Saute flank steak in oil until brown. Add onions, carrots, potatoes and green pepper. Simmer for 30 minutes more. Add tomatoes and seasonings. Cook an additional 30 minutes more.

Memory Enhancer

¼ c. soya milk powder
1 c. spring water
1 t. nutritional yeast
1 T. lecithin powder
2 T. pure maple syrup
1 egg yolk

3 T. fresh wheat germ
2 T. rolled oats
2 T. flaked (rolled) millet or rye
½ T. natural raisins
1 T. Fiber 5

In blender add soya milk powder, spring water, yeast, lecithin powder, maple syrup and egg yolk. Blend well. In cereal bowl add wheat germ, rolled oats, millet, raisins and Fiber 5. Pour blended liquid over dry ingredients and mix well. Allow liquid to soak into cereal, then refrigerate if cooling is desired. Serves 1.

CHAPTER 5

Anemia

One of the telltale signs of every form of anemia is fatigue — often exhaustion. However, each type of anemia has a slightly different cause.

The most widespread and common type is iron-deficiency anemia. Others are pernicious anemia and megaloblastic anemia based on folic-acid deficiency. (An almost unknown or, at least, little-considered type is caused by hypothyroidism, low thyroid function. This sleeper form will be explained later.)

Before charging out of the starting blocks, we might state briefly what this ailment is all about: it is the inability of the body to deliver the amount of oxygen required for its trillions of cells.

Iron Deficiency Anemia

Iron deficiency anemia is probably the most widespread kind, because it can have so many different origins: need for increased iron, limited ability to absorb iron, loss of blood and repeated pregnancies.

The most common symptoms of iron-deficiency anemia, aside from fatigue or exhaustion, are breathlessness after exertion; brittle nails, low attention span, headaches, gastrointestinal upset, pale skin, rapid pulse and loss of sexual interest and desire.

Usually a lack of iron is brought on by a diet heavy in processed foods. A deficiency can come about quite easily, even though the body reuses its iron, losing very little through natural processes — probably less than 10 percent.

It is important to have a ready supply of iron, because this mineral, along with protein and copper, makes up hemoglobin in red blood cells

— the substance which delivers oxygen throughout the body. The most likely groups to have iron-deficiency anemia are menstruating women, teenagers, repeatedly pregnant women and older individuals.

Reasons for iron-shortage in the first three groups seem self-evident. So far as the elderly are concerned, they often secrete too little stomach acid and sometimes need extra hydrocholoric acid and digestive enzymes to process iron properly — 500 to 1,000 mg of betaine Hydrochloride — and vitamin C. Various studies have shown that at least 200 to 500 mg of vitamin C daily helps immeasurably in absorbing iron in any or all age groups.[1]

Foods For Iron Men And Women

A diet of unprocessed foods can supply all the iron needed, if planned with the knowledge that all edibles are not created equal in being absorbable. Meat, fish and poultry contain a form of iron called heme, of which almost 40 percent can be absorbed.[2] Eggs, dried beans, nuts and whole grains, and other non-flesh sources contain a form of iron called ionic, of which about 10 percent can be absorbed.[3] Spinach, which supposedly gave Popeye the Sailor his tremendous strength and turned him into an iron man, is a real fraud. Only about two percent of its ionic iron can be absorbed.[4]

Best Sources Of Iron

The prime food sources of iron in terms of milligrams in a less than four ounce portion are: kidney, 13; soy lecithin, 12; caviar, 12; pumpkin seeds, 11; sesame seeds, 10; wheat germ, 9.4; blackstrap molasses, 9.1; liver 8.8; pistachios, 7.2; egg yolk, 7.2, sunflower seeds, 7.1; chickpeas, 6.9; millet, 6.8; lentils, 6.7; walnuts, 6.0; parsley, 5.0; almonds, 4.7 and oats, 4.5.

The Little-Known Kind Of Anemia

The book, "Solved: The Riddle of Illness" (Keats Publishing) by Stephen E. Langer, M.D. and James F. Scheer tells the fascinating story of how Broda O. Barnes, M.D., Ph.D, a world-renowned thyroid expert, discovered a virtually hidden form of anemia, which affects many people without their knowing it.[5]

When Dr. Barnes was a physiology instructor at the University of Chicago some years ago, he witnessed a demonstration that normal body temperature is a "must" to assure production of sufficient blood cells.

A Ph.D candidate wasn't quite sure why both red and white blood cells are formed only in the marrow of certain specific bones: the long bones nearest the body, the pelvis, ribs and spine. Suspecting that it was a matter of termperature — the body organs being warmer than the extremities, the arms and legs — he carried out an animal experiment to test his theory.

Important Discovery

Sure enough, he proved to be right! Many years afterward, Dr. Barnes, then in medical pratice, remembered this revealing demonstration and understood why some women remain anemic — pale, fatigued and depressed even after iron supplementation. These hypothyroids with their characteristic subnormal temperature could not produce enough blood cells until he gave them thyroid supplementation, which raised their body temperature to normal and increased their ability to produce blood white and red blood cells. Remember that red blood cells carry that all-important oxygen to our cells.

As stated in the Low Thyroid section of this book, Dr. Barnes found that first generation hypothyroids were often able to correct their condition by a daily 225 mcg of kelp, which contains iodine, the major food of the thyroid gland. Second generation hypothyroids and beyond generally need prescription thyroid supplementation to normalize themselves and to get rid of this little-known form of anemia.

Pernicious Anemia

Because pernicious anemia is caused by a deficiency of vitamin B-12 — found only in animal products: meat, milk, cheese and eggs—mainly strict vegetarians and those religiously pursuing a low fat-low cholesterol diet are its victims.

Symptoms

Symptoms of pernicious anemia are similar to those of iron-deficiency anemia with these additions: apathy, periodic constipation and diarrhea and occasional abdominal pain, appetite and weight loss, confusion, hallucinations and memory loss.

This disorder lives up to its name "pernicious," which means very severe or fatal. Unless the condition is corrected in time with vitamin B-12 shots or supplements, it can be fatal. Very little vitamin B-12 is needed, as expressed in micrograms, but that tiny amount must be supplied.

Super Food Sources

The best offense against pernicious anemia is prevention — eating the foods richest in vitamin B-12. Here they are in terms of milligrams in a less than four ounce portion: liver, 0.086; sardines, 0.034; mackerel and herring, 0.0100; flounder, 0.0064; salmon, 0.0047; lamb, 0.0031; Swiss cheese, 0.0021; eggs, 0.0020 and, among others, haddock, 0.0017.

Internal Problems

It is not only vegetarians and low fat-low cholesterol dieters who have problems getting enough vitamin B-12 for protection against pernicious anemia. Paradoxically, even people who eat B-12 rich foods or take a B-12 supplement may not absorb it.

This is because vitamin B-12 requires a stomach secretion called "the intrinsic factor," to bind with and help its absorption through the intestinal walls. Some of us produce too little intrinsic factor, so there's trouble.

Now health food stores stock two types of vitamin B-12 to solve this internal problem: a form of the vitamin called sublingual, because it is placed under the tongue to be melted and drawn right into the bloodstream and a kind blended with the intrinsic factor.

The old-fashioned way of bypassing the intrinsic factor is to get shots of B-12, still successful in warding off or defeating pernicious anemia, which, if left to run its course, can destroy the protective myelin sheaths around nerves of the brain and spinal cord.

Megaloblastic Anemia (Based on Folic Acid Deficiency)

A deficiency of any major nutrient essential to making red blood cells can cause anemia. Too little folic acid can bring on this form of biochemical sabotage, as can a shortage of copper, iron, protein and vitamins B-12 and C.

Revealing Symptoms

Aside from the fatigue or exhaustion common to all anemias, this type is characterized by breathlessness after exertion, decreased attention span, headaches, inability to concentrate, irregular menstrual periods, gastrointestinal discomfort, a sore and shiny tongue and diminished interest in sex.

Why It's Hard To Get Enough

Vegetarians usually ingest enough folic acid (which gets its name from the Latin, folium, meaning leaf), because its main source is green, leafy vegetables. Both brewer's yeast and torula yeast are high in folic acid content. Folic acid is also produced by bacteria in the intestine, but, sometimes, not enough to satisfy the body's needs.

Richest food sources in terms of milligrams per less than four ounces are: alfalfa, 0.80; soybeans, 0.69; endive, 0.47; chickpeas, 0.41; oats, 0.39; lentils, 0.34; beans, 0.31; wheat germ, 0.31; liver, 0,29; split peas, 0.23; wheat, 0.22; barley, 0.21, rice, 0.17, asparagus, 0.12; green peas, 0.11 and, among others, sunflower seeds, 0.10.

However, just brief cooking of vegetables or grains at higher than boiling temperatures can destroy almost 65 percent of the folic acid.

Even with enough intake of folic acid, there still can be problems. Oral contraceptives block the body's ability to utilize folic acid.[6] Antibiotics such as streptomycin and aminoperin destroy folic acid.[7] Alcohol interferes with folic acid absorption, so alcoholics sometimes need more than the 400 mcg daily supplement that nutrition-oriented physicians usually recommend.[8] Patients on anticonvulsants such as phenobarbitol, primidone and phenytoin and those going through dialysis also require additional amounts of this vitamin.[9]

Pregnant and lactating women require a higher than normal intake of folic acid. Adding a raw vegetable or fruit to the daily diet sometimes supplies the deficient amount of folate. However, nutrition-oriented doctors usually recommend a 400 mcg tablet of folic acid as a measure of safety, 800 mcg for pregnant women and 600 mcg for nursing mothers.

Recovery from megaloblastic anemia can be rapid when based on regimes mentioned above — within several weeks or months.

Skier's Delight
(great to take skiing in thermos)

2 lbs. chuck steak,	1½ c. sliced carrots
cut into 2 inch strips	1 c. onion, chopped
3 lbs. chicken wings	4 c. cooked beans
2 T. olive oil	2 c. chick peas or garbonzo
1 can (16 ounces) tomatoes in puree	beansize chunks
2 c. spring water	1 c. sliced spanish pimiento-
3 T. liquid garlic	stuffed green olives
⅛ t. ground black pepper	¼ t. jalapeno peppers, chopped
3 T. parsley, chopped	

In large sauce pan, brown beef strips in oil. Add tomatoes,water, garlic and pepper. Heat to boiling. Reduce heat to low and cover. Simmer 1 hour, stirring occasionally. Add chicken, parsley, onion, carrots and jalapeno peppers. Cover and simmer 30 minutes longer, or until chicken is tender. Stir in cooked beans, chick peas and olives. Simmer 10 minutes longer. Serves 8 to 10.

Sauteed Green Peas

1 lb. (2 c. shelled) fresh peas	1 T. whole wheat flour
½ c. sea salted, boiling spring water	½ c. milk (raw certified)
¼ c. butter (raw certified)	1 T. parsley, minced

Simmer peas in water for 5 minutes. Drain. Saute in butter until tender (5 to 15 minutes). Dust with flour, stir in milk. Bring to a boil. Add parsley. Peas may also be sauteed with other vegetables, i.e., carrots, kohlrabi, cauliflower, lettuce hearts, etc. Serves 2 to 3.

CHAPTER 6

Anorexia Nervosa (Starvation For Thinness)

One of the strangest human ailments is anorexia nervosa.

Victims are mainly young girls so intent upon losing weight that they literally starve themselves to death. This is no exaggeration. One-third of the victims die. Anorexics are now classified as psychotics, not neurotics.[1]

Some psychotherapists claim there's much more involved than a mania to continue losing weight, that anorexics are subconsciously rejecting their puberty, their sexual development, that they are trying to shrink away their breasts and other secondary sexual traits to return to infantile dependency.[2]

This reminds me of a peculiar experience I had a few years ago in Egypt, where feminine beauty is accented by well-padded hips and thighs and full-blown, pendulous breasts. Learning that "an American nutritionist" was a guest of the U.S. Ambassador, an Egyptian couple came to me to find out how they could get their pale, skin-and-bones, 14-year old anorexic daughter to eat.

"Even when I beat her, she won't eat," the father informed me. And the squat, huge-busted mother nodded assent. For an instant, I was fascinated by the mother's wretched skin with such huge pores that it was as if I were viewing them with a magnifying glass.

"Don't beat her. Just give her 30 mg of zinc and a 50 mg capsule of vitamin B-complex daily," I advised.

It is difficult to find vitamin-mineral supplements in Egypt, so I gave the parents part of my personal supply.

I later learned that anorexia is common there and that parents beat young girls, because non-eating causes thinness, which makes them bad marriage candidates.

43

This reminded me of a study which Dr. Jonathan Wright reported at a doctors' workshop held in conjunction with one of our National Health Federation conventions. The findings illustrated that if the female rat is zinc-deprived, her offspring to the third and fourth generation will be undersize, thin and with a poor appetite—some to the point of starvation.

Egypt's notoriously zinc-deficient soils, the girl's anorexia and the mother's poor complexion all seemed related.

Before leaving Egypt, I heard that the young girl was taking her supplements and eating better every day. Several months later, she was back to normal and filling out.

Unaware of or ignoring studies showing that nutrients have helped anorexics, a well-known psychotherapist calls anorexia "a non-classic psychophysiological disorder," in which it's hard to find a biological factor.[3]

In many areas of human illness, the patient is in the middle, claimed by both the psychiatrist and the medical doctor, a rope in a tug of war. Not so in anorexia nervosa.

Biological Factors Coming Up

Until recently, there have been few double-blind studies showing a biological factor in this bizarre illness. M.S. Robboy and associates in the department of obstetrics at the University of California at Los Angeles compared a group of anorexics with two groups of normal age-matched patients malnourished for causes other than anorexia and found the blood levels of beta-carotene extremely high in anorexics 90 to 20 to 8.[4] Why? More research is needed to get the answers.

Several researchers then discovered a zinc deficiency in a group of anorexics. This is significant, because a zinc deficiency can reduce appetite, mainly by diminishing the ability to taste and smell foods to the fullest extent. Thirty hospitalized anorexic patients, deficient in zinc, were hardly able to taste bitter or sour foods, as reported in the Section on Taste and Smell.[5]

Given 30 mg of zinc daily, the anorexics found their ability to taste improved, along with their appetite. As yet, researchers are uncertain if a zinc deficiency causes anorexia or whether it is just related to the disorder's symptoms.

On the basis of much research, Melvyn R. Werbach, M.D., author of *Nutritional Influence on Illness,* p.34. (Third Line Press, Inc.) states that zinc deficiency is well known to depress taste and smell, that anorexia nervosa can, of course, be brought on by too low an intake of zinc, by using oral contraceptives or by deficient absorption of food.

Dr. Werbach, assistant clinical professor in the School of Medicine, UCLA, Los Angeles, states that an experimental study indicates the appropriate nutrient for anorexia nervosa is 50 mg zinc sulfate, three times daily with meals. He cites two other studies of anorexics in which zinc supplementation helped the recovery of patients.

Friends who are natural healing doctors are now using a phosphorus tablet, which, when dissolved in water, tastes delicious to the zinc-deficient patient and abhorrent to those with an adequate zinc supply.

Undoubtedly, zinc makes a positive contribution to coping with anorexia nervosa. For this reason, I'll follow with a list of richest foods in zinc per milligram in a unit of less than four ounces: herring, 110; wheat germ, 14; sesame seeds, 10; torula yeast, 9.9; blackstrap molasses, 8.3; maple syrup, 7.5; liver, 7.0; soybeans, 6.7; sunflower seeds, 6.6; egg yolk, 5.5; lamb, 5.4; chicken, 4.8; regular molasses, 4.6; brewer's yeast, 3.9; oats, 3.7; bone meal, 3.6; rye, 3.4; whole wheat, 3.2; corn, 3.1; coconut and beef, 3.0; beets, turkey and walnuts, 2.8; barley, 2.7; beans, avocados, 2.5; peas, 2.3; bleu cheese, 2.2; eggs, 2.2 and buckwheat, 2.0.

Jack's Carnitine Chops
(BBQ Lamb Chops)

1 can (8 ounces) tomato sauce
½ c. green onions, minced
2 garlic cloves, chopped
6 lemon wedges (3 squirts
    liquid garlic extract - optional)
1 t. brewers yeast
2 T. olive oil
3 T. Black Strap Molasses

2 T. maple syrup
2 T. vinegar (preferably Tarragon)
1 t. steak sauce
1 t. sea salt
½ t. powdered mustard
Dash of hot pepper sauce
4 shoulder lamb chops
    (at least 1 inch thick)

Combine all ingredients, except chops. Cook over low heat, stirring occasionally for about 15 minutes. Brush lamb with sauce. Broil 3 to 4 inches from heat for 3 to 5 minutes on each side. Brush frequently with B.B.Q. Sauce. Makes 4 servings.

NOTE: Be sure to trim all fat from lamb as with all meats. That is where the toxins are stored.

Grated Beet Salad

1 bunch small young beets
    (tops removed for a tossed salad
    bowl), peeled
2 c. red cabbage, shredded
1 c. carrots, shredded

½ c. lemon juice
¼ c. olive oil
Sea salt or vegetable salt to taste
¼ c. sesame seeds

Grate beets finely into a salad bowl. Add cabbage and carrots. Beat together the lemon juice, honey, oil and salt and pour over beet mixture. Toss and chill well. Sprinkle seeds over top. Yield: eight to ten servings.

CHAPTER 7

Appendicitis

"The typical American diet is an open invitation to appendicitis!"

This is what I overheard a physician say to a group of doctors during a coffee break at a medical society's annual meeting, where I was one of the speakers.

The more I thought about it, the more I agreed. With the accent on so much processed food containing so little fiber, Americans are some of the world's most appendicitis-prone individuals.

This troubles me, because many authorities feel appendicitis can almost be wiped out with a medium to high fiber diet. A couple tablespoons of bran, a handful of peas, or a small carrot daily could turn out to be reasonable insurance against inflammation of the appendix, which is what appendicitis is.

I take a fiber product derived from the whole grain and whole vegetables and fruit.

Warning Signals

A sudden attack of appendicitis is not fun and games. Acute pain strikes in the lower right-hand area of the abdomen (called the right hypogastrium, if you'll pardon the expression). It is incredible that an appendage so small can cause so much pain. A dead-end, two to six inch long tube a bit thicker than a pencil, the appendix offshoots the upward turn of the large intestine, ideally located for collecting waste matter and bacteria and becoming infected and inflamed.

Pain centers around the appendix and the navel, the person usually becomes nauseated and may vomit and experience a rapid pulse and rising temperature. Muscles over the appendix may tighten in what's called a protective spasm. Abdominal rigidity is the sign of acute appendicitis and the signal to call the ambulance for a siren-screaming, tire-squealing race to a hospital emergency room.

Well-intentioned individuals sometimes try to relieve the victim's pain with a laxative or purgative and only increase the risk of the appendix bursting, making the case more hazardous for the patient and more complicated for the surgeon.

The Secret Of Prevention

How can a high-fiber diet prevent an attack of appendicitis?

The fiber keeps the stool soft, moist, compact and quickly and easily movable. On the other hand, the waste matter of the constipated person is hard and slow-moving and tends to break into hard balls, some of which become lodged in the appendix.

It pays to keep your appendix, if possible, say some authorities, even if it seems useless. Several epidemiological studies indicate that it may protect against cancer, although researchers can't prove it.

A study by the Medical College of Ohio (Toledo) revealed that 67 percent of 1,165 patients who had developed bowel cancer before the age of 50 had had their appendixes taken out.[1]

George Padanilam, M.D., one of the researchers suggests that the appendix may produce antibodies which keep cancer-causing viruses from attacking the colon. He advises against permitting doctors performing other surgery in that area to remove a normal appendix.

Howard R. Bierman, M.D., of the Institute for Cancer and Blood Research, warned a meeting of the American College of Surgeons, against removing the appendix prematurely, stating that it may perform some immunologic functions, protecting against leukemia.[2]

Dr. Bierman's study of 549 persons who died of some kind of cancer showed that 34.8 percent of them had had their appendixes surgically removed, compared with 23.4 for the group which didn't develop cancer. Nearly half of the persons who had died of colon or rectal cancer had had their appendixes removed. Dr. Bierman, too, cautioned surgeons about taking out normal appendixes while doing other surgery.

Other researchers, also, have found that various kinds of cancer seem to be more prevalent in patients who have had their appendixes removed — particularly colon cancer.

Fabulous Fiber

Vegetarians have a super-low rate of colon cancer and appendicitis, mainly because they get so much fiber from their diet. Along with bran, buckwheat groats and flour, the following are the richest food sources of fiber with a ratio of their percentages of fiber:

Raspberries, 47; pears, 25; melon, 22; strawberries, 19; cabbage, 18; asparagus, 17; cucumbers, 14; apples, 10; carrots, 8.8; green peas, 8.7; spinach, 8.1; onions, 5.0; beans and lentils, 4.1; potatoes, 3,1; whole wheat, 2.9 and brown rice, 1.7.

Fresh Asparagus

Sauce:

3 T. cider vinegar	raw spinach and watercress,
½ c. olive oil	finely chopped
¾ t. prepared mustard	1 medium onion, minced
3 T. mixed parsley,	

Combine all ingredients and blend thoroughly. Makes about ¾ Cup sauce.

Asparagus:

To boil asparagus, arrange washed stalks in a skillet or wire-bottomed pan. Pour in about ½ inch of "boiling" water. Sprinkle with sea salt if you wish. Cover pan. Bring quickly to a boil then lower heat to medium, or low. Cook for 10 to 12 minutes.

Banana Performance Shake

1 ripe banana

1 T. dried skim milk

1 T. honey

1 T. brewers yeast

1 c. raw certified milk

1 T. oat bran

Mix thoroughly in blender until smooth and creamy. Can be semi-frozen for a thicker consistency and eaten with a spoon.

Lightly Steamed Carrots And Peas

3 c. peas

3 c. carrots, cut in ¼ inch pieces - cross ways

Steam lightly and cover with avocado dressing (see below).

Avocado Dressing

2 avocados, pureed

1⅓ c. sour cream

1½ t. sea salt

½ t. chervil

½ t. tobasco

4 t. lemon juice

1 T. onion, minced

Combine all ingredients and chill 30 minutes. Makes 3 cups.

CHAPTER 8

Appetite (Poor)

In this land where too many people have too big an appetite and eat too much, there are many individuals who have too small an appetite and eat too little.

The latter group would like to know why their appetite is poor and how to develop a better one. So here goes.

Many studies indicate that appetite loss can be caused by several factors:

Underlying Reasons

(1) Eating too little to supply the nutrients which tend to generate hunger.

(2) Inability to experience the full range of tastes.

(3) Taking of prescription drugs

(4) Influence of celiac disease, a condition which prevents absorption of fat and calcium, often treated with apples and banana pulp.

In the event of too little food intake, appetite has been stepped up by increasing the eating of the best supplement and food sources of vitamin B-1 and B-12. (See end of this section.) Jonathan Wright, M.D., of Kent, Washington usually recommends a vitamin B-complex tablet with a potency of 50 mg for vitamin B-1 and other major B family fractions and 2,000 mcg of vitamin B-12, as an appetite stimulant.

Inability to taste and smell properly limits the appetite and desire to eat. This usually results from zinc deficiency, which may well tie into the item above: insufficient food intake to supply all necessary nutrients.

Thirty female patients hospitalized for anorexia nervosa, extreme aversion to food, were discovered to be unable to taste bitter and sour tastes, two important parts of the taste spectrum.[1]

Given 30 mg of zinc daily increased their ability to taste and their appetite, as well. (See Section on Taste and Smell.)

Drugs are notorious for decreasing appetite — particularly the chemotherapy drugs which can bring on nausea and vomiting. The most prominent are Methotrexate, mithramycin (Mithracin), carmustine (BICNU), doxorubicin (Adriamycin), cyclophosphamide (Cytoxan), asparaginase (Elspar) and daunorubicin (Cerubidine). Radiation of tumors often reduces appetite, too.[2] Digitalis, when used in large dosages to treat heart disease, can bring on anorexia. So can the antiarthritic drug, d-Penicillamine (Cuprimine), which curbs appetite by causing deficiencies of zinc and copper.

A sharp decrease in appetite develops in alcoholics, due to depletion of vitamin B-1, protein and zinc. Cirrhosis of the liver, gastritis, hepatitis, ketoacidosis, milk intolerance, and pancreatitis can also kill appetite.[3]

Various researchers restored appetite by treating children with celiac disease (faulty absorption of food accompanied by diarrhea and malnutrition) with two to three bananas daily. This disorder also responds to eliminating wheat and rye products from the diet. They contain a protein called gluten, which triggers celiac disease.

One of my doctor friends told me about a study he had read in which emaciated children who constantly threw up and had no appetite were fed one to four bananas, mashed and strained into their milk and whey formula. They stopped vomiting, kept down this food, developed an appetite and began gaining weight.

Foods That Heal

Richest supplement and food sources of vitamin B-1 in milligrams per less than four ounce unit are: brewer's yeast, 16; torula yeast, 15; sunflower seeds, 2.2; wheat germ, 2.0; royal jelly, 1.5; pinon nuts, 1.3; peanuts, 1.2; soybeans, 1.10; sesame seeds, 0.98; brazil nuts, 0.96; bee pollen, 0.93; pecans, 0.86; alfalfa and peas, 0.80; millet, 0.73; beans, 0.68; buckwheat and oats, 0.60; hazelnuts, 0.46; rye, 0.43; lentils and corn, 0.37; brown rice, 0.34; walnuts, 0.33; egg yolk, 0.32; chickpeas, 31: blackstrap molasses, 0.28; liver, 0.25; almonds, 0.24; barley and salmon,

0.21; eggs, 0.17 and lamb and mackerel, 0.15.

The best food sources of vitamin B-12 in milligrams per less than four ounce units: are liver, 0.086; sardines, 0.034; mackerel and herring, 0.0100; red snapper, 0.0088; flounder, 0.0064; salmon, 0.0047; lamb, 0.0031; swiss cheese, 0.0021; eggs, 0.0020; haddock, 0.0017; muenster cheese, 0.0016; swordfish and beef, 0.0015; blue cheese, 0.0014 and halibut and bass, 0.0014.

Zinc is most plentiful in the following foods and supplements in milligrams per less than four ounce units: herring, 110; wheat germ, 14; sesame seeds, 10; torula yeast, 9.9; blackstrap molasses, 8.3; maple syrup, 7.5; liver, 7.0; soybeans, 6.7; sunflower seeds, 6.6; egg yolk, 5,5; lamb, 5.4; chicken, 4.8; brewer's yeast, 3.9; oats, 3.7; bone meal, 3.6; rye, 3.4; wheat, 3.2; corn, 3.1; coconut and beef, 3.0; beets, turkey, and walnuts, 2.8; barley, 2.7; beans and avocados, 2.4; peas, 2.3; bleu cheese, 2.2; eggs, 2.1; buckwheat, 2.0, mangoes, 1.9 and millet, brown rice and almonds, 1.5.

Stuffed Flounder

1 lb. flounder fillets	½ c. cooked brown rice
1 T. olive oil	1 c. tomatoes, pureed
4 T. onions, finely chopped	2 T. wheat germ
⅓ c. raw spinach, chopped	¼ c. whole wheat bread crumbs
¼ c. almonds, sliced	⅛ c. parmesan cheese
4 T. parsley, finely chopped	2 T. sesame seeds
1 t. oregano	Fresh parsley and lemon slices
4 T. cheddar cheese, shredded	as garnish

Brush fillets with oil. Combine onion, spinach, parsley, oregano and almonds. Place on top of fillets and top with cheese. Place rice on top of cheese. Roll each fillet, starting with narrow end. Fasten with toothpicks and place side by side in oiled baking dish. Pour pureed tomatoes over rolls and sprinkle with mixture of wheat germ, bread crumbs, cheese and sesame seeds. Bake 30 minutes at 350 degrees. Remove toothpicks. Place on platter with parsley and lemon slices. Serves 4.

Maureen's Mint Apricots

⅓ c. honey

⅓ c. fresh lime juice

2 T. fresh mint, chopped

3 c. fresh apricots, sliced

Fresh mint for garnish

1 T. brewers yeast

Combine honey, lime juice, brewers yeast and mint in saucepan. Bring to boil. Strain and cool. Add apricots. Chill 2 to 3 hours. Serve in sherbet glasses, garnished with fresh mint. Serves 6.

Orange Turkey Salad

2 oranges

3 c. cooked turkey, diced

1 c. celery, diced

1 c. seedless green grapes

½ t. sea salt

½ t. curry powder

½ c. mayonnaise (home-made, see below)

½ c. toasted slivered almonds

Peel and section oranges over a bowl to reserve 2 tablespoons juice. Combine turkey, celery, grapes, orange sections, juice and sea salt. Cover and refrigerate 1 hour. Combine curry powder and mayonnaise; blend thoroughly. Add to turkey mixture and toss to coat evenly. Sprinkle with almonds. Serve in lettuce cups. Serves 8 to 10.

Mayonnaise

1 egg

½ t. sea salt

¼ t. cayenne pepper

2 T. honey

4 t. apple cider vinegar

7 t. lemon juice

1¼ c. safflower oil (cold pressed)

Blend all ingredients in blender, except the safflower oil. When blended, very slowly add safflower oil. Soon mixture will become thickened. If sweetness desired, add honey.

CHAPTER 9

Arthritis, Rheumatoid and Osteoarthritis

Although an estimated 35 million Americans suffer from the two major forms of arthritis — rheumatoid and osteoarthritis — they get little help from orthodox medicine. The typical stance of traditional medicine and the Arthritis Foundation is, "There's no known cause and no known cure."

Tired of pain-killing medicines and drugs and their side effects, many patients who have heard about successful treatments — some of them double-blind tested — ask their doctors about them and are usually told:

"There's no evidence that they work."

Well, there's no evidence that establishment medicine has any evidence that there's no evidence.

Blanket dismissals of something that might bring relief without side effects — recklessly and irresponsibly depriving the patient of hope and possible help is cruelty on a par with the agony of crippling arthritis.

Oh, Hippocrates, where are you when we need you?

Many Causes

As for there being no known cause, there are many known causes of arthritis, one discovered by the late and brilliant Roger Wyburn-Mason, M.D., Ph.D, the English physician who was first in discovering a viral basis for human cancer. Dr. Wyburn-Mason found amebas in rheumatoid arthritis patients. When he used a therapy to kill these microorganisms, symptoms of arthritis disappeared.

Other causes pinpointed by reputable researchers are: digestive disturbances, malnutrition, too much fat in the diet, chemicals in our foods and the environment, the gamut of stressors, and food sensitivities and allergies.

Before delving into causes, let's have a better understanding of the two major types of arthritis: rheumatoid and osteoarthitis. (Gout, related to arthritis, is covered in its own section.)

Rheumatoid arthritis is a chronic, inflammatory disorder bringing stiffness, deformity and pain to joints and muscles. Immune system defenders attack the tissues as if they are a threat to the body. Three times as many women have it as men. It sometimes strikes young mothers right after they give birth, apparently from attendant physiological, biochemical and emotional stresses.

Osteoarthritis is a wearing-away ailment. Cartilage (gristle) in the joints wastes away, calcium spurs may form on surfaces which contact bones. Synovial tissues which hold a lubricating fluid and insulate the contact of bone with joint cavities thicken, making movement difficult and painful.

This condition usually occurs in people who put their limbs through unusual uses and stresses: the obese and other heavyweights, as well as postmen, contact sports athletes, weight-lifters, stevedores, and, among others, sandhogs.

Conditions That Bring On Arthritis

Underlying these types of arthritis are the causes mentioned above, starting with digestive disturbances. Obviously, digestive problems could lead to nutrients lost through poor digestion and absorption and to undigested food fermenting in the intestinal tract and toxins entering the bloodstream. (See the sections on Constipation and Colon Complications.)

Yucca, a folk medicine used for more than a thousand years by American Indians of the great southwest desert, appears to correct digestive tract disorders and relieve symptoms of both kinds of arthritis, as shown by two double-blind studies conducted by arthritis specialist Robert Bingham, M.D., of Riverside, California.

Indians ate the flowers, fruit, leaves, roots, seeds, seed pods and stalks of yucca and extracted its juice (saponin) for many medicinal purposes by steaming or boiling the plant. Native Americans found yucca juice particularly effective for arthritis, by swallowing and applying it to painful areas.

Revealing Studies

In a 12-month, controlled, double-blind study of 68 rheumatoid arthritis and 97 osteoarthritis patients—all continuing their customary medication —half of the group was given yucca tablets daily (a total of 300 mg) and the other half, look-alike "nothing" (placebo) tablets.[1]

Not quite a quarter of the placebo group reported benefits. More than 60 percent of the yucca-pill takers reported gradual relief from the usual arthritis symptoms: pain, stiffness and swelling with no side effects and unexpected bonus values: better blood circulation, more clear skin and healthier hair and relief from persistent headaches.

In a second double-blind study, 88 rheumatoid and 124 osteoarthritis patients received yucca tablets (300 mg daily) or a placebo.[2] Yucca and placebos were alternated, with the average patients taking yucca for from six to 12 months. (They all continued their usual medication.) Results were almost the same as in the first study: more than 60 percent showed definite relief from arthritis, plus a significant drop in cholesterol, blood triglycerides and blood pressure.

Since then, numerous alternative doctors have helped patients gain relief from arthritis with yucca, a health food store item.

How does yucca help arthritis sufferers? John W. Yale, Jr., Ph.D, a botanist-biochemist, one of the first researchers to suggest saponin for human use, says that this product is not absorbed. However, it appears to protect friendly, intestinal bacteria, which keep under control microorganisms causing fermentation and toxins and prevents these poisons from entering the bloodstream and causing an allergic reaction.[3]

Malnutrition Can Do It, Too!

A peculiar kind of malnutrition assails some rheumatoid arthritis (RA) patients, as revealed by a study at Salisbury General Hospital in Wiltshire, England.[4]

When RA patients were compared with an equal number of non-arthritis patients, 25 percent were found malnourished, with significantly low blood levels of folic acid (a B-vitamin) protein and zinc. The non-arthritis patients showed normal levels of these nutrients. The more severe the symptoms of RA, the more malnourished were the patients.

The researchers were surprised by the deficiencies, because the RA patients seemed to be eating a balanced diet. Finally, they concluded that the malnourishment did not result from an inferior diet, but to the stress of RA and the drugs, which brought about an increased need for specific nutrients.

Another dietary factor, excessive fat, seems to contribute to rheumatoid arthritis.[5] Dr. Charles Lucas and fellow researchers at Wayne State University Medical School in Detroit put six suffering RA patients on a fat-free diet, Within seven weeks, all of them had lost their symptoms.

Then either animal or vegetable fats were given to them, and, in 72 hours, all of their symptoms returned. More investigation of this phenomenon is now in progress. Obviously, one cannot exist indefinitely on a totally fat-free diet without harm. However, follow-up research may show that even a low-fat diet can contribute positively. Time will tell.

Food Sensitivities And More

Fatty foods are not the only dietary factors which contribute to arthritis, as discovered by Dr. Lucas and associate researchers.[6] Obese patients, many of whom develop arthritis, lost symptoms of the condition when put on weight-reduction fast. Credit for this was given to the lessening of strain on joints, due to appreciable weight loss.

However, another key factor should be considered. In eating nothing, patients eliminate foods to which they are sensitive or allergic. As long ago as 1934, medical doctors have found a relationship between food sensitivities and arthritis. Abstaining from offending foods brought an end to most symptoms. (The Section on Allergies tells how to discover food sensitivities.)

Rheumatoid arthritis is commonly called an "autoimmune disease," because the body's immune system makes the error of attacking its own tissues.

Encino, California's James Braly, M.D., a noted clinical ecologist, observes that a more current viewpoint is that rheumatoid arthritis may result from a local inflammatory response when food-containing immune complexes are deposited in and around joints and related tissues, causing the release of painful chemicals (Dr. Braly's Optimum Health Program, Times Books, p. 326).

Arthritis develops in some individuals sensitive to a whole category of foods, nightshade plants: eggplant, peppers—red and green, but not black —Irish potatoes and tomatoes.

Unmasking Nightshade Plants

Many years ago, Dr. Norman F. Childers, of Rutgers University, discovered that nightshade plants can contribute to arthritis in certain individuals.[7] After drinking large amounts of tomato juice daily over a few months, he experienced excruciating pain in joints and muscles. Figuring that other nightshade plants might do the same, he tested them on himself and found his theory was correct. By eating nightshade vegetables, then avoiding them, he could turn arthritis symptoms on and off.

An alternative doctor told me about a hard-to-solve arthritis case. A middle-aged male patient sensitive to nightshade plants eliminated them without showing improvement. Finally, his wife revealed the answer. The man was secretly continuing to smoke, masking his breath with mouthwashes and mints. TOBACCO IS A NIGHTSHADE PLANT!

When he stopped smoking, his arthritis began to improve.

Nightshade foods are often hidden ingredients in processed canned and packaged foods—for instance, potato starch. This is also used as a stiffener for low-cost yogurt. A nightshade seasoning like paprika is often hidden under the blanket term "spice". Rather than strain your eyes reading labels and trying to understand the double-talk terms, it is best to avoid the labels, the containers wearing them and the alleged food within them.

The Worst Is Yet To Come

However, nightshade ingredients are not even the worst part of processed foods with their inflated prices and deflated food values. Chemical additives

—colorings, flavorings, preservatives, emulsifiers—are an open invitation to arthritis, as discovered in many cases by Dr. Theron Randolph, one of the world's leading clinical ecologists.

The same goes for pesticides, herbicides and fungicides used on and in many of our growing foods and other noxious chemicals that pollute our planet and us. Dr. Randolph found that arthritis symptoms disappeared when patients skipped chemicalized foods and avoided environmental pollutants.

Dr. Braly, a disciple of Randolph, indicates that "leaky gut syndrome" accounts for much food sensitivity and allergy. Repeated assaults of problem foods lead to possible arthritis.[8]

Three thousand chemical substances in foods, plus 10,000 chemical-environmental contaminants make the intestinal lining more prone to leak partially digested macromolecules into the bloodstream.[9]

These molecules are far larger than those of the usual nutrients transported by the blood, so immune system defenders regard them as enemy invaders or allergens and battle to get rid of them.

Alcohol, coffee and cigarette-smoking can also contribute to leaky gut syndrome—and, later, arthritis—as much as do problem and chemicalized foods.[10]

How can one find unchemicalized foods? It isn't always easy. Some health food stores carry them. Some farmers grow them. Do a little investigating. Another alternative is to grow your own. If you haven't got the land, work a cooperative deal with a neighbor or friend. He or she furnishes the land and water, and you furnish the seeds and labor and share the crops.

Does Stress Father Arthritis?

Alien and poisonous chemicals in food and environment are just a few of the hundreds of stressors that assail us physically, emotionally and mentally. (See the Section on Stress.) Whatever the form of stress or its degree of intensity, if it persists, we wear down the adrenal system and develop nutritional deficiencies.

Many studies document that severe stress comes before the onset of arthritis and, with it, low blood levels of vitamins C, pantothenic acid and

B-6. An arthritis-like ailment was induced in rats by making them deficient in pantothenic acid, a condition which seemed to keep blood levels of vitamin C depressed.[11] Making up the pantothenic acid deficiency corrected the condition.

When arthritic patients were given a supplement of 25 milligrams of pantothenic acid daily—their only dietary addition—some lost their pain and stiffness within two weeks.[12] (It is possible to get this amount daily from food supplements and food.)

Guinea pigs stressed by low intake of vitamin C and the injection of bacteria developed arthritis. Other animals of the group, given a super high intake of vitamin C, were protected from developing arthritis.[13]

Rats fed foods with high amounts of phosphorus and low amounts of calcium became arthritic.[14] Given two times as much calcium as phosphorus, they lost their arthritis. Much research has established two-to-one as a proper ratio of calcium to phosphorus.

Some individuals believe that the answer to arthritis is cutting down on calcium-rich foods. Stress, which often precedes the development of arthritis, draws calcium out of the bones, as does a dietary shortage of calcium or magnesium. Therefore, calcium needs to be taken in, rather than reduced.[15] Remember, the pain and physical limitations imposed by arthritis are stressors, too, stealing bone and tooth calcium.

Various studies have shown that a liberal intake of calcium seems to decrease the sensitivity to arthritis-caused pain.

At the end of this section are foods richest in the critical nutrients mentioned above.

Spectacular Research Results

An exciting experimental regime of Drs. Charles M. Brusch and Edward T. Johnson, of the Brusch Medical Center, Cambridge Massachusetts, led to 92 out of 100 rheumatoid and osteoarthritis patients showing marked reduction of pain, reduced swelling, greater range of motion and many bonus improvements: more energy, better complexion and skin luster and greater mental alertness. Here it is:[16]

1. Limiting water intake to an hour prior to breakfast, but drinking room-temperature whole milk and soup at meals.

2. Cod liver oil at bedtime or one or more hours before breakfast. Taken at the latter time, it must be 30 or more minutes after the water intake.

3. Daily intake of calories between 1,800 and 2,400.

4. No junk foods — cake, cookies, candies, sweet rolls and other products containing white sugar and/or flour—ice cream and soft drinks.

The Bingham Regimen

Still another successful regime is that of Robert Bingham, M.D., a board certified orthopedic surgeon (mentioned earlier) who operates an arthritis clinic in Desert Hot Springs, California.[17]

While orthodox medicine says nothing can be done about arthritis, Dr. Bingham keeps doing it and has thousands of rheumatoid and osteoarthritis case histories to prove it. (18) This is the regimen for patients in his clinic:

1. 16 hours of daily bedrest.

2. Additional water—eight or more glasses daily.

3. High protein diet: poultry, fish, meat, eggs, dairy products, nuts, whole grains and seeds.

4. Organically grown fruits and vegetables eaten raw and fresh.

5. Special vitamin-mineral-hormone-enzyme regime. (Most new patients are deficient in vitamin B-complex, C, and D—the latter essential to absorption and utilization of calcium, magnesium and iron.)

6. No tobacco, alcohol or refined carbohydrates (junk food).

7. Gradual decrease of drugs and corticosteroid medications to the level tolerable by the patient without excessive pain.

8. Two thousand milligrams of vitamin C daily.

9. Three glasses of raw certified milk daily for protein and calcium. Non-hospitalized patients are permitted to drink pasteurized milk, because certified is permitted in only a few states.

10. 1,000 I.U. of vitamin D from fish liver oils, as well as 25,000 I.U. of vitamin A daily, both particularly helpful for osteoarthritics—levels regarded high by conservative medicine. Half these amounts are recommended by Dr. Bingham for prevention.

The only failures the Bingham therapy has met are patients who refused to abstain from tobacco and alcohol and to follow doctor's orders to reduce pain-killers and tranquilizers and hypnotic drugs.

Another Angle Of Attack

An article by Drs. E. Abrams and J. Sandson (Annals of Rheumatic Diseases) attributes some joint stiffness and pain of arthritis to thickening of synovial fluid, a natural lubricant of the joints. High blood levels of vitamin C make synovial fluid thinner, contributing to easier and greater range of motion, they write.

Here, in the order mentioned above are key nutrients for guarding against arthritis:

Richest supplements and foods in folic acid in milligrams per less than four ounce units are:

Torula yeast, 3.0; brewer's yeast, 2.0; alfalfa, 0.80; soybeans, 0.69; endive, 0.47; chickpeas, 0.41; oats, 0.39; lentils, 0.34; beans and wheat germ, 0.31; liver, 0.29; split peas, 0.23; whole wheat, 0.22; barley, 0.21; brown rice, 0.17; asparagus, 0.12; green peas, 0.11; sunflower seeds and collard green, 0.100; spinach, 0.080; hazelnuts and kale, 0.070; peanuts, soy lecithin and walnuts, 0.060; corn, 0.059; and brussels sprouts, broccoli, brazil nuts, and almonds, 0.050.

Best sources of zinc in milligrams per units of less than four ounces are:

Herring, 110; wheat germ, 14; sesame seeds, 10; torula yeast, 9.9; blackstrap molasses, 8.3; maple syrup, 7.5; liver, 7.0; soybeans, 6.7; sunflower seeds, 6.6; egg yolk, 5.5; lamb, 5.4; chicken, 4.8; regular molasses, 4.6; brewer's yeast, 3.9; oats, 3.7; bone meal, 3.6; rye, 3.4; whole wheat, 3.2; corn, 3.1; coconut and beef, 3.0; beets, turkey and walnuts, 2.8; barley, 2.7; beans and avocados, 2.4; peas, 2.3; blue cheese, 2.2; eggs, 2.1; buckwheat, 2.0; mangoes, 1.9; millet, rice and almonds, 1.5 and salmon, 1.4.

Here are supplements and foods with the highest amounts of pantothenic acid in milligrams per portions of less than four ounces:

Royal jelly, 35; brewer's yeast, 11; torula yeast, 10; brown rice, 8.9; sunflower seeds, 5.5; soybeans, 5.2; corn, 5.0; lentils, 4,8; egg yolk, 4.2; peas, 3.6; alfalfa, 3.3; whole wheat, 3.2; peanuts, 2.8; rye, 2.6; eggs, 2.3; bee pollen and wheat germ, 2.2; bleu cheese, 1.8; cashews, 1.3; chickpeas, 1.2; avocado, 1.1; chicken, sardines, turkey, and walnuts, 0.90 and perch and salmon, 0.080.

Supplements and foods richest in vitamin C in milligrams per less than four ounce units are:

Rose hips, 3,000; acerola cherries, 1,100; guavas, 240; black currants, 200; parsley, 170; green peppers, 110; watercress, 80; chives, 70; strawberries, 57; persimmons, 52; spinach, 51; oranges, 50; cabbage, 47; grapefruit, 38; papaya, 37; elderberries and kumquats, 35; dandelion greens and lemons, 35; cantaloupe, 33; green onions, 32; limes, 31; mangoes, 27; loganberries, 24; tangerines and tomatoes, 23; squash, 22; raspberries and romaine lettuce, 18, and pineapple, 17.

Best bets for vitamin D in International Units per less than four ounce portions are:

Cod liver oil, 20,000; sardines, 500; salmon, 400; tuna, 250; egg yolk, 160; sunflower seeds, 92; liver, 50; eggs, 48; butter, 40; cheeses, 30; cream, 15; corn oil, 9.0; human milk, 6.0; cottage cheese and cow's milk, 4.0; bee pollen, 1.6 and bass.

CHAPTER 10

Asthma

The following words characterize asthma: "A paroxysmal attack narrowing airways and causing shortness of breath with wheezing and a frightening feeling of suffocation."

This disorder can be brought on by many causes: food and beverages (and sulfites in them) or environmental allergens—fresh paint, perfumes, spray deodorants, cigarette smoke, gasoline or car exhaust fumes, grain, wood, coal or chalk dust, various chemicals such as cleaning solvents, household cleaners, insecticides, pollens and molds—the latter sometimes originate in home or auto air conditioners — viral respiratory disease, vigorous exercise, change in moisture content of the air, sudden inhalation of extremely cold or hot air, emotional stress or other stress.

Although this condition can be controlled by drugs, physicians who practice alternative medicine have several ways of treating the disorder without the risk of the side effects of drugs.

Avoid And Conquer

The first method is helping the patient determine foods or environmental allergens or conditions which trigger asthma—and then avoiding them.

One of the key categories of foods to avoid is dairy products, as Israeli researchers discovered.[1] When twenty-two asthma sufferers were taken off milk and related producrs, 15 responded with dramatic improvement. (See the Section on Milk Intolerance.)

Then the fortunate 15 were challenged with dairy products, and five experienced severe asthma attacks. Again taken off these foods, they were able to breathe more freely, sharply reduce their medication and decrease the need for hospitalization.

Something Else To Avoid

A little-known contributor to asthma is a high intake of polyunsaturated fatty acids (PUFAs), present in various vegetable and nut oils: corn, safflower, soy, sunflower seed, peanut and walnut, among others.[2]

The cholesterol craze and the frenzied promotion of polyunsaturated fats over saturated fats such as butter and lard have caused many individuals to overdo the bit—like taking four tablespoons of vegetable oil once recommended by the American Heart Association. Without additional vitamin E, PUFAs can destroy cells, including those of lung tissue. tissue.

Animal experiments show that, in such a circumstance, red blood cells tend to accumulate in arteries and reduce or block blood flow and oxygen delivery, a serious occurrence when coupled with air pollution in most metropolitan areas and stress.

Other Enemies Of The Asthmatic

MSG (monosodium glutamate) — a flavor enhancer — sulfites, preservatives in processed foods, dried fruits and some wines and restaurant salads, where not prohibited by law, as well as the yellow food dye tartrazine (FD and C yellow dye number 5) in many processed foods, can bring on asthma attacks.[3]

Chinese restaurants, notorious for their use of MSG, are slowly giving up the practice—some even advertising that they don't flavor food with MSG. Although banned in some states and nations, sulfites are still applied to keep salad greens looking fresh and crisp in many salad bars and in restaurant kitchens.

Sulfites are a good reason for an asthmatic person to avoid processed foods such as dried fruits—a good reason for everybody to stay with fresh foods, when possible. (4) (Health food stores carry unprocessed dried fruits.) Artificial food colorings are suspect in contributing to a number of ailments — the most prominent, hyperactivity. (See Section on

Hyperactivity.)

Processed foods with their array of additives, colorings, flavorings, and preservatives, are good foods to leave on the shelf — that of the supermarket.

Folk Remedies

Inasmuch as avoidance is not always possible, various alternative therapies are said to help—the first of which are folk remedies such as foods and herbs.

Honey with pollen has its followers among asthma sufferers, although detractors say it could never get through the digestive plumbing and enter the bloodstream.

A researcher at the Heidelberg University Children's Clinic (Germany), U. Wahn, M.D., made a study of seventy children with hay fever and allergy-related asthma who drank a solution of bee pollen and honey each day during the yearly hay fever period and three days per week in winter.[5]

Most of them showed fewer symptoms after this regime, indicating to Dr. Wahn that the pollen somehow had made it into the bloodstream.

A second folk remedy for asthma is chili pepper, noted for burning mouth and throat.[6] Cayenne pepper (capsicum) is an expectorant, say some alternative doctors. Not only does it sting in the sinuses and sometimes bring smarting tears to the eyes, it temporarily irritates the stomach and sets up a sympathetic reaction in the bronchial tubes and in the lungs to discharge secretions, making them less thick and sticky and more open for breathing.

Helpful Herbs?

Now for some more folk medicine. Several herbs are said to help alleviate asthma. Mr. Big among them is mullein, a tall plant of the figwort family with spikes of white, lavender or yellow flowers. Its soft, fuzzy leaves make an excellent tea which, supposedly, helps in two ways: in the drinking and in the inhaling of its steam.

Elecampe, ephedra, eucalyptus, horehound, lungwort and pleurisy root made into a tea individually or in combinations are reputed to relieve symptoms of asthma.

Sometimes honey, chili peppers, and other folk remedies don't do the job, so reinforcements have to be brought in — vitamins with a higher potency than natural foods can provide, when we consider the limitation of stomach capacity.

Exciting Research

Nobel Laureate Dr. Linus Pauling indicates that recent studies show that vitamin C may offer relief in asthma.[7] In three experiments, reduced ability to breathe brought about by inhaling the histamine aerosol, flax dust, or textile dust were controlled to a degree for three or four hours by ingestion of 500 mg of vitamin C. Yale University researchers exposed six healthy, young male subjects to methacholine, a drug which tightens the bronchi and decreases breathing ability in both asthmatics and healthy individuals by approximately 40 percent. When they ingested 1000 mg of vitamin C an hour before exposure to methacholine, their airlow was reduced by just nine percent — a more than four-fold improvement.

Double Blind Study

In a double-blind study of forty-one Nigerian asthma patients over fourteen weeks during the rainy season when prevalent respiratory infections make asthma attacks more severe, twenty-two were given 1000 mg of vitamin C daily and nineteen were given a look-alike pill (a placebo) with no nutritional value.[8]

Takers of vitamin C had fewer than one-fourth the asthma attacks as those on placebos and these were not as serious. Thirteen vitamin C takers experienced not a single attack in the fourteen week interval, but suffered at least one asthma attack in the eight week span after quitting the vitamin C.

In a six month South African study of ten white children with bronchial asthma, the test subjects were administered 1000 mg of vitamin C daily.[9] Not one of them had a severe attack of asthma, and they all showed improved lung function and an enhanced immune system.

Exaggerated Need For Vitamin B-6 (Pyridoxine)

Early studies revealed that many asthma patients are dependent on vitamin B-6 — that is, they do not have a deficiency as such, but an exaggerated need, due to an error in metabolism.

On this basis, five New York physicians designed a five-month, double-blind experiment with seventy-six youthful patients with moderate to severe asthma.[10] Half of the patients were given two 100 mg tablets of vitamin B-6. The other half received placebos. Neither the patients nor the doctors knew which individuals were receiving the vitamin B-6 so that results would not be influenced by human beings.

One month passed, and there was almost no difference between the two groups. However, with the start of the second month, the patients receiving the vitamin B-6 had fewer asthma attacks and less breathing difficulty, wheezing and coughing.

The differences continued to be even more marked between the second and fifth months, with the researchers concluding that vitamin B-6 reduces the severity of asthma attacks with no side effects, compared with devastating side effects of prednisone, a steroid drug frequently used to manage asthma: convulsions, glaucoma, peptic ulcer and psychic disorders.

A Lesser Amount Works, Too!

Even smaller amounts of pyridoxine — 50 mg twice daily — appear to lessen the duration, frequency, and severity of attacks of asthma. Dr. Robert Reynolds, a U.S. Department of Agriculture biochemist, reported that symptoms of every asthmatic on this daily regime were relieved.[11]

However, the same phenomenon occurred as in the previous study. There was no improvement in symptoms until test subjects had taken pyridoxine for more than a month.

Often it is impossible to get the required amount of nutrients from food, because, according to the Dr. Roger Williams' theory of biochemical differences, some individuals have a far greater need for certain specific nutrients than average. Then it may be necessary to buttress the regular diet with food supplements.

The main point is this. It is important to win the war against a tough and frightening physical disorder such as asthma, even if we have to bring up the biggest and best weapons available.

Carl Junior's Green Salad

1 garlic clove, mashed
1 head Bibb or Romaine lettuce,
   torn into bite size
5 radishes, sliced
1 avocado, chopped
2 green onions, chopped

1 c. alfalfa sprouts
2 T. fresh lemon juice
2 T. unrefined olive oil
Sea salt to taste
¼ t. cayenne pepper

Rub salad bowl with mashed garlic clove. Discard garlic. Sprinkle sea salt into bowl. Mix vegetables and pour lemon juice and oil over all. Season with herbal seasoning if desired.

CHAPTER 11

Athlete's Foot

Non-athletes seem to have a monopoly on athlete's foot, fungus-caused reddish, cracked and itchy skin between toes—mainly between the little toe and its too-close neighbor.

This is because athletes know how to protect themselves from the fungus among us, wearing sandals when walking on damp floors of athletic club shower rooms and steam rooms, around inside public swimming pools or on the much-traveled carpeting of motel and hotel rooms.

As with so many human disorders, prevention is easier than cure.

Less than 10 Commandments can help you to avoid athlete's foot for a lifetime, starting with:

Thou Shalt Not:

1. Walk barefooted in damp, public places where the athlete's foot fungus (ringworm) thrives.

2. Wear shoes made partially or wholly from synthetic materials. (They are called "Man-Made Materials." Leather lets your feet breathe.)

3. Wear the same shoes on consecutive days. Let them air and dry.

4. Put on socks made of synthetic fabrics. (Wool or cotton permit better air-circulation in the shoes and lessen the chance of sweat accumulating.)

5. Wear sweat-soaked socks. (Don't give the ever-ready and eager fungus a break.)

6. Fail to dry your feet thoroughly after swimming, bathing or showering—even at home. (Same reason as Number 5.)

Getting Rid Of The Stuff

The husband of a dear friend had real complications from his athlete's foot. He proved to be allergic to the salve given him by the doctor, and his feet swelled to almost twice their size. The cracks between his reddened and puffy toes migrated to the top of his feet, and the fungus worked its way under his toenails.

He refused my advice to go back to his doctor.

"Then try an alternative doctor," I recommended.

"No way!" he responded. "Marion borrowed a folk medicine book, and I'm going to try one of the remedies."

"Like what?"

"Vinegar."

"Dabbing vinegar between the toes with balls of cotton?"

"No. I'll soak my feet in a diluted vinegar bath."

"His feet were so swollen and raw looking, I was afraid the fiery burn of the vinegar would launch him through the roof."

However, he poured a cup of apple cider vinegar and a few quarts of warm water into a white enameled basin, sat on a chair, and gingerly lowered his feet into the basin. Somehow, he was able to stand it for fifteen minutes. Strangely, his feet felt better.

That night he repeated the process, and the swelling began to go down. He did the same thing every morning and night for a week. Apparently the warm water had opened the pores and permitted the vinegar to penetrate. Each time he would blot his feet dry with a clean Turkish towel. After another week of his self-medication, he was healed, and the fungus was gone—even from under his toenails.

Underneath It All

Later I learned that this man had had a persistent infection treated by his doctor with a lengthy series of antibiotic shots, which eventually killed the harmful bacteria and, with them, the friendly, intestinal organisms which synthesize various vitamins of the B family.

Without those B vitamins, he couldn't build up his resistance and beat back the fungus. I recommended a local nutrition-oriented physician, who had him eat a quart of high quality yogurt daily to colonize his intestines with beneficial organisms—that and a diet heavy in B vitamins: beef liver, two bowls of wheat germ cereal (eaten cold), and three tablespoons of brewer's yeast in raw certified milk (which he enjoyed).

He looked and felt great—better than he had in years!

Others victimized with athlete's foot have followed this formula with success. Most of them didn't have to dunk their whole feet into a dilute solution of vinegar. They merely dabbed diluted vinegar between their toes each morning and night.

Open sandals helped keep their feet dry of perspiration. One person I know made tiny cotton ball wedges between all his toes and left them there to assure constant dryness. Still others washed their feet with soap and water, dried them thoroughly and then spread on cornstarch to keep them dry.

Success I have seen brought about by these methods is indeed encouraging.

CHAPTER 12

Bad Breath (Halitosis)

Nobody has died from bad breath, but this disorder—if persistent — can be the death of a person's relationships, so it deserves some attention.

If one looks for the solution only in the obvious place—the mouth — he or she isn't looking far enough, because, it usually originates far below: in the stomach or intestinal tract, due to poor digestion and assimilation.

Often there's not enough hydrochloric acid in the stomach for complete digestion, so undigested food passes into the intestines, putrifies, and gives off foul gases which rise up as foul breath.

Solving The Problem

Nutrition-oriented doctors often suggest that patients deficient in hydrochloric acid take a tablespoon of apple cider vinegar just before each meal. This helps digestion and often does away with bad breath before bad breath does away with the patient's social life.

If this home remedy fails to work, the doctor usually has the patient visit his or her health food store and buy 500 mg tablets or capsules containing hydrochloric acid, betaine and pepsin, to be taken just before the meal.

Constipation Could Be The Culprit

Constipation can also contribute to bad breath. (See the Section on Constipation.) One of the listeners to my national "Accent on Health" television program wrote to tell me about her husband's problem with halitosis:

"The odor is strong. His breath is so bad it would curl the armorplate on

74

a battleship. I can't sleep in the same room with him, and nobody at the shipyard wants to work with him—even outdoors. I'm afraid he'll lose his job.''

I directed her to an alternative physician in her area. It turned out that her husband had a bad case of constipation, caused mainly by a low fiber diet, not drinking enough water, and an army of putrefactive bacteria at work on the accumulated waste matter in him.

(For a referral to a nutrition-oriented doctor, see the list in the back of the book. If there's none in your area, check with your nearest health food store.)

A daily ration of eight tablespoons of oat bran spread on top of his whole wheat cereal, mixed into his juice, or baked into muffins, plus three glasses of water more than he habitually drank soon regularized him. A 32-ounce container of high grade yogurt each day for a week—one-third of the contents before each meal—soon implanted friendly bacteria (lactobacillus acidophilus) in his intestines to colonize and take over.

Within ten days, his breath "was sweet," his wife wrote: "Thanks, Maureen, for returning my bedmate to me."

A Certain Vitamin

An experiment showed that patients deficient in vitamin B-6 often exhaled offensive breath. When this vitamin was added to their diet, the foul breath soon disappeared.[1]

Vitamin B-6 is not plentiful in foods. However, here are the foods and the milligrams of this vitamin per less than four ounce units: brown rice, 3.6, whole wheat, 2.9; royal jelly, 2.4; soybeans, 2.0; rye, 1.8; lentils, 1.7; sunflower seeds, 1.1; hazelnuts, 1.1; alfalfa, 1.00, salmon, 0.98; wheat germ, 0.92; tuna, 0.90; bran, 0.85; walnuts, 0.73; peas and liver, 0.67; avocados, 0.60; beans, 0.57 and oats, chicken and beef, 0.40.

Carbohydrates And Bad Breath

Experiments by Dr. Seizo Kawasaki, of Japan, as reported in "Dental Abstracts," revealed that the type of food consumed contributes to breath odor due to how that type of food alters the chemistry of the saliva.[2]

Dr. Kawasaki found that, within three hours, the saliva will pick up odors of food. The saliva odor is strongest after the eating of carbohydrates — sugars, starches and cellulose. It is not quite as strong after proteins are eaten. Fats do not cause a mouth odor and actually block any from forming.

Just as food can putrefy in the intestines, so can it rot in the mouth, if proper oral sanitation is not practiced. This means that teeth should be brushed and flossed to make sure there's no collection of putrefying food to give off foul odors.

Certain malformed teeth and poor relationships between teeth create hollows and traps for food. Dentists can correct these food debris collection areas to make mouth hygiene easier and to assure no odoriforous breath from this source. Decaying teeth and swollen gums also collect foods which putrefy and give off unpleasant odors. (Usually swollen gums are caused by deficiencies of vitamin C and niacin, as many studies indicate.)

All of us know individuals who excuse themselves at frequent intervals to gargle mouthwashes to assure a sweet breath. An article in the journal Dental Abstracts blasts the notion that mouthwashes are an efficient way of insuring against halitosis.[3]

Using a toothbrush effectively can do much to reduce or eliminate mouth odors for at least two hours. A mouthwash will mask odors for only about a half hour.

Other Breath Polluters

Tobacco and alcohol breath are hard to conceal — as is that for onions and garlic. Fortunately, there's now a sociable, odorless garlic food supplement on the market.

However, if garlic and onions are your thing, you may still be able to cover their odor by chewing on parsley or various other pleasantly fragrant herbs: basil, mint, rosemary or thyme.

Most dental authorities frown on sugary mints and chewing gum to cover bad breath. Some of them could be harmful to the teeth and the body, because they contain either sugar or an artificial sweetner.

Two herbs are excellent breath cover-ups until the basic causes are corrected. You just chew on some peppermint or wintergreen. That's straight out of folk medicine. If you don't believe it, just check with the folk.

Sometimes correcting bad breath can be a successful do-it-yourself project. However, there are times when professionals—the dentist and/or the doctor—need to be called in to help. It may cost a little to get the problem solved and to be welcomed back into society, but the reward could be worth more than the price.

Almond Milk

Soak 3 ounces almonds overnight in 5 ounces apple juice. In morning, add 3 to 5 ounces spring water and blend in blender for 2 to 3 minutes. Flavor with honey and a banana.

Susan Porter's Oat Bran Muffins

2 c. whole meal stoneground flour	1 T. apple juice concentrate
½ c. oat bran	1 egg white (yolk discarded)
1½ c. spring water	¼ t. ginger powder
½ c. dates, pitted and chopped	Pinch of ground cloves

Preheat oven to 400 degrees. In a sauce pan, simmer dates and water for 5 minutes and cool. Combine all ingredients and thoroughly mix to a cake consistency. Place large spoonfuls into non-stick muffin tins that have been lightly dusted with oat flour. Bake muffins for 15 minutes, or until golden brown. Remove from oven.

Wagner's Spiked Sprouts

1 bunch green onions	1 cup celery, sliced (slanting slices)
1 large dry onion	1 green pepper, cut in thin slices
½ cup water chestnuts, sliced	Seasoning salt (spike)
¾ cup spring water	1 tablespoon honey
½ pound bean sprouts	½ bunch parsley, chopped

Cut green onions in 1-inch lengths, using most of the tops as well. Peel dry onion, cut in half, then slice in slanting slices. Sprinkle with kelp or vegetable seasoning salt. Heat in large heavy skillet along with water chestnuts, bean sprouts, water and honey. Mix well and add celery. Steam for 2 to 3 minutes. Add pepper. Toss gently a time or two. Serve hot on rice. Scatter blanced and toasted almonds or toasted sesame seed and parsley over the top. Serves 4 to 6.

CHAPTER 13

Baldness

"Hair today and gone tomorrow."

This sentence sums up the negative future for many men and, sadly, for an ever-increasing number of women.

"What upsets me is that there's nothing much we can do about hair-loss but regret it," a semi-bald man at one of my health seminars told me.

"Sorry, but you're wrong," I responded. "Male pattern baldness gives little room for optimism — except for toupee-makers and hair-transplanters. However, there are many kinds of baldness, some of which respond to improved diets."

This person did not display the usual male pattern baldness—an evenly retreating hairline and a circle of shining scalp at the crown of his head, typical of individuals who were dealt the wrong genes. So I made him aware of encouraging animal and human studies.

Remarkable Results

Researchers controlled the thinning and thickening of animal hair by withdrawing essential amino acids from their diets, then restoring them.

Magnesium-deficient rats lost hair in bunches.[1] On diets low in biotin or inositol (B vitamins), they became hairless.[2] Men deficient in vitamin B-6 often lost their hair.[3] Men shorted on folic acid sometimes became totally bald. However, a normal intake of this vitamin restored their hair, in most instances.[4]

Heavy doses of vitamin B-complex have revved up human hair growth in some cases.[5]

Medical doctor friends tell me that a diet rich in the nutrients mentioned above have on occasion fulfilled the high nutritional needs of some semi-bald men and brought on a new crop of thick hair.

One nutrition-oriented medical doctor sometimes encourages hair growth with a diet accenting protein—calf's liver, brewer's yeast, wheat germ, and two tablespoons of granulated lecithin.

Unsuspected Causes Of Hair Loss

Persons losing large amounts of hair rarely realize that certain drugs or medicines could be victimizing them: blood thinners like dicumarol, heparin and heparinoid; carbimazole—used to temper hyperthyroidism — and certain antibiotics such as penicillin, sulfonomides and mycin drugs.[6]

Once these drugs are discontinued, hair usually grows back. Severe illness, pregnancy, or stress can bring on temporary hair loss — even baldness. Stress can contribute to permanent hair loss, because often it is never-ending, inasmuch as the person never learns to manage his or her daily stress. (See the Section on Stress).

Probing to find the root causes of stress, eliminating or minimizing it, and learning how to turn it into a challenge helps to lessen its ravages and increase hair growth. Regular, vigorous exercise is a secondary but, still, an effective way of coping with stress, because physical activity uses up the surplus hormones and energy generated by the stress response.

In "Let's Get Well," (Harcourt, Brace & World, page 165), the late Adelle Davis confesses that stressful work on her book with many sleepless nights led to an alarming condition—her hair falling out and receding at the temples.

Immediately, she slept more and went on her anti-stress program: 500 mg of vitamin C, 100 mg of pantothenic acid, and two mg each of vitamins B-2 and B-6 with each meal, between meals and every three hours during the night, when awake. (Today it is difficult to buy vitamins B-2 and B-6 in potencies of less than 25 mg.)

Additionally, Adelle took a half teaspoon of inositol, five mg of folic acid, 50 mcg of biotin and 300 mg of PABA. New hair came in thick and vigorously and even went back to its original natural color.

Why Women Lose Their Hair

Women lose hair or even go bald for more reasons than men do. With greater career opportunities in business and industry, women now meet new and continuous horrendous stress. Further, the Pill—actually, its aftermath—produces a similar physiological stress and hormonal changes as in pregnancy. And, as at the end of pregnancy, when the Pill is no longer taken, hair falls out either subtly or obviously—and frighteningly. The Pill is notorious for stealing vitamin B-6, a critical nutrient for healthy hair growth.[7]

However, within a half year, it grows back as before. Rigid dieting, too, can cause serious hair loss. Dr. Frank A. Evans brought back hair growth of dieting women with a supplement of para-aminobenzoic acid (PABA).[8]

Use of rollers and bobby pins, tight coiling or braiding of hair, permanents, waving, straightening and coloring solutions, hair appliances and shampoos all contribute to hair loss—sometimes, baldness.

Regimes like the Davis anti-stress formula occasionally correct what is brought on by the physical stresses mentioned in the above paragraph.

Correcting The Deficits

A sluggish thyroid gland (See the Section on Low Thyroid Function: Hypothyroidism) often causes hair to become thin and fall out profusely.[9] In first generation hypothyroids, this condition can usually be corrected by taking a kelp tablet daily. Kelp has a healthy helping of iodine, the thyroid gland's favorite food. In second generation hypothyroids or beyond, thyroid hormone, a prescription item, is necessary to rectify this ailment.

Following are the key nutrients needed for normal hair growth: protein, magnesium, vitamin B-6, folic acid, inositol, biotin and PABA.

Protein-rich foods in addition to those mentioned a few pages back are: cheese, eggs, fish, meat, milk, soy flour, tofu, yeast and yogurt.

Prime food sources of magnesium in milligrams per less than four ounce units are: kelp, 740; blackstrap molasses, 410; sunflower seeds, 350; wheat germ, 321; almonds, 270; soybeans, 240; brazil nuts, 220; bone meal, 170; pistachio nuts and soy lecithin, 160; hazelnuts, 150; pecans and oats, 140;

walnuts, 130; brown rice, 120; chard, 65; spinach, 57; barley, 55; coconut, 44; salmon, 40; corn, 38; avocados, 37; bananas, 31, cheese, 30; tuna, 29; potatoes and cashews, 27 and turkey, 25.

These are highest rated food sources of vitamin B-6 in milligrams per less than four ounce units: brewer's yeast, 4; brown rice, 3.6; whole wheat, 2.9; royal jelly, 2.4; soybeans, 2; rye, 1.8; lentils, 1.7; sunflower seeds and hazelnuts, 1.1; alfalfa, 1; salmon. 0.98; wheat germ, 0.92; tuna, 0.90; bran, 0.85; walnuts, 0.73; peas and liver, 0.67; avocados, 0.60; beans, 0.57; cashews, peanuts, oats, beef, chicken, and turkey, 0.40; halibut, 0.34; lamb and banana, 0.32; blackstrap molasses, 0.31 and corn and egg yolk, 0.30.

Best foods for folic acid in milligrams per less than four ounce units are: torula yeast, 3; brewer's yeast, 2; alfalfa, 0.80; soybeans, 0.69; endive, 0.47; chickpeas, 0.41; oats, 0.39; lentils, 0.34; beans and wheat germ, 0.31; liver, 0.29; split peas, 0.23; whole wheat, 0.22; barley, 0.21; brown rice, 0.17; asparagus, 0.14; green peas, 0.11; sunflower seeds and collard greens, 0.10; spinach, 0.080; hazelnuts and kale, 0.070; peanuts, soy lecithin, and walnuts, 0.060; corn 0.059; brussel sprouts, broccoli, brazil nuts, and almonds, 0.050.

It is impossible to supply the potency of the Adelle Davis Anti-Stress Formula in foods. Supplements are necessary.

Foods richest in inositol in terms of milligrams per less than four ounce units are: soy lecithin, 2100; chickpeas, 760; brown rice, 700; wheat germ, 690; lentils, 410; barley, 390; veal and liver, 340; oats, 320; torula yeast, 270; beef, 260; beans, 240; oranges and alfalfa, 210; peanuts, 180; blackstrap molasses and whole wheat, 170; peas, 160; grapefruit and sunflower seeds, 150; strawberries and cantaloupe, 120; cauliflower and cabbage, 95 and human milk, 92.

Best food sources of biotin in milligrams per less than four ounce servings are: rye, 0.33; royal jelly, 0.29; brewer's yeast, 0.20; soybeans, 0.19; liver, 0.12; torula yeast and butter, 0.10; split peas, 0.082; sunflower seeds and brown rice, 0.070; rice bran, 0.060; rice germ, 0.058; egg yolk, 0.052; green peas and lentils, 0.042; walnuts and peanuts, 0.040; chickpeas, 0.032; barley, 0.031; alfalfa, tuna, cashews and pecans, 0.030; whole wheat, 0.027; oats and sardines. 0.024; corn, 0.021; mackerel, wheat germ, eggs, blackstrap molasses and bee pollen, 0.020.

Highest rated foods for PABA content in milligrams per less than four ounce units are: sunflower seeds and liver, 0.62; brewer's yeast, 0.49 and wheat germ, 0.037. Only a small number of foods has been tested for PABA content. PABA supplements are available in health food stores.

Mama's Carrot Salad

4 c. cole slaw	1 fresh pear, mashed
⅓ c. plain yogurt	6 c. carrots, grated
Juice of ½ lemon, squeezed	¾ c. raisins

Mix all ingredients together and chill. Best if served within a couple hours of preparing. Serves six.

Sunflower Seed Milk

Soak 3 ounces sunflower seed overnight in 5 ounces apple juice. In the morning add 3 to 5 ounces spring water and blend in blender 2 to 3 minutes. Flavor with honey and a banana, or carob powder to taste. Delicious over cereal or just to drink. Add one egg for extra nutrition.

Milk Fed Salmon

4 salmon steaks	½ c. lemon juice
2 c. whole milk	1 T. kelp
3 garlic cloves, minced	1 t. brewers yeast
2 T. olive oil	

Marinate salmon steaks in milk, garlic and brewers yeast. Drain. Brush with olive oil and grill on broil slowly (do not over cook, just warm up). Before serving, sprinkle with lemon, kelp and pepper and top with chopped parsley.

Bell Pepper Salad

3 green bell peppers	⅓ c. vinegar
3 red bell peppers	¼ c. sesame seeds
⅓ c. olive oil	Vegetable seasoning

Cut red and green peppers into very thin slices. Toss in oil, vinegar and seasoning. Serve with rose hips tea.

CHAPTER 14

Bedwetting

On several occasions, I had the rare pleasure of talking at length with the late Adelle Davis, perhaps the most knowledgeable nutritionist of this century.

An item she mentioned that interested me least at the time has turned out to be one that interests young mothers most. (My nutrition-oriented doctor friends and their patients have appreciated it, too.)

I'm talking about coping with bed-wetting.

Adelle Davis told me she had read an article in the American Journal of Clinical Nutrition which "might well have revealed the underlying cause for many—if not most—cases of bed-wetting."

Test subjects in an experiment were unable to control the containment of urine when made deficient in the mineral magnesium. Today I'm far more impressed with this research than I was then. Just imagine! A few bottles of magnesium supplement may be all that separates a bed-wetter from being normal! Perhaps it's just a matter of eating some of the magnesium-rich foods to be mentioned at the end of this section.

Can't They Get Enough In Food?

As I look at the top 25 foods on the list of magnesium-richest foods, I see only three that are the type eaten everyday and only three others eaten occasionally. On the basis that 1200 mg of calcium is considered a good daily intake and that the calcium-to-magnesium ratio should be roughly two to one, this would make the daily requirement for magnesium around 600 mg—possible to obtain from food.

Because most parents don't know which foods are magnesium-rich and, therefore, don't feature them often in meals or snacks, it is easy to see why many children could be deficient in magnesium and therefore be bed-wetters.

The feedback I get from physician friends is that added magnesium doesn't work all the time—what does?—but that it works enough of the time to justify a trial for bed-wetting cases.

A Matter Of Capacity

Parents sometimes don't have enough patience with the bed-wetter, thinking that the child has more to do with the problem than he or she does. Let me explain. A study of 223 non bed-wetters and 75 bed-wetting children by Dr. John W. Gerrard, professor of pediatrics at the University of Saskatchewan, disclosed that bed-wetters usually have only half the bladder capacity of non bed-wetters![1]

Authorities say that most bed-wetters overcome their problem by the time they are five—either through enlargement of the bladder or through receiving stronger physical signals to wake up and go to the bathroom.

Still other authorities claim that food allergens make the child's bladder over-sensitive so that he or she automatically voids the urine to get rid of the offending food's residue. The child's most-repeatedly eaten foods are usually the offenders. (See the Section on Food Allergies.)

From Negative To Positive

Too great expectations from the child, obvious displeasure, outbursts of temper, or punishment may delay his or her progress and may even lead parents to the desperate measure of resorting to prescription medicines.

Such drugs are a mixed blessing or a mixed curse, however you want to look at them. Deaths have resulted from overdoses, so they must be carefully used or not used at all.

Not long ago at a dinner party in northern California, I met a prominent medical doctor from Mexico, who told me he deals with bed-wetting by having parents urge the child to gain greater bladder control by urinating only partially, stopping, starting again, stopping, and then completely voiding.

"This not only strengthens the control muscle, but also gives the child confidence that he or she has greater power over urinating than previously believed. It sometimes carries over to increased confidence that there won't be "another 'accident' at night," he explained.

A second point he made was that, in the daytime, the child should not run to the bathroom at the first urge, but should try to delay and expand the interval between voidings. His position is that the bladder usually has greater storage capacity than believed and has to be retrained for greater retention for longer times.

Both of these recommendations, when carried out, have helped his patients.

A Folk Medicine And More

Some folk medicines have been mentioned in the literature, but one seems to give better results than the others. That's raw, unfiltered, unprocessed honey. Those who know folk medicine best suggest a teaspoon right before bedtime.

I wondered whether the honey treatment is supposedly effective because it rates among the foods with a high magnesium content. If so, it would bring us right back to the Adelle Davis finding.

A quick check of magnesium-rich foods shows that honey, although with an appreciable magnesium content, rates far down the list.

Here is a partial list of the best-rated magnesium foods in terms of milligrams per less than a four ounce serving: kelp, 740; blackstrap molasses, 410; sunflower seeds, 350; wheat germ, 320; almonds, 270; soybeans, 240; brazil nuts, 220; pistachios and soy lecithin, 160; hazelnuts, 150; pecans and oats, 140; walnuts, 130; brown rice, 120; chard, 65; spinach, 57; barley, 55; coconut, 44; salmon, 40; corn, 38; avocados, 37; bananas, 31: cheeses, 30; tuna, 29; potatoes and cashews, 27 and turkey, 25.

Lillian's Rice Pilaf

1 large onion — chopped	½ t. kelp
¼ c. butter	⅓ c. raisins
2 c. cooked brown rice	¾ c. almonds (toasted), sliced
2 c. beef bouillon	4 T. patsley, chopped

Saute onion in butter in large skillet until tender, but not brown (about 3-4 minutes). Add rice and saute for 3 minutes. Add bouillon, sea salt and raisins. Bring to a boil. Remove from heat, cover and let stand 5 minutes. Stir in almonds and parsley and fluff with a fork. Makes 6 servings.

CHAPTER 15

Birth Control

In his Bestways magazine column several years ago, my collaborator Jim Scheer, wrote an item to the effect that strenuous exercise like long-distance or marathon running shuts off monthly periods and often prevents women from becoming pregnant.

One of his pixyish, female readers responded by letter, observing that strenuous marathon running was anything but reliable for birth control. She commented:

"However, there is one athletic method that is foolproof: running faster than your mate."

All right, girls, lace up those Addidas!

Actually, numerous studies have shown that long-distance running does tend to reduce the chances of conceiving. Many gynecologists have, as patients, female marathon runners who have tried to become pregnant and have failed, despite taking fertility drugs. After stopping running for a few months, they usually conceive.

Body Fat Signal

From running or from any other cause such as illness, an in-built body mechanism of a woman acts as a birth control system if she becomes too thin and drops to within 10 percent of total body fat.

It is as if body wisdom recognizes extreme malnutrition and decides if there aren't enough nutrients to support the body as is, there just won't be enough to sustain a fetus, too.

Like too little body fat, too little of a certain nutrient—vitamin B-6— seems to shut off fertility in many women.[1]

In fact, one woman complaining to her gynecologist about newly-occurring premenstrual syndrome (PMS), confided that she had found a natural way of birth control and had eliminated the Pill:

"I don't take vitamin B-6 and skip most of the foods I know contain it."

He had to point out that such a measure isn't infallible and, besides, it is a two-edged sword. Thus far, she has avoided becoming pregnant, but has brought on a host of painful and stressing PMS problems.

A Dangerous Anti-Fertility Food

About as hazardous a method of birth control as eliminating vitamin B-6 is the one mentioned by Jean Carper in her fascinating book, "The Food Pharmacy" (Bantam): eating a lot of green peas for their anti-fertility ingredient.

Here's evidence cited by Jean of green peas' efficacy:

1. The no-gain in Tibet's population in 200 years—a population that goes heavy on green peas and barley.

2. Experiments in India with male and female rats, which became sterile when their diets were 30 percent green peas.

3. Identification by Dr. S.N. Sanyal, of the Calcutta Bacteriological Institute, of the anti-fertility factor in the peas, synthesizing it and feeding it to human beings. The pregnancy rate of women nosedived by 50 to 60 percent. The sperm count of men was reduced by half.

After a near lifetime of work to curb India's population explosion with the green pea anti-fertility factor, Dr. Sanyal came in second to the Pill, because he could not equal its performance.

Natural ways of avoiding pregnancy are not reliable. Even running long and hard cannot guarantee non-fertility — unless you can outrun your mate.

Minted Green Peas

2 c. Fresh Peas, Shelled	½ c. Cold Water
¼ t. Sea Salt or Kelp	2 t. Fresh Mint Leaves, Chopped
½ t. Honey	1 T. Butter

Place peas in saucepan and add cold water, salt and honey. Cook tightly covered for 5 to 7 minutes over moderate heat. Just before serving add butter and mint. Shake pan to distribute evenly. Remember when shopping that it takes 3 pounds of unshelled peas to serve 4. OR JUST SAY NO!

CHAPTER 16

Bladder Infection (Cystitis)

A strange fact about bladder infection (cystitis) is that it is common to opposite age and sex groups—young women and older men, causing them to urinate often and bringing on a burning feeling when voiding the bladder and right after.

Inflammation makes the bladder feel full even when empty. In extreme instances, many ulcers spread over the bladder walls, causing widespread scars and contraction, reducing the storage capacity.

How does cystitis develop?

Infection usually starts in the urethra, the tube through which urine is voided. Cystitis is more frequent in women than men, because of their short urethra—about one and a half inches long—near the rectum and sexual organs, from which bacteria enter and have only a short distance to spread to the bladder.

Bladder infection in men is less frequent, mainly because the male urethra is roughly nine inches long—a much greater distance for infection to move—and its opening is far from sources of infection. Cystitis strikes the elderly male due to blockages of the urinary tract, including an enlarged prostate. (See the section on Prostate Problems.) Blockages permit harmful bacteria to colonize and spread.

Plan Of Attack

Recurring cystitis signals that a basic problem is not being corrected. This calls for a medical examination of the inside of the urethra and bladder, a cystoscopy.

The traditional way to treat cystitis is with antibiotics, which usually work, but—in the process—destroy friendly bacteria in the intestines and B vitamins made there.

Folk medicine is particularly rich in home remedies for bladder infection: cranberry juice, fresh cranberries, cherry juice, corn silk tea, and garlic cloves or liquid, deodorized garlic.

Gary Gordon, M.D. of North Highland, California (near Sacramento) has helped patients with most of these folk medicines: a half cup of cranberry juice every two hours—even upon waking up at night.

Taken every few hours, one half to three quarters of a cup of whole, fresh cranberries put through a food processor and eaten straight or with a bit of honey brings relief to some of Dr. Gordon's patients.

More Folk Fare

A half cup of cherry juice every two hours often helps his patients as well as cranberry juice.

In Miracle Medicine Foods (Warner Books), Rex Adams tells that corn silk tea appears to flush poisons from the urethra, bladder and kidneys and brings about healing. It can be made easily by boiling a handful of dried, brown corn silk for 15 minutes to assure sterility. After some cooling, it is drinkable.[1]

Corn silk can be stored indefinitely unrefrigerated. Those who do not have corn planted in the backyard or a farmer friend can buy corn silk from the following source: Indiana Botanic Gardens in Hammond, Indiana 46325.[2]

I mentioned another folk medicine remedy to a friend with cystitis: garlic. She began chopping and eating four to six cloves of garlic a day, despite the odor. Not long ago, she wrote me a note, saying:

"After a week of eating four to six cloves of garlic daily, my cystitis has disappeared. And so has my husband."

One way I assure getting my garlic and still keeping my friends is by taking liquid, deodorized garlic from a squeeze bottle. Six to eight squirts in a half glass of water three times daily have cleared up my rare bouts with cystitis within several days. Another effective treatment is vitamin C.

For Cystitis: C.C., Senorita!

Beyond the realm of folk medicine is the vitamin C therapy for cystitis and other genito-urinary ailments, discovered by the late Dr. Irving Stone during his 40 years of experiments with this particular vitamin.

Two grams — 2,000 milligrams — taken by mouth every two hours permit the vitamin C to accumulate in the urine, where it soothes and heals inflammation and detoxifies poisons, Dr. Stone once told me.

Foods that heal — folk remedies mentioned earlier — and Dr. Stone's heavy intake of vitamin C have helped relieve many a person's cystitis.

Puffed Breakfast

1 bowl puffed millet (found at health food store)
2 c. fresh or unsweetened cherry juice

Add all ingredients in bowl and serve. Cherry juice makes a great substitute for milk.

Hans' King Kolic Salad

½ c. olive oil   1 head Romaine lettuce
⅛ t. thyme   Kelp to taste
1 T. odorless garlic

Mix ingredients and pour over lettuce. Serves 4.

CHAPTER 17

Body Odor

Sometimes even frequent bathing or applications of deodorants won't banish body odor entirely—or at all.

Then, another approach must be taken, one used by alternative medical doctors. Jonathan V. Wright, M.D., of Kent, Washington, in his best-selling book, "Dr. Wright's Book of Nutritional Therapy," describes a case of extreme body odor that six showers daily could not help.

"The basic cause was magnesium deficiency, because the patient avoided eating fresh vegetables. Lack of fiber from vegetables—from other sources as well—contributed to constipation, which did not help the cause either," he told me.

Magnesium: The B.O Banisher

"In just about any case, a magnesium supplement reduces the odor," says Dr. Wright.

Richest food sources of magnesium per slightly less than four ounces are the following in terms of milligrams: sunflower seeds, 350; wheat germ, 320; almonds, 270; soybeans, 240; brazil nuts, 220; pistachios, 160; soy lecithin, 160; hazelnuts, 150; pecans, 140; oats, 140; walnuts, 130. Among the vegetables with highest marks for magnesium are chard, spinach, corn, avocados, potatoes and various greens.

Several studies indicate that a low intake of magnesium can bring on body odor. No one knows exactly why. However, magnesium is involved in a great number of metabolic reactions.

Our Telltale Odor

A byproduct of cell metabolism, the odor of our body, is as distinctive as our fingerprints. This unique odor is the means by which bloodhounds track down individuals and by which a baby identifies its mother.

When nutritional shortages make the metabolic process less efficient, the byproducts develop a stronger odor. Sweat—perspiration in refined circles—has no odor. It is water with a miniscule amount of salt. However, when confining clothing or humidity slows down evaporation, this moisture joins with skin bacteria, which themselves produce waste products with an odor.

Perspiration under the arms and in the genital area is especially attractive to skin bacteria and, consequently produces more concentrated odors. Feet sometimes develop a strong odor because they are tightly enclosed —particularly in today's "non-breathing" synthetic footwear— with trapped moisture for skin bacteria.

Unfortunately even regular bathing with soap and water, changing to clean dry clothing, and using antiperspirants and deodorants can control only normal body odors. Imbalances of metabolism must be coped with in different ways.

Zinc May Get You In Sync

Dr. Wright and numerous other alternative doctors often recommend increased zinc intake — along with magnesium — to manage unpleasant body odors. Thirty mg of zinc daily has overcome offensive body odors.

Zinc-rich foods are herring (110 mg per less than a four ounce serving); liver (7 mg per less than four ounces) wheat germ (3.5 mg per ounce serving); sesame seeds (2.5 mg per ounce); soybeans (3.5 mg per two ounces); egg yolk (2.7 mg per large egg); lamb (5.4 per less than a four ounce serving); chicken (4.8 mg per four ounces); oats (3 mg per three ounce serving); rye, wheat or corn (1.5 mg per two ounce serving).

Even this abbreviated list illustrates how easy it is to add thirty mg of zinc to the diet each day.

Other Means Of Deodorizing

The late B.F. Hart, M.D., of Fort Lauderdale, Florida, mentioned on two occasions his pet formula for coping with body odor: magnesium, zinc, vitamin B-6 and para-amino benzoic acid (PABA, one of the B-vitamins). He never did specify the potencies. However, Gary Gordon, M.D., of Sacramento, California, often recommends that his patients use the same combination of vitamins and minerals in these potencies to correct body odor: magnesium: 220 mg; zinc, 30 mg; PABA, 100 mg, and vitamin B-6, 100 mg.

In the Journal of Pediatrics (June, 1979), a case of body odor like "putrid fish" was covered in depth. This was banished by eliminating foods containing large amounts of choline: among them are eggs, fish, liver and legumes.

Some individuals have defective ability to metabolize a substance called trimethylamine, and this handicap shows up in a fishy odor.

Peculiar and strong body odors which resist bathing and deodorants can often be managed by adding nutrients mentioned or by excluding choline-rich foods.

Yogurt Wheat Germ Rolls

1 c. warm yogurt (110 degrees)	1 egg
1 T. dry active yeast	¾ c. wheat germ
¼ c. butter	2½ c. whole wheat flour
1 t. kelp	½ c. non-instant dry milk powder
3 T. black strap molasses	

Place yeast in yogurt and let stand for a few minutes. Add butter, kelp, molasses, egg and wheat germ and stir quickly. Add flour and milk powder and combine well. Beat 10 minutes with electric mixer, or 200 strokes by hand. Cover bowl and put in a warm place until size doubles (approximately 1 hour). Shape in rolls and bake at 350 degrees for 20 minutes. Yields 20 2 inch rolls.

Lemon-Avocado Dressing

2 medium avocados, diced
1 T. fresh lemon juice

1 t. chives, chopped

Peel and dice avocados. Place all ingredients in blender and blend slowly for a few seconds only. Remember that avocado breaks down very quickly.

Potato-Avocado-Celery Sandwich

2 T. mashed potatoes
1 T. avocado

2 slices homemade bread
¼ stalk celery, finely chopped

Mix potato and avocado. Spread thickly over bottom slice of bread. Spread celery over surface and top with second slice of bread. Cut for eating. Makes 1 sandwich.

CHAPTER 18

Breast Ailments (Fibrocystic Disease)

A feeling of horror came over her!

My friend had just discovered a large lump in her breast.

"Is it cancer? I'll have to have a biopsy. Maybe a mastectomy!" she sobbed.

Despite her worst fears, her growth turned out to be non-cancerous, a symptom of a benign breast disorder that nearly 50 percent of American women experience. Fortunately, the growth was regressed by dietary changes, and my friend is well and relieved.

Growth of lumps caused by fibrocystic breast disease can usually be stopped and, in most cases, reversed. But, first, it is important to know what the complex of three non-cancerous breast abnormalities is: a super-abundance of fibrous tissue; small, round, firm and painful cysts—bags or sacs of membrane, containing fluid—and excessive growth of milk-transporting ducts.

Symptoms And Times Of Arrival

Fibrocystic disease usually shows itself in three stages. I accent the "usually," because there are individual variations. Premenstrual swelling of the breast, accompanied by pain and tenderness, which subsides after the menstrual cycle, comes in the latter teens and early twenties.

Next come a number of small nodes, often with a large lump, easily mistakable for cancer. Yet there's a marked difference. Unlike cancer, such a mass has only two dimensions. It is high and wide, rather than tri-dimensional This stage happens in the late twenties or early thirties.

Last comes full-blown cystic breast disease—usually many cysts forming in and blocking the milk ducts, causing a dull pain and a feeling of being milk-filled, and a burning sensation, along with one or more lumps. Occasionally the breast and nipples sting. A watery discharge may issue from the nipples. This stage often arrives after the mid-thirties.

What To Do About It?

In the typical nutritional treatment, it is not so much what you take as what you stop taking that relieves or even dissipates this condition.

Studies by Dr. John Minton, professor of clinical oncology at Ohio State University, reveal that eliminating coffee, tea, chocolate, cola drinks, certain over-the-counter medicines as well as prescription drugs will control fibrocystic disorders in most women.[1]

These beverages and foods contain a family of chemicals called methylxanthines: caffeine, in coffee, some tea, chocolate and cola drinks; theophylline in tea and theobromine in chocolate. Just cutting them out of the diet usually eliminates the breast lumps and pain and the need for a biopsy.

Some patients have tried to rid themselves of this condition merely by cutting down on products containing methylxanthines. It didn't work. This is an all-or-nothing-at-all therapy. If the patient rids herself of the lumps and pain and resumes ingesting methylxanthines, the negative condition will often return.[2]

Another Enemy: The High Fat Diet

Several studies implicate a high fat diet in contributing to fibrocystic disease. In order to make the hormone estrogen, the body needs fat. The theory holds that, inasmuch as estrogen hypes up cell production — especially in the breasts—reducing the amount of dietary fat helps to lower estrogen levels and, therefore, the possibility of developing fibrocystic disease.

Thus far, we have dealt with eliminating certain nutrients to deal with this disorder. Now here's something to be added to the diet: vitamin E. A double-blind study by Dr. Robert London resulted in clinical improvement in three-quarters of the patients due to the administration of 600 I.U of vitamin E (alpha tocopherol acetate) daily through two menstrual cycles.[3]

The trace mineral selenium, which works closely with vitamin E, also helps win the war against fibrocystic disease. As in its usefulness for breast cancer, selenium can be a major factor.

Foods Richest In Vitamin E And Selenium.

To keep fibrocystic disease under control with vitamin E, it is virtually impossible to get enough of this vitamin in the daily intake of food. However, the following food sources of vitamin E offer a good foundation on which to base the supplement. Here are the foods richest in this vitamin in terms of International Units per less than four ounce portions: wheat germ, 160; safflower nuts, 35; sunflower seeds, 31; whole wheat, 30; sesame oil, 26; walnuts, 22; hazelnuts, 21; almonds, 15; olive oil, 14; cabbage, 7.8; brazil nuts and peanuts, 6.5; cod liver oil, 5.4; cashews, 5.1; soy lecithin, 4.8; spinach, 2.9; asparagus, 2.5; broccoli, 2.0; butter, 1.9; parsley, 1.8; oats, barley and corn, 1.7 and avocados, 1.5.

Richest sources of selenium in terms of milligrams per less than four ounce units are: corn, 0.40; cabbage, 0.25; whole wheat, 0.13; beans and peas, 0.12; vegetable oils, 0.100; onions, 0.080; chicken, 0.070; beets, 0.065; barley, 0.062; tomatoes, 0.060; soybeans, 0.054; salt water fish, 0.053; fresh water fish and liver, 0.050; seaweeds, 0.043; brown rice, 0.039 and alfalfa and peanuts, 0.038.

Salmon Loaf

⅔ lb. Canned Salmon	½ c. Wheat Germ
2 T. Lemon Juice	¾ c. Whole Wheat Cracker Crumbs
¼ c. Chopped Green Pepper	⅔ t. Vegetable Seasoning
1 Medium Onion, Diced	½ c. Dill Weed
½ c. Celery, Chopped	½ c. Whole Milk
½ c. Fresh Parsley	¼ c. Liquid from Fish
½ c. Sunflower Seeds, Ground	2 Eggs, Beaten

Mix all ingredients together. Pack into greased loaf pan. Bake for 1 hour at 325 degrees, or until firm. Serves 4.

SPINACH SALAD

½ lb. fresh spinach, torn   2 t. wheat germ
3 farm fresh eggs, hard boiled and diced 1 avocado, chopped
1 green onion, diced   ¼ c. raw milk cheese, grated

Mix ingredients in large bowl. Mix the following ingredients and pour over the salad:

⅛ c. unrefined sesame oil   ¼ t. dry parsley
⅛ c. apple cider vinegar   ¼ t. marjoram
⅛ c. water   ¼ t. turmeric
¼ t. sea salt   ¼ t. dry mustard
¼ t. dill weed

Garnish with chopped parsley. Serves four to six.

CHAPTER 19

Breast-Feeding Problems

Physicians specializing in pregnancy and childbirth (obstetricians) are still surprised at the number of mothers, who, despite poor health and undernourishment, expect that, by some miracle, their breast milk will sustain their infant in good health.

It won't. Again, it's a case of depositing money in the bank in order to draw it out, an increased intake of protein, vitamins, minerals and unsaturated fatty acids for pregnant and nursing women.

Good nutrition will produce good mother's milk, and poor nutrition will produce poor mother's milk.

The following guidelines for daily nutrient intake from nutrition-oriented obstetricians will help assure excellent quality and sufficient quantity of mother's milk:

Vitamin A, 25,000 I.U.; a vitamin B-complex capsule with 50 mg of the major vitamin B fractions; (much, if not most mother's milk, is deficient in B vitamins); vitamin C, 500 mg; (this minimal amount boosts the percentage of iron assimilated; 25 to 50 I.U. of vitamin E (Alpha tocopherol, the natural form); vitamin K from three or four brussels sprouts, a bowl of oatmeal, or several ounces of spinanch, cabbage or broccoli and iron — 18 to 20 mg — from organic sources: three or four ounces of pumpkin seeds and a bowl of wheat germ cereal. Inorganic iron can destroy much-needed vitamin E.

Calcium And Protein Critically Important

During nursing, calcium requirements are higher than at any other time of life. The lactating mother must supply her own needs and those of the infant. Numerous authorities say that, unless she takes in at least 1200 mg of calcium daily, she runs the risk of honeycombed bones (osteoporosis) after menopause, because a certain level of calcium constantly needed in the blood will be drawn out of her bones.

To assure absorption of calcium, she will need at least 400 I.U. of vitamin D and 600 to 700 mg of magnesium, say nutrition-oriented obstetricians. A tablespoon of cod liver oil or several ounces of sardines or salmon will supply the required vitamin D. Less than four ounces of sunflower seeds and a bowl of wheat germ cereal can more than supply this daily allowance of magnesium. An alternative is a magnesium supplement or a calcium-magnesium supplement at a two to one ratio in favor of calcium.

A tablespoonful of safflower, sunflower, corn or soy oil in salad dressing —or a handful of walnuts, pecans, brazil nuts or hazelnuts—will usually supply the essential fatty acids needed daily.

Protein intake upped by 10 percent in pregnancy should be raised another 10 percent during nursing, say nutrition-oriented physicians. An extra slice of whole grain bread and a few ounces of almonds, cashews, or sunflower seeds will provide the added protein.

Advantages Of Mother's Milk

Assuming a well-fed mother, mother's milk has numerous advantages: colostrum, more zinc than in cow's milk, more easy assimilability and less chance of the infant developing celiac disease, a disorder characterized by a defect in digestion, preventing absorption of fat and calcium.

The baby bottle can't match the breast. Colostrum, the first milk from the mother's breast, makes the suckling infant immune to a vast assortment of human ailments, from which cow's milk can't protect him or her: the flu, polio, staph infections and, among others, viruses.

Mother's milk has a higher level of the mineral zinc, so important to a strong immune system, to rapid healing, to proper sexual development, and to working as a vitamin A helper.

Better assimilability of mother's milk has been a well recognized fact established for years. Now we learn from the U.S. Department of Agriculture's Children's Nutrition Research Center at Baylor College of

Medicine in Houston that, contrary to popular belief, healthy breast-fed infants take in fewer calories and grow at a different rate than healthy bottle-fed babies.[1]

Dr. Cutberto Garza and Janice E. Stuff, researchers there, stated that "By eight months, breast-fed infants have consumed 30,000 fewer calories than reported intakes for bottle-fed infants.[2]

"Breast-fed infants use their calories a lot more economically, but we don't know why or how."

Obstetricians at St. James University Hospital, Leeds, England, claim that with the dramatic increase in breast-feeding, the number of children's celiac disease cases has dropped, probably due to the delay of giving cereals to infants until the fourth or sixth month.[3] Gluten, a protein in cereals, is the villain behind celiac disease. The longer grain is withheld, the less chance of gluten intolerance in the babies, state the doctors.

Milk Supply For Full-Term Babies And Preemies

It is not uncommon for the milk supply to decline in some, if not many —women. What to do? Sometimes more frequent feedings can prime the pump. If that doesn't work, check into other possible causes: the Pill, which can prove harmful to milk and infant; heavy smoking of cigarettes or marijuana; an elevated fever; low thyroid function, over-fatigue, or pregnancy.[4]

There's good news for mothers of premature infants who can't seem to produce enough milk to satisfy their newborns—at least for mothers who don't smoke.[5] This comes from the U.S. Department of Agriculture's Nutrition Research Center at Baylor College of Medicine in Houston.

Physiologist Judy M. Hopkinson instructs mothers who delivered eight to 12 weeks early to empty both breasts at least six times a day. Twenty-three of the 30 nonsmoking—80 percent—maintained an adequate milk supply after the infants went home, she said. However, only three of 11 smoking mothers—just 27 percent—continued producing enough milk.

"Smokers have a significantly lower milk volume than nonsmokers," she stated. The 11 smokers averaged 18 percent less milk during the first two weeks after giving birth and 40 percent less milk by the fourth week.

Although preemies have to be tube fed, because they are too immature to suck and swallow, "Mothers want to give them their milk," she said. "It's one of the few things they can do, and it's a very emotional issue."

More About Increased Milk Supply For Preemies

Many women who deliver prematurely don't have the appropriate information to produce enough milk, and their volumes further decline by about the fourth week.[6]

Actually most of these mothers can increase milk production by pumping more frequently. Five times a day is enough to maintain milk volume, and eight to 10 times a day will increase milk volume within a week or two.

"It's important to empty both breasts thoroughly at each pumping," advises Hopkinson. "That takes between eight and 12 minutes per breast."

Although pointing out that mother's milk is preferred over formula or donor milk, she still advises that mother's milk be fortified with extra protein and minerals—namely calcium and phosphorus—for the very low birthweight infant.

She realizes that milk from these mothers is naturally fortified with extra protein for about a month after premature delivery. However, the levels are so variable that protein is added to ensure that the tiny infant always gets enough.

Common Breast-Feeding Complications To Avoid

Another problem with breast-feeding is passing along effects of drugs, medicines and other substances in the milk, jeopardizing the baby's health, states the Harvard Medical School's Health Letter.[7]

Even when a drug isn't especially toxic, it could bring on allergies or drastic changes in friendly, intestinal tract bacteria. Here's a list of the most commonly used drugs and how they could possibly harm the breast-fed infant.[8]

Alcohol should be eliminated or used sparingly, because, if it is at a high level in the mother's bloodstream, it will be at a high level in breast milk.

Amphetamine passed along in mother's milk disturbs the baby's sleep and makes him or her irritable. Antibiotics pass easily into breast milk and could upset the balance of friendly and unfriendly bacteria in the large intestine.

Antihistamines, decongestants and medicines for bronchitis or asthma may, in certain cases, bring on crying, irritability and sleeplessness.

Aspirin could interfere with the baby's blood-clotting. So breast-feeding should be delayed for at least an hour after taking the aspirin.

Barbiturates and certain sleeping pills enter the breast milk and affect the infant as the adult.

Caffeine in coffee and other beverages has difficulty passing into breast milk, but that which does can make the baby irritable and unable to sleep.

Many of the cough syrups have an iodine ingredient and could influence the infant's thyroid function. For this reason, The Harvard Medical School Health Letter advises avoiding them.

Hazard Of Bottle-Feeding

Bottle-feeding is not without risks, indicates health columnist Dr. Stephen Jaksha.[9] It can cause baby to have crooked teeth. Artificial nipples with too large holes permit milk to flow through too fast and force the baby's tongue forward to reduce the flow. Frequently, this brings about the habitual pressing of the tongue against the teeth upon swallowing.

If this tendency is not detected before it hardens into a habit, it could cause developing teeth to move outward and become crooked.

An artificial nipple with too small holes is just as bad, causing the baby to suck too hard and making the dental arch collapse and, again, producing crooked teeth.

Your doctor or dentist can help you select the proper nipple, which, at best, cannot match nipples provided by nature.

Although, as stated above, there are major problems connected with breast-feeding, they can all be avoided with a little forethought and planning.

Peggy's Salmon Patties

1 can (1 lb.) salmon
3 T. water-ground cornmeal
1 T. all-purpose whole wheat flour
2 T. vinegar
Sea salt and pepper to taste
Olive oil for frying

Flake salmon, but do not drain. Add remaining ingredients except olive oil. Shape into 8 flat patties. Fry on both sides in ½ inch hot oil skillet. Drain on absorbent paper. Makes 4 Servings.

Mother's Salad

2 avocados, peeled and sliced
2 stalks celery, chopped
1 cucumber, diced
1 red bell pepper, chopped
1 T. wheat germ

½ small green cabbage, shredded
2 medium carrots, grated
3 lettuce leaves, torn into pieces
2 c. alfalfa sprouts

Place all chopped vegetables, with exception of avocados, in a salad bowl. Add avocados last and slowly stir into salad, being careful to keep the mixing to a minimum as they thin down quickly.

CHAPTER 20

Bruises

A physician friend recently told me about an overweight patient who said she was, "Blue about black and blue bruises all over my body."

To make sure she was not an abused wife, the doctor asked how she got her bruises.

"I don't know," she replied. "It seems if I even look at myself, a new set of bruises appears."

Bruising, which is bleeding under the skin, is one of the commonest conditions to walk into a doctor' office and one of the easiest for the nutrition-oriented physician to manage.

Various studies show that a deficiency in any one of several nutrients —or all of them—can encourage bruises: vitamin C, bioflavonoids, (See the Section on Miscarriages), vitamin K and the mineral zinc.

Likewise, adding one or more of these nutrients to the diet by means of natural foods and/or by supplements seems to correct easy bruising.

Why Deficiencies Of Vitamin C Occur

Many reasons exist for the fact that the body may signal its need for vitamin C by bruising easily: (1) eating too few fresh fruits and vegetables —a common omission by the elderly; (2) being exposed to pollutants, allergens, or heavy metals; (3) taking one or more drugs which destroy or use up huge amounts of this vitamin; (4) long-time stress such as a severe illness, frustration or depression or (5) frequent emotional outbursts such as anger, and (6) smoking.

Pollutants drain away vitamin C, because this vitamin reacts with toxic substances to cancel or lessen the harm they can do: benzene, carbon tetrachloride, fluorine and lead. Vitamin C joins with allergens and drugs — anesthetics, atropine, ammonium chloride, aspirin, barbiturates, estrogen, stilbestrol and sulfonamides, among others—and is used up and thrown off in the urine.[1]

So the need for vitamin C is upped. Smoking one cigarette has been found to use up 25 mg of vitamin C, a nutrient which is non-storeable. Imagine the deficit created by the smoking of a whole package of cigarettes! When this deficit isn't overcome, spontaneous bruising often takes place.

Heavy Weight Loss: Another Stress

When the obese start to melt off appreciable poundage, a strange condition sometimes occurs: wholesale bruising. Even the bind of tight clothing or the slightest touch brings on another black and blue bruise.[2]

Doctors explain this by the fact that tiny capillaries, once supported by fat, are suddenly on their own and rupture.

In many instances, a diet high in fresh fruits and vegetables will banish bruises by supplying both the needed vitamin C and a related nutrient, bioflavonoids—especially concentrated in the white pulp of citrus fruit.

Here is a list of best sources of vitamin C in terms of milligrams per less than a four ounce serving: rose hips, 3,000; acerola cherries, 1,100; guavas, 240; black currants, 200; parsley, 170; green peppers, 110; watercress, 80; chives, 70; strawberries, 57; persimmons, 52; spinach, 51; oranges, 50; cabbage, 47; grapefruit, 38; papaya, 37; elderberries and kumquats, 36; dandelion greens and lemons, 35; cantaloupe, 33; green onions, 32 and limes 31.

Although the Food and Drug Administration (FDA) considers bioflavonoids inessential in human nutrition, many nutrition-oriented physicians have seen incredible feats achieved by bioflavonoids.

Studies on which the FDA bases its judgment have not been conducted long enough and with high enough potencies of this nutrient, claim many nutrition-oriented medical doctors. Listing of best food sources of bioflavonoids by the number is not available. However, bioflavonoid supplements in various potencies can be bought at any health food store.

Vitamin K And Zinc

Noted for helping blood to clot, vitamin K, although made in the intestines, is sometimes needed from the outside to reverse unsightly bruising. Along with harmful bacteria, antibiotic therapy kills friendly bacteria which synthesize vitamin K, limiting the available supply of this vitamin.[3]

Green, leafy vegetables are a good source of vitamin K to draw upon — with special accent on the following foods whose rating is stated in milligrams per less than a four ounce serving: cheddar cheese, 22; camembert cheese, 16; brussel sprouts, 1.5; soy lecithin, 1.2; alfalfa, 0.52; oats, 0.49; spinach, 0.33; soybeans, 0.30; cauliflower, 0.28; cabbage, 0.25; broccoli, 0.20 and liver, 0.10.

Numerous surveys have shown that elderly adults are particularly low on the mineral zinc—hardly any age group escapes, thanks to the nation's well-documented zinc-deficient soils.

Several studies indicate that zinc-deficiency may be at least partially responsible for bruising in older adults. In one study, half of forty patients 65 to 99 years of age showed numerous bruises, with the worst ones belonging to the most zinc-deficient.[4]

Best sources of zinc per 100 milligrams per less than a four ounce serving are: herring, 110; wheat germ, 14; sesame seeds, 10; torula yeast, 9.9; blackstrap molasses, 8.3; maple syrup, 7.5; liver, 7.0; soybeans, 6.7; sunflower seeds, 6.6; egg yolk, 5.5; lamb, 5.4; chicken, 4.8; brewer's yeast, 3.9; oats, 3.7; rye, 3.4; whole wheat, 3.2; corn, 3.1 and coconut and beef, 3.0.

Hanley's Egg Cakes

6 eggs, beaten
½ lb. bean sprouts
1 bell pepper, chopped
2 cans Franco American Beef Gravy
½ bunch watercress, chopped
6 green onions, chopped
½ c. sesame seeds

4 celery stalks, chopped in ¼-inch strips
1 pepper - mature red hot,
    finely chopped
½ c. water chestnuts, cut in half
2 T. olive oil
½ t. sea salt
⅛ t. pepper

Saute vegetables in olive oil and seasonings. Remove from skillet and combine with eggs which have been beaten. Add olive oil and cook as you would a pancake. Warm gravy in saucepan and pour over pancakes. Makes 10-12 servings. Stores well and can be rewarmed in oven.

Karl Rolfes' German Cole Slaw

1 head cabbage, grated
3 carrots, grated
3 green onions, thinly sliced
6 T. mayonaise
    (home-made — see below)

1 bunch broccoli, chopped
1 green pepper, chopped
1 bunch radishes, chopped

Combine ingredients and add dressing. Sea salt and pepper to taste.

Home-Made Mayonnaise

2 eggs
2 T. fresh lemon juice

¾ c. vegetable oil (cold-pressed)
¾ t. fine mixed herbs

Place eggs, herbs and lemon juice in blender. Add oil very slowly as you blend. Chill in refrigerator until ready to serve. Delightful on either a cold vegetable salad or on hot steamed vegetables.

CHAPTER 21

Bulimia (Binge-Eating, Then Purging)

All eating disorders are bizarre—particularly bulimia, characterized by binge-eating, then vomiting or using cathartics or diuretics. A relatively new name on the psychological scene, bulimia actually means "ox or bull hunger".

An estimated 30 percent of high school and college age girls use this method to stabilize their weight, and then it firms into a fixed pattern of conduct.

Underlying this desperate measure is a personality bedeviled by emotional stress: frustration, emptiness, feelings of low self-esteem, self-consciousness, loneliness, depression and perfectionism, striving to lose weight to gain approval to elevate self-esteem.

Although bulimics do their best to hide their eat-and-run-to-the-bathroom conduct, they eventually reveal themselves by certain actions and by physical appearance: disappearance to the bathroom or restroom soon after eating; at least a faint odor of gastric juices from throwing up, despite a mouthwash; a constant, strong cover-up odor, which might in itself be a give-away; puffy face, irregular menstrual cycles or absence of them; sore throat from the food's two-way traffic; mottled or stained teeth (erosion from powerful gastric juices) and hair loss (insufficient key nutrients and emotional stress).

The Rankin Method

So far, the greatest success in turning bulimics around has been with much psychology and some nutrition. And one of the foremost persons in normalizing bulimics is psychologist Howard Rankin, clinical director of the Hilton Head Health Institute, Hilton Head Island, South Carolina.[1] Prior to coming to the Institute, Dr. Rankin headed the eating disorders unit at St. Andrews, Britain's largest and oldest psychiatric hospital.

Rankin deals with the bulimic basics, changing behavior, not curing symptoms.

"We help people understand about good nutrition, exercise and the value of sensible, structured eating," he explains. "Bulimics are terrified that if they consume a thousand calories a day, they're going to put on weight. We show them they won't.

"What many times causes the binges in the first place is a combination of strenuous dieting and irregular meals. We change all of that.

"We start with a level of caloric intake we know will not put on weight. We add exercises. This is a critical component. In a week's time, bulimics start to discover they really can maintain weight and that the nutritious, structured meals actually can help them," says Rankin.

"We also help people reassess their expectations about their bodies, their appearance, themselves. We help them become realistic about weight goals. Some people whose normal weight might be 140 pounds think their 'perfect weight,' in terms of appearance and social pressure should be 115 pounds.

"What happens is they starve themselves and then their bodies, trying to protect the normal weight and caloric intake, and react with those excessive urges. Our educational approach — that's what it is — helps modify their behavior," states Rankin.

How To Stop Binges?

One of the most emotionally shattering happenings to bulimics—roughly 19 percent of the female population and five percent of the males—is to fall off their meal plan, binge and purge. This is because they tend to be perfectionists.

"...We show them how to stop a binge well before it gets out of control. We do that with a technique we used in England called 'craving control,' he explains.

"This technique allows a bulimic to have a small amount of, shall we say, ice cream, and showing that just because she's started doesn't mean she has to finish the whole gallon. It's crucial to treatment that the bulimic understands this."

Dr. Rankin admits the process is slow, but claims this is the only way treatment can be successful.

"We help people build confidence through self-paced, graded exercises and good nutrition. We're changing habits. That takes time, but we know it's worth it."

Do certain nutritional deficiencies contribute to the making of a bulimic? Or are certain emotional factors at the bottom of this disorder? Or is this condition a blend of the nutritional and emotional?

Probably, the latter? The deficiency of one nutrient may contribute: that of copper, say some authorities. If this is so, perhaps supplying this mineral may help to hurry the healing process. So let's consider the use of additional copper in the diet.

Remember that copper is a trace mineral and that the bulimic just shouldn't load up on it the way she might on vitamins. It just might be that she will need to eat only a small amount of only two or three of the copper-containing foods to get the required additional amount. Only two or three milligrams may be all that's needed. (WARNING: It may be hazardous to the health to take in much more than this.)

Here are high-content-of-copper foods in milligrams per less than four ounce units: liver, 3.7; wheat germ, 2.9; thyme, 2.4; blackstrap molasses, 2.2; honey, 1.7; hazelnuts, 1.4; regular molasses, 1.2; brazil nuts, 1.1; walnuts, 0.90; kelp and salmon, 0.80; cashews, 0.76; ginseng, 0,75; oats, 0.74; lentils, 0.71; barley, 0.70; almonds, 0.68; bananas, 0.51; tuna, 0.50; avocado and coconut, 0.39; brown rice, 0.36; bee pollen, 0.32 and egg-plant and kale, 0.30.

Liver And Pineapple

¼ pineapple (about 1½ c. — sliced)	1 c. chicken stock
1 large green pepper, thinly sliced	1 lb. calf liver, cut in thin strips

Remove skin from pineapple and core. Slice pineapple and cut slices into matchstick-size strips. Steam-stir green pepper slices in a few tablespoons of the stock until it begins to become tender. Add liver strips and cook over medium heat, stirring occasionally until liver is still pink on the inside and juicy, adding more stock as needed to keep mixture from sticking. Add pineapple strips and heat thoroughly, with enough stock to provide a sauce. Serve over brown rice. Makes 4 servings.

CHAPTER 22

Burns

Treat burns right—and right away!—to prevent pain and to promote quick, scarless healing.

And what's the right way? It isn't smearing them with butter or lard, in the old folk medicine manner, because their later removal could cause pain and damage the healing.

Authorities agree on immediate treatment of burned hands or feet in this way: immersing them in a basin full of ice-chilled faucet water and holding them there until, upon removal, the pain is gone. The severity of the burn determines how long this should be done—minutes or hours. A clean, ice-water soaked sheet or towel may be applied to other body parts. If caustic acid has caused the burn, the body part should be cooled and cleansed with running tap water.

How To Tell The Degree Of Burn

Certain definite signs tell you the degree of the burn: (1) redness and irritation without broken skin for the first degree burn, like ordinary sunburn; (2) blisters and mild skin destruction for the second degree burn; (3) dry yet firm parchment-like skin with deep-layer destruction—sometimes to the bone—for the third degree burn and (4) a scorched or charred appearance for the fourth degree.

Third and fourth degree burns demand a quick trip to an emergency hospital, because they can bring on a form of shock, sometimes with bleeding profuse enough to lower blood pressure. They can also severely narrow arteries. Both conditions require skilled medical attention.

Alternative Treatment

Some years ago, David H. Klasson, M.D., at Greenpoint Hospital in Brooklyn brought pain-relief and quicker healing to serious burn cases by spraying burns with a one percent solution of vitamin C (ascorbic acid). He also had patients take more oral vitamin C than they could possibly derive from food: 200 to 500 mg four times a day.[1]

Why does this treatment work? Animal experiments at New Jersey Medical School add to already well established findings that ascorbic acid boosts immune system function.[2] This is especially important in burn victims, because their immune system is already depressed. Vitamin C seemed to prevent second degree burns from becoming third degree.

Right Diet Can Help

In addition to using the Klasson spray of vitamin C, many alternative doctors like to reach the Klasson daily intake level of ascorbic acid by means of a natural nutritional supplement—like rose hips, with a potency of 3,000 mg for less than four ounce units—or any of the following fruits with high milligram ratings: acerola cherries, 1,100; guavas, 240; and black currants, 200.

Other high C foods to help reach the daily total are: parsley, 170; green peppers, 110; watercress, 80; chives, 70; strawberries, 57; persimmons, 52; spinach, 51; oranges, 50; cabbage, 47; grapefruit, 38; papaya, 37; elderberries, and kumquats, 37; dandelion greens and lemons, 35; cantaloupe, 33; green onions, 32 and limes, 31.

The Klasson treatment is important because ascorbic acid—outside and inside—brought rapid pain relief so that habit-forming, pain-killing narcotics such as morphine could be stopped, among other benefits: no side-effects such as those which sometimes come with sulfa; ability to discontinue antibiotics, which destroy friendly intestinal bacteria, and less fluid pooled under the skin, permitting quicker skin-grafting and lowering the chance of infection.[3] The late Fred Klenner, M.D., of Reidsville, North Carolina, a pioneer in clinical use of intravenous and oral ascorbic acid, achieved startling success with burns by means of a three percent solution vitamin C spray on burned areas every two to four hours over a five day period, along with the daily regime of three or four grams orally and 30 or more grams given intravenously.[4]

OTHER VITAMINS MAY CONTRIBUTE

Apparently the stress of severe burns depletes vitamin A, because patients in this condition have lower blood serum levels of this vitamin than non-burn patients.[5]

Supplemental vitamin A brings them up to normal. Studies have found vitamin A-deficient individuals with a weakened immune function and, therefore, more infection-prone. High doses of vitamin A promoted higher immune system effectiveness.[6]

Noted for poor wound-healing and vulnerability to infections, diabetic surgical patients with wounds and burns healed faster with vitamin A supplements.[7]

Vitamin A-Rich Foods May Help

Some nutrition-oriented physicians bolster the daily diet with 5,000 to 25,000 I.U. of vitamin A by means of the following natural foods, listed in milligrams per less than a four ounce serving: calves' liver, 22,000; dandelion greens, 14,000; carrots, 11,000; yams, 9,000; kale, 8,900; parsley and turnip greens, 8,500; collard greens and chard, 6,500; watercress, 5,000; red peppers, 4,400; winter squash, 4,000; egg yolk and cantaloupe, 3,400; endive, 3,300; persimmons and apricots, 2,700; broccoli, 2,500; pimentos, 2.300; swordfish, 2.100; whitefish, 2,000; romaine, 1,900; mangoes, 1,800; papayas, 1,700; nectarines and pumpkin 1,600; peaches and cheeses, 1,300.

Let me add that vegetables and fruits mentioned here supply beta carotene, a vitamin A precursor which depends upon an efficient thyroid and liver to be translated into vitamin A.

Fascinating Case History

Remembering the exciting results achieved on serious burns by Drs. Evan V. and Wilfrid E. Shute, pioneers in clinical treatment with vitamin

E, I was able to direct a friend's son to the proper alternative medical doctor for treatment. A freak accident had created a crisis. Tim, a teen-aged boy had been standing at the kitchen stove. One of his brother's had thrown a big, hard rubber ball to another brother. The ball had ricocheted off the brother's fingertips high, over Tim's head, bounced against the wall and hit the handle of a stirring spoon in a huge pot of boiling lentil soup. The soup splattered all over Tim's face, fortunately missing his eyes.

Tim's mother had done the right thing, applying cold water-soaked towels to his face. Then she had rushed him to a doctor friend, who had given Tim the Klasson vitamin C spray therapy.

Several days later some ugly scars began to show. Immediately, the doctor followed the Shute formula, putting Tim on 600 International Units of vitamin E daily and giving him vitamin E ointment to apply generously and with a light touch.

Within several weeks, Tim's face looked smooth and clean, as if he had never had the burns.

It is virtually impossible to reach the 600 I.U. level with foods. So the supplement seems to be the only means of using the Shute therapy effectively.

CHAPTER 23

Bursitis
(Pain In
Joint Areas)

Many individuals think that pain, limited range of upper arm movement, and tenderness in the shoulder socket tell the whole story of bursitis.

Actually, that's 140th of the story!

Throughout the body are 140 bursas, pockets designed to encase the ball end or rounded part of a bone to make a moveable joint—at the knee, the ankle, and elbow, among others.

However, bursitis, a form of arthritis, does occur most often in the shoulder. Supposedly, the bone can move easily — with little friction — in the pocket's fluid next to the pocket's tissue. And "supposedly" is the right word, because the fluid thickens and becomes resistant, and inflammation swells the tissue. Sometimes, razor sharp calcium deposits develop there, making movement of the joint excruciating.

What's The Cause?

All sorts of opinions have been launched as to the whys of bursitis: accident or injury, stretched muscles, infection, stress-related inability to absorb necessary nutrients, and the rigors of hard and repetitious physical labor.

Writing in the Journal of The American Medical Association, based on examination of 314 bursitis patients, N.W. Paul, M.D. states that this disorder was not brought on by occupation or injury, but by a metabolic problem: the patients were not being fed the right food or they were not using it with efficiency.[1]

I.S. Klemes, M.D., Medical Director of the Ideal Mutual Insurance Company and the J.C. Penney Company, subscribed to the same theory

— that patients were deficient in key nutrients.[2]

So Klemes administered vitamin B-12, because this vitamin had been effective in making nucleoproteins, is important in the metabolism of nervous tissue and has given relief to patients with a certain form of neuralgia.

Klemes injected a daily dose of 1 cc. of vitamin B-12 for seven to 10 days, followed by the same injection three times weekly for the next two to three weeks, then one or two weekly for two to three weeks, depending on the patient's progress. Relief came quickly. Calcium deposits, if any, were absorbed.[3]

Although it is impossible to derive this vast amount of vitamin B-12 daily from food, a diet rich in vitamin B-12 over a long period might forestall the development of bursitis and would supply a nutritional backdrop to injections given for active bursitis.

These foods in terms of milligrams per less than four ounce units are the richest sources of vitamin B-12: liver, 0.086; sardines, 0.034; mackerel and herring, 0.0100; red snapper, 0.0088; flounder, 0.0064; salmon, 0.0047; lamb, 0.0031; swiss cheese, 0.0021; eggs, 0.0020; haddock, 0.0017; muenster cheese, 0.0016; swordfish and beef, 0.0015; bleu cheese, 0.0014, and halibut and bass, 0.0013.

Zonelle's "Stuffed" Salmon

4 baking potatos	3 T. parmesan, grated
1 can salmon	¼ t. sea salt
2 T. butter	⅛ t. pepper
1 egg, beaten	3 T. green onion, minced

Scrub potatoes and bake in a 300 degree oven for 1 hour and 15 minutes or until tender. Cut in half lengthwise, scoop out pulp and mash. Drain and flake salmon, reserving liquid. Add cream to liquid to make ¼ Cup. Combine potato pulp with butter, liquid, egg, cheese and seasonings. Fold in salmon and onion, and spoon into potato shells. Bake at 200 degrees for 40 minutes, or until filling is lightly browned. Makes 4 Servings.

Slim 'N Trim Salad

3 hard boiled eggs, chopped
¼ lb. fresh spinach
½ lb. fresh apricots, halved and pitted
⅓ lb. white chicken meat, cut in pieces

⅓ lb. lean roast beef, thinly sliced
⅓ c. sliced scallions,
  cut in 1-inch pieces
⅓ c. celery, sliced Paprika dressing

Arrange spinach, apricots, chicken, beef, scallions, and celery on large platter. Serve with Paprika Dressing (see below).

Paprika Dressing

¼ t. dry mustard
¼ t. paprika
¾ t. sea salt
1 t. honey

1 egg, beaten
¼ c. mild vinegar
2 T. olive oil

Combine above ingredients in top of double boiler. Cook, stirring constantly, over simmering water until mixture thickens. Remove from heat and cool.

CHAPTER 24

Cancer

A recent pronouncement by the General Accounting Office (GAO) — that's the branch of federal government which keeps statistics — scathed the government's cancer establishment, charging them with juggling figures and misleading the American public.[1]

They try to justify the billions of dollars poured into their research by giving the impression that they are gaining on cancer. The sad fact is: cancer is gaining on them.

How they perpetrate this is reminiscent of what Abraham Lincoln used to say about statistics and statisticians:

"A dog has four legs and a tail. You can call the tail a leg, but a dog still has four legs and a tail."

No matter how hard they work to create a statistical five-legged dog for us, we are still getting the tail-end of things. Here's how they do it, the inside story turned inside-out.

Statistics Look Better Under Cosmetics

The incessant campaign for early reporting of cancer is working right and working right into the hands of statisticians, making the figures look a lot better than they really are. The establishment counts as "cured" anyone who lives five years from the first reporting date. Even if the patient died the day after five years, he or she would technically be among the cured. The earlier the reporting date, the better looking the statistics.

Now for a second device. The debilitating nature of orthodox cancer treatment — "cut, burn, and poison" — would give a well person an 88 percent chance of surviving one year.

When toxic chemicals are poured into the bodies of dying cancer patients, the already lowered immune system is decimated, and they fall victim to myriad diseases—such as pneumonia and heart disease. So then deaths are shifted to another category of cause, and cancer statistics improve.

From the GAO's report, it seems entirely possible that if statistics were accurately calculated, cancer of the colon would be the nation's primary killer. As presently recorded, more people will die of cancer in a year than died in both the Korean and Vietnamese wars.

The Unholy Three Of Therapy

Still the cancer establishment doggedly—five leg doggedly—pursues the same methods: surgery, radiation and chemotherapy.

I started the first edition of my book, Nutrition: The Cancer Answer (Statford Publishing) with the following observation—that every new idea goes through three phases:

(1) It is ignored. (2) It is ridiculed. (3) The establishment claims it as their very own.

For many years, knowledgeable health professionals have recognized that, in many instances, cancer can be prevented and controlled by nutrition. Orthodox medicine has continually rejected and ridiculed the idea that cancer can have nutritional causes.

Finally, in 1982, the prestigious National Academy of Science published a report recognizing the vital connection of diet and cancer cause and prevention. Only then did the American Cancer Society, along with the governmental, industrial and medical complex admit what prevention-minded health professionals were shouting for more than 40 years — timidly, grudgingly at first and, today, as if they had discovered it.

Now they campaign with full-page ads, featuring vegetables containing beta carotene, that nutrition may, in fact, be the cancer answer.

All The Time In The World

Still cautious, cancer research organizations warn that a food regimen will not be available for another 20 years. Do you know what 20 years means? Eight million more dead Americans! Can we wait that long to apply a full armamentarium of nutritional information? Apparently, the cancer establishment can.

Most of us don't realize that the American Cancer Society, founded in 1913, described itself as a "temporary" organization that would cease to exist once cancer was eradicated. Almost seven decades later, the Society is the richest private charity in the world.

How goes the battle?

Patrick Quillin's Healing Nutrients, page 15 (Contemporary Books), states that a Harvard professor has compiled statistics, showing that "we have lost the war against cancer."

Within the last few decades, an unorthodox school of thought has emerged which considers cancer a preventable metabolic disease. This new wave of medical practitioners has proven to its own satisfaction that cancer is a chronic, systemic, metabolic imbalance. And nutritional deficiency tilts it even more, sapping the immune system.

Then cancer, like a beast seeking its prey, strikes at the weakest and most stressed organ and assumes the identity of cells peculiar to that organ.

The medical establishment daily battles the non-orthodox school, trying to suppress its methodologies, with warfare raging in the newspapers, medical journals, doctors' offices and in courts.

Differences Spell Apartness

Underneath it all, are opposite-pole interpretations of the nature of cancer. Orthodox medicine assumes that because each type of cancer is biologically distinctive and there are many types of cancer cells, that there are many varying causes and treatments.

In direct contrast, proponents of the metabolic approach, embrace various internal change concepts, based on the fact that a cancer cell is an aberration of a naturally-occurring cell, one that exists as a part of the life cycle. Deficiencies of specific vitamins, minerals and free-floating enzymes—plus stressors—cause these cells to malfunction, disabling their ability to be protected by normal body defenses.

Inherent in these opposing belief systems is the alternative physicians' deep-seated confidence in the wisdom of nature and the conviction that the God of nature knew how to heal in its fruits, vegetables, grains, legumes, nuts and herbs.

Orthodox medicine holds a stubborn belief in man-made chemicals which interrupt natural body functions and try to kill the cancer cell, while destroying the body's ability to rid itself of the disease.

Robert Atkins, M.D., in his brilliant book, Dr. Atkins' Medical Revolution, telling about his transition from drug treatment to natural healing, writes: "Once medicine was my God. Now God is my medicine."

Proper Foods: A Biochemical Barrier To Cancer

As a cancer prevention measure, many individuals now eat broccoli, cabbage, spinach and cauliflower, among a host of fresh vegetables and fruits containing beta carotene, the precursor to vitamin A, which is the nutrient noted for preventing degenerative diseases, including cancer. (See list below.) Some authorities find vitamin C-rich foods helpful for the same purpose.

Several research projects of Dr. Walter Troll, of New York University have indicated that in cultures which eat liberal amounts of seeds, the incidence of cancer is low or non-existent.[2] The theory is that seeds contain all the elements needed for growth and continuity of life and, therefore, are highly nutritious and tend to prevent cancer.

Vitamin B-17 (amygdalin) is found in seeds—in other foods, too—and is recommended by some alternative doctors for various kinds of cancer. Please see a list of vitamin B-17 foods below.

Twelve years of research ended in my book, Nutrition: The Cancer Answer, which has sold more than 150,000 copies and was named "the best health book," by the American Book Exchange. While it is impossible for me to compress all of the life-saving information gathered, I will mention that this book lists 164 foods with cancer-blocking agents. In following sections, I will offer pointers on the various kinds of cancer.

However, basic to it all, is the fact that robust health, a strong immune system, unshakable faith and a stubborn resistance are the best weapons for prevention and, often, for cure.

These are the foods with the highest beta carotene content in terms of

International Units per less than a four ounce portion:

Dandelion greens, 14,000; carrots, 11,000; yams, 9,000; kale, 8,900; parsley and turnip greens, 8,500; spinach, 8,100; collard greens and chard, 6,500; watercress, 5,000; red peppers, 4,400; squash, 4,000; cantaloupe, 3,400; endive, 3,300; persimmons and apricots, 2,700; broccoli, 2,500; pimentos, 2,300; mangoes, 1,800; papayas, 1,700; nectarines and pumpkins, 1,600; peaches, 1,300; cherries and lettuce, 1,000, tomatoes and asparagus, 900; soybeans, 700; kumquats, 600 and watermelon, 590.

Vitanmin C-rich supplements and foods in milligrams per units of less than four ounces follow:

Rose hips, 3,000; acerola cherries, 1,100; guavas, 240; black currants, 200; parsley, 170; green peppers, 110; watercress, 80; chives, 70; strawberries, 57; persimmons, 52; spinach, 51; oranges, 50; cabbage, 47; grapefruit. 38; papaya, 37; elderberries and kumquats, 36; dandelion greens and lemons, 35; cantaloupe, 33; green onions, 32; limes, 31; mangoes, 27; loganberries, 24; tangerines and tomatoes, 23, squash, 22; raspberries and romaine lettuce, 18 and pineapple, 17.

Best sources of vitamin B-17, better characterized as amygdalin, nitriles and nitrilosides, in milligrams per units of less than four ounces are: black lima beans, 5,100; bitter almonds, 4.200; white lima beans, 3,600; bean sprouts, 2,000; green lima beans, 1,700; wild cherry bark, 1,300; bitter cassava, 940; quince seeds, 680; buckwheat, 340; guava seeds, 190 and kidney beans, navy beans and black eyed peas, 34.

CHAPTER 25

Bladder Cancer

A stunning setback for cancer of the bladder occurred in the late 1960s, when a pair of Tulane University scientists—Dr. Jorgen U. Schlegel, head of the Urology department, and biologist George Pipkin—discovered that vitamin C (ascorbic acid) can destroy cancer-producing substances that precede bladder cancer in smokers.[1]

Schlegel and Pipkin administered 1,500 mg of vitamin C in three time-spaced doses of 500 mg each. (This was before timed-release vitamins were on the market.)

The success rate was so phenomenal that Schlegel recommended such a regime for "individuals who, due to age, cigarette-smoking or other factors may be prone to bladder cancer formation." (Bladder cancer is twice as prevalent in smokers than in non-smokers.)

How This Regime Works

Ascorbic acid enters the bloodstream, creating a buildup beyond the body's normal needs, so that it spills over into the urine, stored in the bladder. Before the bladder can discharge the vitamin C-saturated urine, the second 500 mg dose of this vitamin enters the bloodstream.

Later, the third dose follows, keeping the ascorbic acid concentration in the urine so high that it prevents cancer cells from forming.

Dr. Linus Pauling reports that a later Schlegel study indicates that bladder cancers in cigar smokers often regress if the patient takes 1,000 mg of vitamin C or more daily.[2]

As a nutritional base for vitamin supplementation, here are supplements and foods richest in vitamin C in milligrams per less than four ounce units:

rose hips, 3,000; acerola cherries, 1,100; guavas, 240; black currants, 200; parsley, 170; green peppers, 110; watercress, 80; chives, 70; strawberries, 57; persimmons, 52; spinach, 51; oranges, 50; cabbage, 47; grapefruit, 38; papaya, 37; elderberries and kumquats, 36; dandelion greens and lemons, 35; cantaloupe, 33; green onions, 32; limes, 31; mangoes, 27; loganberries, 24; tangerines and tomatoes, 23, squash, 22 and raspberries and romaine lettuce, 18.

CHAPTER 26

Cancer, Breast

Numerous studies show that a great deal can be done with nutrition to prevent breast cancer.

A survey by Dr. J.G.C. Spencer, of Frenahay Hospital in Bristol, England, revealed a higher than average cancer rate in goiter belts in fifteen nations on four continents—areas where the soil has only about one-seventh the amount of iodine needed to prevent low thyroid function (See the Section Low Thyroid Function.)[1]

Lower than normal thyroid function seems to invite cancer, as shown by many animal experiments. Cancerous tissue from rats grafted onto other rats took hold readily in animals whose thyroid glands had been removed, but hardly ever in those with normal thyroid function.[2]

Studies of thousands of laboratory rats and human beings by Dr. Bernard Eskin, director of endocrinology in the Department of Obstetrics and Gynecology at the Medical College of Philadelphia, show that a lack of iodine, the thyroid gland's most essential nutrient, encourages breast cancer.[3]

The Peril Of Iodine-Poor Soils

Dr. Eskin learned that the highest incidence of breast cancer—also deaths from it—are in the Goiter Belts of Austria, Poland, Switzerland and the United States. (Goiter Belts, as described in the section on Low Thyroid Function, are in mountainous areas and environs as well as in a nation's central flat lowlands.

The United States Goiter Belt is in the level Great Lakes states and the northern area of the country from the mountains of the New England

States across the country to Washington and including provinces in Canada following this path along the border.

The Great Lakes area reveals the highest death rate in the United States from breast cancer. Just the opposite, iodine-rich Japan and Iceland boast the world's lowest rates of goiter and deaths from breast cancer.[4] As a matter of fact, the breast cancer death rate in Japan, where iodine is generously supplied in seafood and seaweed eaten daily, is just one-fifth that of the United States.[5] Kelp is the best source of iodine and available in any health food store.

Supplements and foods supplying the most iodine in milligrams per unit of less than four ounces are: kelp, 180; cod liver oil, 0.84; haddock, 0.31; cod, 0.14; chard and beans, 0.10; sea salt, 0.095; perch, 0.074; sunflower seeds, 0.070; herring, 0.052; turnip greens, 0.047, halibut, 0.046; peanuts and cantaloupe, 0.020; liver, 0.019; soybeans, 0.017; pineapple, 0.016; potatoes, 0.015; cheeses, 0.011 and lettuce 0.010.

Selenium: A Cancer Preventer?

The story about the mineral selenium in relation to breast cancer is similar to that of iodine. Healing Nutrients (Contemporary Books) by Patrick Quillin, Ph.D, tells that authorities mapped the soil selenium levels across the United States, then overlaid a map of number of cancer cases in each state.

The correlation amazed the experts! States with the lowest levels of soil selenium — consequently crops grown on them were selenium-deficient — correlated with highest incidence of cancer cases.[6]

South Dakota, with the highest amount of selenium in the soil, had the lowest number of cancer cases. And Ohio, with the lowest amount of selenium in the soil, had the highest incidence of cancer — 200 percent higher than that of South Dakota.[7]

Quillin mentions that cancer patients often have a lower-than-normal blood level of selenium and that this finding meets criticism on the basis that cancer might have brought on the low selenium levels.[8]

A second study involving 10,000 American test subjects answered that criticism. Blood samples were taken and frozen. As individuals developed cancer, their blood samples were thawed out for checking. Those with cancer turned out to be the ones who, at the start of the study, had the lowest blood selenium levels. Scientists conducting the study found that low blood selenium levels doubled the chance of developing cancer![9]

Special Protection Against Breast Cancers!

Spearheading the discovery that selenium may be particularly useful in protecting against breast cancer was Gerhard N. Schrauzer, Ph.D, of the University of California at San Diego.

Schrauzer found that, by adding trace amounts of selenium to drinking water of mice susceptible to breast cancer, the incidence of such cancer dropped from 82 percent to 10 percent.[10]

One of his prime contributions was analyzing selenium levels in blood samples from blood banks in 17 nations. Schrauzer found that selenium blood levels were three times as high in Asian and Latin American nations compared with the United States and Europe and that death rates from breast cancer were two to five times higher in the United States and in Europe than in Asia and Latin America.[11]

Best Food Sources

Most nutrition-oriented medical doctors set an upper limit on selenium intake at no more than 200 mcg daily. So beneficial at moderate intakes, selenium can be a poison at high levels.

It is estimated that most diets—particularly in the western states where soil selenium is plentiful—contain about 100 mcg of this trace mineral. Here are many of the selenium-richest foods in terms of milligrams per less than four ounce servings. (Remember a milligram is one-thousandth of a gram, and a microgram — the measurement used in relation to selenium — is one-millionth of a gram.):

Corn, 0.40; cabbage, 0.25; whole wheat, 0.13; beans and peas, 0.12; vegetable oils, 0.100; onions, 0.080; chicken, 0.0.70; beets, 0.065; barley, 0.062; tomatoes, 0.060; soybeans, 0.054; saltwater fish. 0.053; freshwater fish and liver, 0.050; brown rice, 0.039; alfalfa and peanuts, 0.038; meat, 0.022; garlic and rye, 0.020; egg yolk, 0.018 and grains, 0.015.

Other Defenses Against Breast Cancer

Researchers in numerous projects have discovered that, over and above assuring sufficient iodine and selenium, women can reduce the incidence of breast cancer by cutting their fat intake from 40 to 45 percent of total calories to 20 percent or less.

Other studies say, "Reduce fat intake and also add a lot of fiber and you will slash the amount of breast cancer by 50 percent."[12]

Also, reduce weight. There is some evidence that overweight individuals tend toward breast cancer. Stanford University researchers have found that women who were overweight in their college years are more prone to develop breast cancer.[13]

A fourth preventive measure is breast-feeding. One study indicates that women who breast-fed their first or second child for one to six months reduced their breast-cancer risk by 10 to 25 percent. Those who nursed for seven or more months reduced their risk by 50 to 75 percent.[14]

The fifth preventive measure is breast self-examinations. This effort hasn't been as effective as it might be, because most women don't know how to do it properly. So says Jean Richardson, a University of Southern California assistant professor of preventive medicine, who tested 540 women with a foam rubber breast model.[15]

Only one percent of the women found the five lumps present.

"Even when the women were told to press hard on the model and try to find the lumps, almost half of them didn't find a single one," says Dr. Richardson.

Inasmuch as early detection is a important, some authorities advise that women have periodic mammograms, an X-ray technique for detecting cancer. Some women object on the grounds that there may be a radiation hazard. The American Cancer Society claims that a cancer risk from such radiation is negligible, if it exists at all.

Rather than take the ACS' word for it, many women are being tested by means of modest-cost nuclear magnetic resonance (NMR)—a device which gives off no radiation, can show which lumps are cancerous or benign and eliminates the need, expense, and discomfort of a biopsy.

Hooray!

Jayne's Salmon Patties

2 c. Red Salmon
2 T. Grated Onion
⅛ c. Capers

2 T. Tomato Puree
1 t. Lemon Juice

Flake salmon and add lemon juice, onion, capers and tomato puree. Let stand for 15 minutes. Drain off any liquid and press fish lightly into small round cakes. Set on buttered baking sheet and cook under broiler for 6 to 7 minutes. Serve with fresh steamed beets and steamed corn on the cob.

Sesame Dressing

½ c. ground sesame seeds
1 c. spring water, approximately
1 t. kelp

Juice of ½ lemon
½ garlic clove

Place seeds and one cup water in an electric blender and blend until smooth. Add remaining ingredients and blend until smooth, adding more water if necessary to give dressing the correct consistency. Yield: About one cup.

NOTE: Add ½ cup chopped onions, ½ cup chopped celery and ½ cup mixed alfalfa, mung bean and lentil sprouts. Blend until smooth for a mock tuna-sandwich spread.

CHAPTER 27

Cancer (Cervix and Vagina)

A mystery!

In girls born a generation ago, cancer of the cervix or vagina was a rarity. Today it is one of the most prevalent kinds of cancer — with any small city in the United States reporting more cases annually than existed throughout the world 40 years ago.

Why?

The major answer seems to be that some mothers of girls and young women who develop vaginal or cervical cancer took the prescribed diethylstilbestrol (DES), a synthetic hormone to prevent miscarriage during the first three months of pregnancy. (See the Section on Miscarriage.)

A study by Dr. Arthur L. Herbst, a Harvard Medical School gynecologist, and associates some years ago brought to light the DES-vaginal and cervical cancer connection. In checking into the strange fact that, within a three year period, seven girls in New England had developed this kind of cancer, he found one thing in common: mothers who had taken prescribed DES during the first trimester of pregnancy.

When the Herbst team followed up with an investigation of 170 reported cases, they found that patients ranged in age from seven to 29 with 100 vaginal and 70 cervical cancers. All of the patients had been exposed to the synthetic hormone in the mother's uterus. Twenty-four of the young people died of the cancer.

Inasmuch as DES had been used to prevent miscarriage for a 26-year period (1950 to 1971) before Herbst's announcement, the Harvard gynecologist made the ominous prediction that more was yet to come as babies born in this timespan reach maturity. He was too right! Thousands of new cases have appeared.

Many lawsuits have been launched against the makers of DES and doctors who prescribed it, but lawsuits have not been known to cure cancer, reassemble the pieces of shattered lives, or bring back the dead.

Certainly pregnant women will not knowingly take synthetic estrogen. However, this won't finish the matter, because pregnant women are still unknowingly taking DES. How? In the meat and poultry they eat.

The Curse Causeless Shall Not Come

DES is used to increase weight of cattle and chickens prior to marketing. Although it is illegal to include DES in animal or chicken feed, the U.S. Department of Agriculture doesn't have the manpower to monitor 50,000,000 cattle or many times that many chickens to determine the residues of diethylstilbestrol in meat.

Implants of DES are permitted in cattle and chickens. Again, who knows how much DES the pregnant women—any of us, for that matter —are ingesting along with that juicy hamburger?

Does this little bit of DES amount to anything? Judge for yourself. The Encylopedia of Common Diseases (Rodale Press) states that this hormone is so potent that just two parts per billion is poisonous in the diets of mice. Only an infinitesimal daily amount, .07 millionths of a gram of DES— a gram is just 1/28th of an ounce—causes cancer in the mice.

Every time the DES issue is brought up, agricultural economists come back with the weary argument that meat and poultry would cost a lot more if it weren't for diesthylstilbestrol. True. So, let's pay it! There's nothing low cost about cancer therapy or health care in general.

Fortunately, an estimated 25 percent of the cattle is raised without DES. This wholesome meat—poultry, as well—is featured by health food stores that have the refrigeration capacity for it.

Highest Risk Candidates

Over and above the DES factor, various studies have shown that cervical and vaginal cancer are most prevalent in the following: lower economic groups, those with virus-caused genital infections — such as warts and possibly Herpes—and individuals who start sex practices at an early age and have numerous partners.[1]

Women who have five or more children have been found to be twice as prone to cervical cancer as those with one to three children.[2] Some authorities agree that wear and tear on the cervix during labor and delivery —also related inflammation in the process—contribute to developing this kind of cancer.

Smoking, a long-suspected contributor to cervical cancer, has now been officially indicted by several studies, most conclusively by that of reseachers at Emory University School of Medicine and at the Centers for Disease Control (Atlanta).[3]

Cancers and other tumorous conditions of the cervix develop more readily in smokers than in non-smokers. The more the person smokes, the greater the hazard. How does smoking contribute to cervical cancer? The researchers believe that the toxic products of the smoke are delivered in the bloodstream to the sensitive surface of the cervix and serve as a constant irritant.

Users of the birth control pill have a higher risk of cervical dysplasia than non-users.[4] Dysplasia is abnormal multiplication of non-malignant cells. Women with this condition are more prone than others to develop cervical cancer. Warning! Cervical hyperplasia should be checked frequently by a gynecologist. (See list of Alternative Doctors in back of book.)

Folic Acid To The Rescue

A nutritional lack may contribute to cervical hyperplasia, feel some authorities—a deficiency of folic acid, one of the B vitamins. Either, the woman is not getting enough of this nutrient or the Pill or antibiotics (sulfonamides) are depleting her supply.

A study of 47 young cervical dysplasia patients by a University of Alabama team led by Charles E. Butterworth, M.D. and Kenneth Hatch, M.D. revealed that 10 milligrams per day of folic acid may be able to arrest or possibly even reverse some early dysplasia in Pill users.[5]

Of 22 women on the folic acid for three months, four were rewarded with complete reversal of their condition. The remaining 18 found their condition arrested. Not one of the takers of the placebo improved. In fact, the hyperplasia of four placebo-takers became worse.

Due to the fact that folic acid is one of the nutrients important to proper cell division, the researchers theorize that with a folic acid deficiency, cell division might be abnormal.

A Big Boost From Vitamins A And C

In a comparative study to discover if the vitamin A precursor beta carotene and vitamin C can help prevent cervical cancer—this one by Dr. Sylvia Wassertheil-Smoller and associates at Albert Einstein College of Medicine—the researchers discovered that the healthy women ingested much more of these nutrients than woman with abnormal Pap smears.[6]

The researchers concluded that women prone to cervical cancer might get protection from these nutrients—particularly a daily minimum of 90 mg of vitamin C.

So far as folic acid is concerned, it is difficult, if not impossible to derive enough of this vitamin from supplements and natural foods to meet the daily requirements of the Butterworth-Hatch study. However, the following folic acid-rich supplements and foods will supply a good base for the actual folic acid vitamin. Here they are in terms of milligrams per less than four-ounce units:

Torula yeast, 3.0; brewer's yeast, 2.0; alfalfa, 0.80; soy beans, 0.69; endive, 0.47; chickpeas, 0.41; oats, 0.39; lentils, 0.34; beans and wheat germ, 0.31; liver, 0.29; split peas, 0.23; whole wheat, 0.22; barley, 0.21; brown rice, 0.17; asparagus, 0.12; green peas, 0.11; sunflower seeds, 0.10; collard greens, 0.100; spinach, 0.080; hazelnuts and kale, 0.070; peanuts, soy lecithin, and walnuts, 0.060; corn, 0.059; brussels sprouts, broccoli, brazil nuts and almonds, 0.050 and beef and bran, 0.040.

These are the best supplement and food sources of the vitamin A precursor, beta carotene, in international units per less than four ounce units: dandelion greens, 14,000; carrots, 11,000; yams, 9,000; red peppers, 4,400; squash, 4,000; cantaloupe, 3,400; persimmons and apricots, 2,700; pimentos, 2,300; mangoes, 1,800; papayas, 1,700 nectarines and pumpkin, 1,600; peaches, 1.300; cherries, 1,000; tomatoes, 900; kumquats, 600; watermelon, 590; pink grapefruit, 440; tangerines and green peppers, 420 and plums, 300.

Relative to the Wassertheil-Smoller study, it is possible with supplements and natural foods to surpass by far the daily 90 milligrams of vitamin C which she found protective against cervical cancer. Here in terms of milligrams per units of less than four ounces are the best bets for vitamin C:

Rose hips, 3,000; acerola cherries, 1,100; guavas, 240; black currants, 200; parsley, 170; green peppers, 110; watercress, 80; chives, 70; strawberries, 57; persimmons, 52; spinach, 51; oranges, 50; cabbage, 47; grapefruit, 38; papaya, 37; elderberries and kumquats, 36; dandelion greens and lemons, 35; cantaloupe, 33; green onions, 32; limes, 31; mangoes, 27; loganberries, 24; tangerines and tomatoes, 23; squash, 22; raspberries and romaine lettuce.

CHAPTER 28

Cancer (Colon)

A middle-aged, male, office-worker during his first visit to one of my medical doctor friends complained of being unable to correct his chronic halitosis. (See the Section on Bad Breath.)

The doctor studied the forms which the patient had filled out about his diet, glanced across the desk at him, and asked:

"How frequent are your bowel movements?"

"Every three or four days."

"That's what I thought," commented the doctor. "Do you ever eat a laxative food like bran?"

"No, doctor. I like to let things happen naturally, to give the bowels a chance to work."

"I'm afraid things won't happen naturally on your diet. Your constipation results from a low fiber diet. There's nothing unnatural about changing to a higher fiber diet—whole grains and more fresh vegetables and fruit—getting daily bowel movements, clearing up your halitosis and protecting yourself against colon cancer. A little physical exercise will help, too."

The new eating and exercise program worked wonders for the patient, who, during his next office visit, asked the doctor why constipation might possibly bring on bowel cancer. As many alternative physicians do, the doctor mentioned research done by Dr. Robert Bruce, director of the Toronto branch of the Ludwig Cancer Research Institute.

The Bruce experiments revealed that the waste matter stored in the large bowel has potential cancer-causing substances, and the longer constipation persists, the longer the bowel walls are exposed to these substances, and the greater the threat of colon cancer, second only to lung cancer as a major killer.[1]

A Fat Chance Of Developing Colon Cancer

In the 1920s, the greatly respected Max Gerson, M.D. was run out of the country for suggesting that the high fat diet contributed to cancer.

A low fiber diet is bad enough. Couple it with a high fat intake, and you've got problems in Colon Country. The validity of Dr. Max Gerson's early research on the low-fat diet for preventing colon cancer is demonstrated daily by the excellent record of the Seventh Day Adventists, mainly vegetarians who eat whole grains, legumes and fresh raw vegetables which include the little-known nutrient, vitamin B-17.

Several studies indicate that the more dietary fat eaten, the more bowel cancer. An experiment showed an increase by 100 times of anaerobic bacteria—those which need no oxygen to exist—in stools of individuals who eat much fat.[2]

If not kept in check by a diet rich in specific nutrients—fiber, vitamins, minerals and all-important enzymes — these organisms are capable of changing bile acids in fecal matter into chemicals which can cause cancer and also of converting bile into estrogen hormone, which could trigger growth of tumors.

Britain's Dr. Denis Burkitt, world-renowned for his expertise in fiber in relation to human waste, has found that abundant refined carbohydrates — sugar and starch — like excess fat, encourage the multiplication of cancer-causing bacteria and, consequently, chemical changes which can invite cancer.[3]

Dr. Burkitt and family eat only fiber-rich, home-made, whole wheat bread and also a heaping tablespoon of bran sprinkled on other foods.

Just as it is important that we eat whole foods, so it is important that our bran be whole bran, rather than a part of a food which is presently in vogue.

I recently discovered a delicious-tasting fiber product which contains the whole seed, fruit and grain, herbs and lactobacillus acidophilus. It is a flavorful addition to my foods.

Accent On Vegetables And Yogurt

Most vegetables contain quality fiber, although not at the bran level, and offer special protection against colon cancer, as underscored by a revealing study made some years ago by Dr. Saxon Graham, chairman of Social and Preventive Medicine at the State University of New York at Buffalo, and co-workers.[4]

The Graham team queried 256 male colon cancer patients at Roswell Park Memorial Institute and 783 non-cancer patients of the same ages as to how often they ate some 19 vegetables, including the now-noted, cruciferous cancer-fighters: cabbage, broccoli, brussels sprouts, cauliflower and turnips and veggies such as beta carotene-rich carrots and tomatoes, among others.[5]

Of course, the colon cancer patients showed little regular intake of vegetables on the list, compared with the others. Those who consumed the most vegetables had the least risk of cancer. The more frequently they ate them, the less likely they were to develop colon cancer.

My book, Nutrition: The Cancer Answer, lists 164 cancer-blocking agents in foods.

Now it turns out that a food quite distant from the vegetable kingdom also helps the cause: yogurt. Yogurt made from milk with lactobacillus acidophilus added — or a health food store, top-grade, chemical and additive-free yogurt made from raw certified milk, if available — is usually well-tolerated by even the milk intolerants and helps reduce waste matter enzymes which can lower the body's defenses against cancer-causing agents.[6]

Two researchers, Goldin and Gorbach, have tested this milk product on fecal enzymes in human subjects and observed changes in them indicating a lower risk of colon cancer.[7]

As indicated earlier, vegetables, fruits and grains are a few of the champions guarding us against this epidemic disease which now claims the lives of one in three Americans. The complete answers are far greater in scope and depth than can be covered in such limited space.

I wrote Nutrition: The Cancer Answer so that you and your family could know the basic problems in greater detail and also the means of coping with them, to help assure that you and those dear to you can avoid becoming another dismal statistic.

Dwight's Fiber Rich Breakfast

1 very ripe banana, chilled   2 T. fiber
1 c. yogurt

This drink can be eaten with a spoon if made by hand...In small bowl, mash banana with fork. Stir in yogurt and fiber, place in a glass and serve with a spoon.

Zonelle's Oat Dollar Pancakes

1 c. rolled oats   ½ t. baking soda
2 T. bran   ⅔ buttermilk
2 T. wheat germ

In medium bowl, combine oats, bran, wheat germ, soda and buttermilk. Let stand for 2 minutes, until oats have absorbed most of the milk. Shape into eight small patties and bake in hot, lightly oiled skillet, turning when browned. Serve hot. Makes 2 servings.

CHAPTER 29

Colon Cancer Precursor (Familial Polyposis)

Even a cancer precursor, familial polyposis—growths on the colon—often responds to heavy daily doses of vitamin C: 3,000 mg of the timed-release product over six months or more.

Surgery is only a delaying action for this inherited condition, because, usually, after the large intestine is removed and the small intestine is connected to the rectum, new growths appear on the remainder of the rectum.

Research by Dr. Jerome DeCosse and associates at the Medical College of Wisconsin (Milwaukee) with eight polyposis patients led to five of them showing a total disappearance of growths or to a marked reduction within six months of the daily treatment.[1]

Dr. DeCosse used vitamin C because he believes that chemicals in the colon combine with oxygen to produce polyps and then cancer in the colon. An anti-oxidant such as ascorbic acid prevents or reverses the hazardous oxidation process, he indicates.

Why Food Alone Can't Do It

Timed release capsules were fed to the test subjects to assure that as much ascorbic acid as possible would reach destination: the large intestine, without being absorbed by the bloodstream.

Dr. DeCosse feels that his vitamin C treatment will eventually be the therapy of choice over surgery in most instances and an excellent preventive measure.

Some alternative doctors who have patients with this ailment also follow a diet high in vitamin C. Following are supplements and foods richest in this vitamin in milligrams per units of less than four ounces:

Rose hips, 3,000; acerola cherries, 1,100; guavas, 240; black currants, 200; parsley, 170; green peppers, 110; watercress, 80; chives, 70; strawberries, 57; persimmons, 52; spinach, 51; oranges, 50; cabbage, 47; grapefruit, 38; papaya, 37; elderberries and kumquats, 36; dandelion greens and lemons, 35; canteloupe, 33; green onions, 32; limes, 31; mangoes, 27; loganberries, 24; tangerines and tomatoes, 23; squash, 22; raspberries and romaine lettuce, 18; pineapple, 17 and tangelos and royal jelly, 16.

CHAPTER 30

Cancer (Eye)

Rising fast in cancer statistics is malignant melanoma of the eyes.

You and I can do something specific to protect ourselves from eye cancer and make those statistics plummet. This is the opinion of Dr. Margaret A. Tucker, who directed a recent study on this subject by the National Cancer Institute.[1]

Beware of excessive exposure to the sun without sunglasses. Take care —and take cover—you all who were born in the South, especially if you have blue eyes. Blue-eyed individuals are particularly prone to eye cancer, states Tucker.[2]

Her words are aimed primarily at youngsters in the family. Exposure to strong sun in early childhood seems to be a major cause of melanoma of the eyes. She warns that babies are most vulnerable for a logical reason: their eye lenses can't filter out as much ultraviolet light as those of an adult. Tucker recommends that parents use sunhats or baby bonnets on toddlers.[3]

Tucker's survey reveals that blue-eyed and green-eyed individuals are at 60 percent greater risk than those with brown eyes. Southern-born persons have a three times higher risk of eye cancer than those born in the north.[4]

A Second Opinion

Thomas B. Fitzpatrick, M.D. and Arthur J. Cohen, of Massachusetts General Hospital, agree on most points with Tucker but add that melanoma of the skin and eyes appears to be caused, not so much by daily sun exposure, as by brief and irregular exposure to intense sunlight.[5]

Highest risk candidates are white professional indoor workers who sun themselves on weekends or during tropical winter vacations. Occasional exposure to powerful rays of the sun appears to increase chances of eye melanoma, they claim.[6]

Can anything be done nutritionwise to protect candidates for eye melanoma from becoming the real thing?

Numerous studies by biochemist Dr. Daphne Roe, of Cornell University, indicate that a healthy daily ration of beta carotene-rich foods is one of the best preventives against melanoma.

Deep yellow and dark green vegetables and fruits are treasuries of beta carotene: carrots—from which the original carotene was derived—sweet potatoes, yams, squash, pumpkin, zucchini squash, cantaloupes, other yellow melons, peaches, and apricots.

Two helpings a day of any of the above should help in preventing melanoma of the eye and skin, says Garry Gordon, M.D., whose Preventive Medicine Clinic is in North Highland, California, near Sacramento.

Maureen's Cream Of Carrot Soup

1 T. wheat germ	⅛ t. pepper
1 onion, chopped	⅛ t. cloves, ground
1 lb. carrots, pared and sliced	1 t. orange rind, grated
3 T. butter	¾ c. orange juice
2 c. water	½ c. sour cream
1 t. sea salt or kelp	

Saute onion and carrots in butter in large sauce pan for 5 minutes. Add water, kelp and pepper. Bring to a boil and lower heat. Cover and simmer 25 minutes or until carrots are tender. Lift carrots and onions from broth with slotted spoon. Place in blender, add wheat germ and 1 cup of the broth. Whiz until smooth. Return mixture to broth in sauce pan. Add cloves, orange rind and orange juice. Heat just to boiling. Stir about ½ cup hot soup into sour cream in a small bowl. Return to sauce pan blended. Remove from heat. Do not boil after sour cream is added. Serve hot in mugs or soup bowls.

CHAPTER 31

Cancer (Lung)

Probably the most frightening cancer statistic in a recent 25-year period is that for lung cancer—a 185-percent increase for men and a shocking 239 percent for women, directly related to more women smoking.[1]

Lung cancer accounts for more than one-third of cancer deaths in men and 16 percent in women. Cancer of the lungs is the most certain killer of any form of cancer. My good friend, Richard A. Kunin, M.D., in "Mega-Nutrition," (McGraw-Hill) states that chain-smokers above age 55, are at 80 times greater risk to develop lung cancer than non-smokers of that age.[2] Further, smokers live shorter lives and die more painful and prolonged deaths.

How "Safe" Can "Safer" Cigarettes Be?

On a few occasions, Dr. Kunin has remarked to me that what the cigarette-makers call a "safer" cigarette is a cruel misnomer. (Not only is it a misnomer, it is a misleader, in my opinion.)

Sure, the amount of tar may be reduced, admits Dr. K., but cigarette smoke contains many other poisons that drastically lower ability of the immune system to defend us from cancer: arsenic (without "old lace"), cadmium, carbon monoxide and, among many others, lead.

The first three build up poisons in the body of the smoker and those who live and/or work with him or her. And carbon mononoxide chokes off the oxygen supply, ever so slowly suffocating and starving body cells.

The world-wide movement to prohibit smoking in public places and in working environments may not set well with smokers. However, second-hand smoke to which non-smokers are often subjected has been proved to be even more harmful than inhaled smoke and can bring on a host of unnecessary and unwanted physical ailments to innocent bystanders, including lung cancer.

Passive smoke is indeed injurious to the health of non-smokers, as numerous studies have indicated — studies done in Louisiana, Pennsylvania, Greece, Japan and Germany: injurious enough to increase the incidence of lung cancer.

Why Should Non-Smokers Take Physical Punishment?

Smokers make the choice to smoke and then become hooked, victims of slow suicide. Non-smokers who opt not to smoke don't need to suffer deteriorated health due to someone who happens to share the same environment. For many decades, non-smokers—in the majority—have quietly and with resignation inhaled offending smoke from smokers — the minority. It's time for a change to majority rule.

In any event, Dr. Kunin is right that when tobacco companies accent "safer" cigarettes with less tar, they divert the attention from the other poisons.

So much for the harm that smoking does to smokers and non-smokers. Let's look at some remarkable foods which can help undo the harm.

Encouraging Research

A monumental, 19-year study of 2,000 middle-aged men's diets by distinguished epidemiologist Richard B. Shekelle and co-investigators at Rush-Presbyterian-St. Luke's Medical Center (Chicago) revealed remarkable information about the value of beta-carotene, a vitamin A precursor from carrots, broccoli, kale, spinach, pumpkin and squash, tomatoes, turnips, sweet potatoes and yams.[3]

Men who ate little carotene had seven times as much lung cancer as those who ate the most carotene. Carotene even protected long-time smokers, but not nearly to the degree that it protected non-smokers.[4]

And how many carrots—for instance—did Dr. Shekelle find necessary to protect against lung cancer—enough to turn a fellow into Peter Rabbit? Not really. Only a half cup daily!

Another study that highlights the incredible protective power of carotene like a flash of lightning is that of the late Dr. Marilyn Menkes, of Johns Hopkins University School of Hygiene and Public Health. Blood level of carotene tells the story.[5]

Dr. Menkes and her associate measured the amount of beta carotene in blood specimens gathered in 1974 and then tracked down the donors nine years later. The ninety-nine individuals who were stricken with cancer of the lungs turned out to have had lower blood levels of beta carotene than those who were cancer-free. Odds for the persons with low beta carotene levels to get cancer were more than two times greater.[6]

Low-Cost Lung Insurance

In her excellent book, "The Food Pharmacy" (Bantam), Jean Carper answers the question as to how much more beta carotene a person would have to eat to realize this protection. On the basis of Dr. Menkes' figures, she states: the amount in one carrot.[7]

What reasonable cost insurance!

Dark green vegetables such as broccoli, spinach and kale—all high in carotenes—were shown in still another study to protect current smokers and those who had quit the habit within the past five years. Persons who ate some of these vegetables three times weekly were twice as prone to develop lung cancer as those who ate them every day.[8]

Then the topper of them all is a 10-year study of diets of 250,000 individuals in Japan. Those who daily ate green and yellow vegetables high in beta carotene had far less cancer — not only of the lungs, but of the colon, cervix, prostate and stomach.[9]

One key point that must be made is that beta carotene cannot effectively help heal past lung and larynx abuse of smoking when the person continues smoking, adding new insults to the body. There's a limit to what beta carotene can do!

Marinated Vegetables

1 head cauliflower, chopped	**Marinade:**
1 lb. broccoli, chopped	½ c. unrefined olive oil
1 lb. zucchini, cubed	½ c. fresh orange juice
¼ to ½ lb. yellow squash, cubed	¼ c. fresh lemon juice
10 cherry tomatoes, sliced in half	½ t. oregano, crushed
½ lb. carrots, sliced	½ t. basil
1 c. artichoke hearts	2 garlic cloves, crushed
¼ c. raw turnips, cubed	1 t. honey

Combine and mix marinade ingredients. Place vegetables in extra large bowl and pour marinade over top. Refrigerate at least two hours. Yield 18-20 servings.

Smoker's Cure from Gentcrewal Areade Launceston Tasmania, Austrailia

Austrailian folk lore has a method of quitting smoking by using colts foot tea:

Roll your own—using ½ colts foot tea and ½ tobacco. After one week, start putting in less tobacco and more colts foot tea. (Also, 3 glasses of fresh carrot juice/day.)

CHAPTER 32

Cancer, Prostate
(See Prostate Problems)

CHAPTER 33

Cancer (Skin)

Give yourself an unusual birthday gift every year!

Strip down to your birthday suit and examine every inch of your skin for cancer. This birthday gift could save your life, indicates Edward Lewis Tobinick, M.D., a Beverly Hills, California dermatologic surgeon and assistant clinical professor of medicine at UCLA.[1]

A near epidemic of skin cancer called malignant melanoma (mole cancer) — an 80 percent increase in the last 12 year period — and also a shocking increase in cell carcinoma in sun-exposed skin areas sound an all-out warning to everyone of us encased in skin.[2]

Dr. Tobinick, who has taught doctors early detection of epidermal cancers, explains how to identify a malignant melanoma.[3]

Warning Signs

A malignant melanoma reveals itself by its surface, border, color and diameter, he says. Normal moles have an even surface—flat or elevated. Melanomas show an uneven surface — flat in one part and raised in another.

Normal moles have a smooth outline in contrast with a melanoma's ragged outline. While normal moles are of one color, melanomas are brown or black, mixed with other colors: red, white or blue. Tiny melanomas are rare, states Dr. Tobinick. The usual melanomas measure larger than one-quarter of an inch, the width of a pencil eraser.

No matter how a mole looks, it is suspect if it bleeds, changes size, or itches, warns Dr. Tobinick.

Another Menace

Each year, between 400,000 and 500,000 individuals in the United States discover basal cell carcinomas (sun cancers) on skin areas now or once exposed to sun, 90 percent on head and neck. Rarely fatal, such cancers respond best to early diagnosis and treatment.[4]

Sun cancers are somewhat harder to detect than melanomas, but they can be readily identified. Although they look much like pimples, they don't go away like pimples. Early sun cancers can bleed after only slight irritation, show a crust or scab, and lose the normal pattern of pores, developing a smooth, shiny or pearly appearance, sometimes displaying small, red blood vessels on the surface.

Even a tiny, firm growth with a raised edge and a shiny, pearly surface can be dangerous. Check this and any other suspicious looking growth on the skin. My book, Nutrition: The Cancer Answer (Statford Publishing) can relieve your mind by giving you a solid foundation for cancer prevention.

Prevention: The Best Medicine

These common skin cancers have one thing in common. They are encouraged by excessive sun-exposure—past or present. A little sunshine is a good thing for activating the development of vitamin D in the skin. However, most sun-worshippers get a lot more than a little sunshine.

A mixture of para-aminobenzoic acid (PABA) in an ethyl alcohol solution has been found by Harvard University medical researchers to furnish an excellent sunscreen for absorbing parts of the ultraviolet rays that bring on sunburn and skin cancers, while permitting tanning.[5] Health food centers carry such effective and protective products.

Animal experiments show that PABA not only guards against skin cancer but also keeps the skin soft, smoothe and youthful. (See Section on Wrinkles.)[6]

Insurance From Vitamin Supplements

Is it possible for anti-oxidant vitamins such as C and E taken by mouth to guard against skin cancer brought on by the sun?

Yes. In about 50 percent of the cases, indicate dermatological researchers Drs. Homer S. Black and Wan-Bang Lo, of the Baylor College of Medicine, Houston, who made a milestone discovery as to how exposure to the sun contributes to skin cancer.[7]

Ultraviolet light from the sun causes oxidation of in-the-skin cholesterol, one of whose by-products is cholesterol alpha-oxide, a well-documented cancer-causative. Black and Lo learned that two-thirds more antioxidant vitamins C and E were indeed delivered to the skin of mice which had received these supplements for two weeks than to the skin of the non-supplemented mice.[8]

The researchers found that as anti-oxidant accumulation in the skin increased, the synthesizing of cholesterol alpha-oxide decreased.

A steady supply of these vitamins is necessary, inasmuch as defense of the skin against cancer-causing chemicals uses them up.

Nutritional Defense Against Melanoma?

While vitamins C and E seem helpful in the prevention of sun-induced cell carcinoma, beta carotene, a vitamin A precursor in orange, red and green vegetables and fruit, has been found by several nutritional researchers, including Dr. Daphne Roe, of Cornell University, to discourage the development of melanoma.

This is no surprise, because this nutrient has been shown in numerous experiments to block lung cancer. The advantage of beta carotene as a supplement is that taking a toxic dose is difficult. At super-high intakes, the skin becomes yellowish or orange colored, the signal to cut down.

Studies by Dr. Walter Troll, of New York University, state that seed-eating people throughout the world have little or no cancer.[9] Vitamin B-17 (amygdalin) found is seeds, as well as other foods, is suggested by some alternative doctors for various types of cancer. A list of vitamin B-17 foods will be supplied below.

For more details on seed foods and amygdalin, obtain a copy of my Nutrition: The Cancer Answer.

Richest food sources of beta-carotene in international units per units of less than four ounces are: dandelion greens, 14,000; carrots, 11,000;

yams 9,000; kale, 8,900; parsley and tuurnip greens, 8,500; spinach, 8,100; collard greens and chard, 6,500; watercress, 5,000; red peppers, 4,400; squash, 4,000; cantaloupe, 3,400; endive, 3,300; persimmons and apricots, 2.700; broccoli, 2,500; pimentos, 2,300; romaine, 1,900; mangoes, 1,800; papayas, 1,700; nectarines and pumpkin, 1,600; peaches, 1,300 and cherries and lettuce, 1,000.

Best supplements and foods for vitamin C, named earlier as a possible preventive of cell carcinoma, in milligrams per less than four ounce units are: acerola cherries, 1100; guavas, 240; black currants, 200; parsley. 170; green peppers, 110; watercress, 80; chives, 70; strawberries, 57; persimmons, 52, spinach, 51; oranges, 50; cabbage, 47: grapefruit, 38; papaya, 37; elderberries and kumquats, 36; dandelion greens and lemons, 35; cantaloupe, 33; green onions, 32; limes, 31; mangoes, 27; loganberries, 24; tangerines and tomatoes, 23; squash, 22 and raspberries and romaine lettuce, 18.

Ideal food sources of vitamin E, also named earlier as a possible preventive of basal skin cancer, in International Units per less than four ounce servings, are: wheat germ, 160; safflower nuts, 35; sunflower seeds, 31; whole wheat, 30; sesame oil, 26; walnuts, 22; corn oil and hazelnuts, 21; soy and peanut oil, 16; almonds, 15; olive oil, 14; cabbage, 7.8; brazil nuts and peanuts, 6.5; cod liver oil, 5.5; cashews, 5.1; soy lecithin, 4.8; spinach, 2.9; asparagus, 2.5 broccoli, 2; butter, 1.9; parsley, 1.8; oats, barley and corn, 1.7; and avocados and pecans, 1.5.

Following are the best foods for vitamin B-17, better characterized as amydalin, nitriles and nitrilosides, in terms of milligrams per units of less than four ounces: black lima beans, 5,100; bitter almonds, 4,200; white lima beans, 3,600, bean sprouts, 2,000; green lima beans, 1,700; wild cherry bark, 1,300; bitter cassava, 940; quince seeds, 680; buckwheat, 340; guava seeds, 190 and kidney beans, navy beans and black eyed peas, 34.

Caroline's Carrot Cake

2½ c. unbleached flour	1¾ c. honey or date sugar
5 t. baking powder	1 c. safflower oil
½ t. cinnamon	1 c. walnuts, chopped
¼ t. orange peel	1 c. raisins
¼ t. lemon peel	1 c. spring water
3 egg whites	2 c. carrots

Grate carrots and chop walnuts. Sprinkle raisins with flour. Sift flour and baking powder. Add orange and lemon peel and cinnamon. In a large bowl, beat honey and oil. In a small bowl, beat egg whites until frothy and set aside. Add water to honey and oil mix. Add flour mixture and mix well. Add raisins, walnuts and grated carrots, mixing after each addition. Fold in egg whites. Place in a 9 x 13 glass baking dish Sprinkle top with raw sugar and chopped walnuts. Place in 350 degree oven for 40 to 45 minutes.

Haus Slaw

1 c. carrots, shredded	Unsweetened shredded coconut
1 c. rutabaga, shredded	Sour cream
1 c. cabbage, shredded	

Toss shredded vegetables together lightly. These vegetables make a delightful flavor combination. Place a tall slender server of unsweetened shredded coconut in the center of a large platter. Pile the shredded vegetables around the coconut. To serve, lift the shredded vegetables off with tongs and sprinkle top with some of the coconut and finish with a spoonful of sour cream. Serves 6.

CHAPTER 34

Candida
Albicans
(Fungus Infection)

One of those difficult-to-diagnose diseases, Candida albicans has many symptoms which could indicate other ailments. However, we know for sure it is a most stubborn fungus (or yeast) that thrives in warm, moist body areas such as the anus, intestines, nose, throat and vagina.

Everybody carries this yeast in the intestinal tract, which is one reason why Candida albicans is so hard to diagnose. In most individuals, it remains under the control of far more numerous, friendly, intestinal bacteria.

Certain special developments of the 20th century transformed it from a quiet, harmless guest to a dominant, fast-spreading enemy bent on taking over and sickening the entire body: antibiotics introduced and increasingly used since World War II; cortisone utilized in high doses; continued increase in consumption of refined carbohydrates — mainly sugar — and widespread use of the birth control pill.

The Candida Take-Over

Let me explain more in depth. Antibiotics kill off harmful bacteria, but they also decimate the friendly bacteria in the intestines. Then the quiet guest strives to dominate the household. Candida albicans thrives in the presence of cortisone and hormones in the Pill. Refined carbohydrates are the favorite foods of this fungus. They multiply and thrive on them.

Symptoms? Feeling drained by fatigue, inability to sleep, poor memory, aching muscles, abdominal discomfort or pain; pain and/or swelling in the joints, premenstrual syndrome and 48 other symptoms, many of them common to half a dozen other physical ailments.

About the only way to know for sure about the diagnosis is to visit an alternative doctor or clinical ecologist experienced in testing for it. Inasmuch as everybody has Candida in the intestines, cultures must be taken in various warm moist body places as an indication of its spread and takeover: anus, armpits, under the breast, in the groin, gum areas, mouth, male sex organs, nose, rectum, vagina and vulva. The cultures are sent to a lab for testing.

Solutions?

Stubborn resistance and a strong offensive are the best answers to defeating the persistent Candida yeast. This means cutting out all refined flour and all types of sugar: white, brown, golden, corn syrup, honey, maple syrup, molasses and sorghum — all processed foods, canned or packaged, because their list of products disguises sugars, and also sweetened soft drinks.

Dr. William Crook, who wrote a smashing best-seller on Candida, The Yeast Connection, told me that he rules out all fruit from the diet of his Candida patients: fresh, canned and dried.

A persistent misunderstanding about Candida is that one cannot eat yeast supplements or yeast in baked goods.

"I have had this point verified by experts, and the yeast you eat has no bearing on Candida albicans," Dr. Crook explained to me while a guest on my "Accent on Health" TV show.

Not By Food Alone!

The Crook anti-Candida diet is heavy on protein and complex carbohydrates with some fat: vegetables, whole grain breads and cereals, chicken and lamb, fish, nuts, butter, cold-pressed oils, and a good quality yogurt without fillers, sweetening or fruit.

In my conversations with John Trowbridge, M.D., of Houston, Texas — one of the prominent persons on our list of alternative doctors in the back of the book— I find that he puts his patients on a diet similar to that of Dr. Crook. I might add that Dr. Trowbridge has written a classic book on Candida albicans, The Yeast Syndrome, and is one of the world's foremost authorities on this subject.

Candida diets like that of Dr. Trowbridge call for yogurt containing the all-important lactobacillus acidophilus and other friendly cultures to colonize the colon. Further, yogurt can be tolerated by many milk-intolerants.

For milk-intolerants who can't handle yogurt, carrot acidophilus, available at health food stores and taken according to directions on the label, may help. Some alternative doctors advise even those who can take yogurt to supplement it with capsules of friendly bacteria to hurry the recolonization process.

Other supplementary items recommended by alternative doctors are odorless garlic — six spurts of the liquid from the plastic squeeze container in a half glass of water; a daily multiple vitamin with minerals; a vitamin B-complex tablet of 50 mg strength to supply vitamins produced by the friendly bacteria before the fungus overwhelmed them; at least 1,000 mg of vitamin C and two cups of Pau D'Arco tea (sometimes called Taheebo tea) and supposedly an enemy of the Candida albicans yeast.

Usually these measures correct the condition, but, if they don't, visit your alternative doctor again. He or she has a stronger therapy.

Lentil Soup Dinner

4 chicken breasts, skinned (cut into 1 inch squares)	1 t. cumin
	1 t. nutmeg
4 c. stock or spring water	1 t. cayenne pepper
1 c. lentils, dried and washed	1 t. celery seed
2 large white onions, quartered	6 garlic cloves, minced
2 celery stalks (including tops), chopped	1 t. thyme
½ green bell pepper, diced	Few sprigs of parsley
6 medium carrots	1 t. sweet basil
1 T. Tamari soy sauce	3 T. olive oil

Brown chicken in oil, turning often. Bring liquid to a boil and add lentils. Reduce heat and simmer for 30 minutes, partially covered. Add remainder of ingredients and simmer for 20 minutes more. Add 1 Tbl of Tamari. Remove half of soup from pan to blender and whiz for a few seconds to obtain a thick, warm lentil puree. Mix back into remaining soup and stir to desired consistency. Serves 6-8 people.

Corky's Pistachio Salad

¾ c. natural seedless raisins
½ c. fresh carrot juice
4 medium carrots
1 medium beet
2 T. cashew mayonnaise
(see below)

½ c. pistachio nuts
4 large or 8 small lettuce leaves
½ c. alfalfa, lentil or mung sprouts
1 stalk celery, finely chopped

Soak raisins in carrot juice for 1 hour, or until plump. Grate carrots and beet and mix with other ingredients. Place in refrigerator until cool. Mix in dash of mayonnaise. Serve on a bed of lettuce leaves.

Cashew Mayonnaise

½ c. cashews
1½ c. boiling spring water

1 t. sea salt
½ t. onion powder

Blend, cook, stirring constantly. Add 2 to 4 tablespoons lemon juice.

CHAPTER 35

Cataracts

A condition in which the lens of the eye becomes milky or dark and reduces or shuts off vision is called a cataract.

Latest research reveals that the deficiency of various nutrients — vitamins C, B-2 and D and the mineral calcium—can contribute to the development of cataract, particularly vitamin C.

Finding that vitamin C concentrates 30 times more in the eyes than in the blood induced Allen Taylor and associates at Tufts University's Laboratory for Nutrition and Cataract Research to determine if adding appreciable amounts of vitamin C would keep cataracts from forming.[1]

How Cataracts Form

Cataracts develop when proteins in the eye lens are exposed to oxidation and light over the years. Then proteins cluster to form a cloudy mass.

The Tufts researchers exposed cultured eye tissue to ultraviolet light to cause oxidation, discovering that the more vitamin C they added to the culture, the longer it took to form cataracts.[2]

Does taking additional vitamin C assure that more of this vitamin will be delivered to the eyes? Experiments with guinea pigs show that it does.[3]

Richest Food Sources Of Vitamin C

The following are the best sources of this vitamin rated in milligrams per less than four ounce servings: Rose hips, 3,000; acerola cherries, 1,100; guavas, 240; black currants, 200; parsley, 170; green peppers, 110; watercress, 80; chives, 70; strawberries, 57; persimmons, 52; spinach, 51;

oranges, 50; cabbage, 47; grapefruit, 38; papaya, 37, elderberries and kumquats, 36; dandelion greens and lemons, 35; cantaloupe, 33; green onions, 32; limes, 31; mangoes, 27; loganberries, 24; tangerines and tomatoes, 23, squash, 22; raspberries and romaine lettuce, 18 and pineapple, 17.

Other vitamin deficiencies which may contribute to cataracts are vitamin B-2, and D—the latter, because it is essential for metabolizing calcium. Insufficient calcium has also been related to development of cataracts.

One of the common symptoms of vitamin B-2 deficiency is cataracts, as has been revealed in several studies. This vitamin is plentiful in only two food supplements and in one food.

The following list shows these and other supplements and foods with appreciable amounts of vitamin B-2 in terms of milligrams in less than four ounce units: torula yeast, 16; brewer's yeast, 4.2; liver, 4.1; royal jelly, 1.9; alfalfa, 1.8; bee pollen, 1.7; almonds, 0.92 and wheat germ. 0.68; mustard greens, 0.64; egg yolk, 0.52; cheeses, 0.46; human milk, 0.40; millet, 0.38; chicken, 0.36; soybeans and veal, 0.31; eggs and sunflower seeds, 0.28; lamb, 0.27; peas, blackstrap molasses, parsley and cottage cheese, 0.25; sesame seeds, 24; egg white, lentils, rye and beans, 0.22 and spinach, turkey, broccoli and beef, 0.20.

Nutrients Which Resist Cataracts

Exposure to sunlight in moderation makes it possible for the body to synthesize vitamin D. (See Section on Wrinkles.) Best supplement and food sources of this vitamin in international units per less than four ounces are: cod liver oil, 20,000; sardines, 500; salmon, 400; tuna 250; egg yolk, 160; sunflower seeds, 92; liver, 50; eggs, 48; butter, 40 and cheeses, 30; cream, 15; corn oil, 9.0; human milk, 6.0 and cow's milk and cottage cheese, 4.0.

Richest food and supplement sources of calcium per milligram in servings of less than four ounces are: sesame seeds, 1,200; kelp, 1,100; cheeses, 700; (See Section on Milk Intolerance); brewer's yeast, 420; sardines and carob, 350; molasses, 290; caviar, 280; soybeans and almonds, 230; torula yeast, 220; parsley, 200; brazil nuts, 190; watercress, salmon, 150 and chickpeas, 150; egg yolk, beans, pistachios, lentils, and kale, 130; sunflower seeds and cow's milk, 120; buckwheat, 110; maple syrup and cream, 100; walnuts, 99 and spinach, 93.

Sesame Salad Dressing

½ c. sesame seeds, ground
1 c. spring water
1 t. kelp

Juice of ½ lemon
2 T. liquid garlic

Place sesame seeds and spring water in blender. Blend until smooth. Add remaining ingredients and blend until smooth, adding more water if necessary to give correct consistency. Yield about 1 cup. Place on your favorite lettuce.

Hanley's Deviled Eggs

¼ bunch parsley, finely chopped
8 hard-boiled eggs,
   cut in half and yolks removed
¼ c. mayonnaise (home-made)
½ t. dry mustard

Sea salt and pepper to taste
1½ T. horseradish
2 T. sweet pickle relish
1 T. paprika

Mash yolks thoroughly with fork. Blend in remaining ingredients. Fill egg white halves with mixture and garnish with paprika and chill. Serves 6 to 8.

Home-Made Mayonnaise

½ t. mustard powder
4 fluid ounces sunflower oil
   (cold pressed)

Juice of ½ lemon
6 T. chopped parsley

Put egg yolk into a bowl. Add mustard powder and beat together. Add 2 tablespoons of oil, drop by drop. Beat in 2 teaspoons of lemon juice and finally the rest of oil, a little at a time. Add extra lemon juice to taste to taste. Put mayonnaise into a liquidizer with parsley. Work to a smooth, green sauce.

CHAPTER 36

Cholesterol (20 Natural Ways To Lower)

Conventional medicine stresses two ways to lower cholesterol—a low-fat, low-cholesterol diet and drugs. Side-effects of the drugs as listed in ads in medical journals are chilling. One drug in particular appears to encourage cancer.

In a $150 million, ten-year study by the National Institutes of Health (NIH), cholestyramine reduced cholesterol slightly better than did no treatment at all. However, consider the horrendous side-effects.

Edward R. Pinckney, M.D., coauthor with Cathey Pinckney of "The Cholesterol Controversy," penetrated the optimistic, rose-colored publicity issued by the NIH about encouraging results in lowering cholesterol and analyzed other aspects of the study.

Underneath The Cosmetics Of The Beautiful Publicity Face

These are the naked facts.[1] Seventy-three percent more gastrointestinal cancers and 800 percent more deaths occurred in the group taking cholestyramine. Those taking this drug had 45 percent more incidence of gallstones than those not taking it and 44 percent more required gallstone-related surgery, with all the risks of that operation.

The anti-cholesterol drug-takers had 22 percent more bile duct disease and 170 percent more heartburn. There were 175 percent more deaths as a result of accident or violence among the drug takers, including 100 percent more suicides, 100 percent more homicides and 220 percent more accidents.

Now the drug-pushers want cholesterol tests and a monitoring of cholesterol levels for everybody from two year olds on up. They seem determined to get us away from good God-given foods—milk, eggs, butter and meat—even though, as some authorities say, only one out of every 500 persons needs to do this, sufferers from familial hypercholesterolemia, an inherited super-high cholesterol condition.[2]

How Accurate Is The Test?

And, speaking of the cholesterol test, this is indeed a foundation of sand upon which to build a house — inaccurate and unreliable. Judge for yourself. The College of American Pathologists sent a blood sample with a 263 cholesterol reading to 5,000 laboratories for testing. Results were frightening, shocking and confidence-destroying, ranging from a low of 101 to a high of 525![3]

Once a person's blood cholesterol goes above 220 — the generally-accepted level indicating increased susceptibility to heart attack — nutrition-oriented medical doctors usually recommend doing what comes naturally—using certain foods and vitamin supplements to lower blood cholesterol.

Here, in alphabetical order, are natural cholesterol-lowering foods and supplements—mostly the former—the most extensive list ever offered for lowering cholesterol:

1. APPLES eaten on a daily basis have been shown in various studies here and in Europe to lower blood serum cholesterol by approximately 10 percent. Several researchers put test subjects on two to three apples a day—one in mid-morning and one in mid-afternoon or—in the event of three—one in the early evening.[4]

In an apple-eating experiment by French researcher R. Sable-Amplis, of the University of Paul Sabatier—two to three apples daily—eighty percent of the group showed reduced cholesterol within a month—about a 10 percent decline. Good Guy HDL cholesterol rose, and Bad Guy LDL cholesterol dropped.[5]

2. BARLEY is a star at reducing blood serum cholesterol levels, says Dr. Asaf Qureshi, a scientist in the U.S. Dept. of Agriculture's Cereal Crops Research Unit in Madison, Wisconsin. Dr. Qureshi feels that barley scores by lowering the liver's ability to produce cholesterol. It can be used several times a week as a cooked cereal or in bakery goods—bread or

muffins.[6]

3. BEANS (pinto or navy)—as little each day as a cup cooked—lowered cholesterol by 19 percent in subjects tested by Dr. James Anderson, fiber expert at the University of Kentucky. Also the ratio of HDL to LDL became more favorable. (Even baked beans help. No sugar, please!)[7]

4. CARROTS (three medium size raw, eaten daily) have been shown to lower cholesterol by almost eleven percent.[8]

5. CHILI PEPPER reduces blood serum cholesterol level by supressing the liver's ability to produce cholesterol, it is believed. Researchers in Bangkok, Thailand made rice flour noodles, adding two teaspoons of freshly ground jalapeno pepper to slightly more than a cup. Those who ate the noodles daily experienced lowered cholesterol and increased ability to dissolve blood clots.[9]

6. EGGPLANT serves a special function in cholesterol control, it was discovered at the University of Texas. Eggplant appears to block blood levels of cholesterol from rising when fatty foods have been eaten.[10]

7. GARLIC (a daily ration of five fresh cloves minced into other food), has been shown to lower blood serum cholesterol by nearly 10 percent in 25 days. An Indian researcher, Dr. M. Sucur fed this amount of garlic to 200 patients. Cholesterol dropped in almost all of this group with super-high blood serum levels. After patients reduced their cholesterol to desired levels, Dr. Sucur kept it stable with only two cloves of raw garlic daily.[11]

Another approach: an odorless, socially-acceptable form of garlic sold in health food stores can accomplish the same thing. Scientists at Loma Linda University in California fed four capsules of liquid garlic extract daily to patients with high cholesterol. Six months later, these individuals had achieved an average cholesterol reduction of 44 points.[12]

8. GRAPEFRUIT PECTIN, that gelatinous stuff that holds jelly together, can lower cholesterol. Dr. James Cerda. a researcher at the University of Florida, fed patients with high cholesterol a little more than a half ounce of grapefruit pectin capsules daily and, in four months, brought their cholesterol down by an average of eight percent. (Most health food stores carry this supplement.)[13]

9. LECITHIN derived from soybeans—slightly more than an ounce daily—reduced blood levels of cholesterol by 18 percent.[14]

10. MILK (skim) lowers cholesterol, as demonstrated by several

researchers.

11. OAT BRAN, a water-soluble fiber is one of the most effective foods for reducing cholesterol. A study by Dr. J.W. Anderson revealed that eating oat bran daily as a cereal or in muffin form can reduce blood cholesterol by up to 19 percent.[15]

12. OLIVE OIL, as demonstrated by Dr. Scott M. Grundy, of the Center for Human Nutrition at the University of Texas in Dallas, can lower or control cholesterol levels. Grundy keeps his blood cholesterol in line by taking two teaspoonsful daily and holds his consumption of fats to between 30 and 35 percent of total calories.[16]

13. ONIONS have scored high in a number of studies for reducing cholesterol levels in human beings and animals, with high grades for raising the beneficial cholesterol (HDL) over the harmful variety, LDL.[17]

14. PLANTAINS (LARGE GREEN BANANAS) — one half to a whole unit daily — have been discovered to lower blood cholesterol dramatically and create a more favorable ratio betweeen HDL and LDL cholesterol. Ripe plantains don't work. (Green plantains are available in many supermarkets and in produce stores.)[18]

15. SEAFOOD eaten several times a week contributes to controlling fat circulating in the blood and keeping cholesterol levels from elevating, indicate many studies.

16. SEAWEED such as kelp lower cholesterol in a manner that researchers can't quite fathom. It seems to remove cholesterol from the intestine. (If you're not into eating seaweed, Japanese-style, you might want kelp tablets from the health food store.)[19]

17. SOYBEANS and products derived from them—soy milk, lecithin and tofu—help break down fatty deposits so that they can be flushed from the body more readily—and, in the process, also lower blood cholesterol. Soybean products seem to work best on patients with extra-high cholesterol, 300 or more. Researchers at the University of Milan, Italy caused cholesterol levels to plummet by fifteen to twenty percent, simply by having patients eat soybeans used in various recipes in place of meat and milk products.[20]

18. SPINACH proved a good cholesterol-reducer in animal experiments by Japanese scientists.[21]

19. YAMS (SWEET POTATOES) which contain much water-soluble

fiber, in addition to beta-carotene, contribute to cholesterol control, if eaten four or five times weekly. In a Japanese experiment, sweet potato fiber proved the best of twenty-eight fruit and vegetable fibers for binding with cholesterol and removing it.[22]

20. YOGURT is a real winner in lowering cholesterol. Three cups a day have caused cholesterol levels to decline by as much as five to 10 percent a week, with the proportion of Good Guy HDL rising in ratio to LDL.[23]

The above list offers the opportunity to alternate and combine. Recipes below will serve as a pattern for doing just that.

Bonus:

Experiments by England's Constance Spittle Leslie, a pathologist at Pinderfields Hospital in Wakefield, Yorkshire, taking vitamin C—1,000 mg daily—led to decrease of her blood cholesterol from 230 to 140. When she discontinued taking this vitamin, her cholesterol returned to its former level. Patients at the hospital experienced a similar reduction on her vitamin C regime.[24]

Bonus 2:

Researcher Josef Patsch, at Baylor College of Medicine, found by experiments, that daily vigorous exercise is one of the best means of lowering blood serum cholesterol, of increasing the ratio of HDL to LDL, and of ridding the blood of excessive fats.[25]

This is no quick-fix. Benefits won't last forever. The program must be continued regularly, insists Patsch.

Gene Arceri's Navy Bean Supper

1 c. dried navy beans	2 c. goat cheese, grated (optional)
½ c. onions, chopped	2 t. herbal seasoning
2 carrots, diced	Sea salt to taste

Wash beans. Cover with water in saucepan and soak overnight (or bring to a boil). Reduce heat and add onions and carrots. Simmer until beans are desired texture (1 hour minimum).

Ruth McAnich Apple-Lamb Curry

1 lb. lamb steaks, boneless
  (or stewing meat)
1 onion, mince
1 garlic clove, minced
2 T. odorless liquid garlic
3 T. olive oil
1 T. curry powder
1 t. paprika

½ t. ginger, ground
1 t. jalapeno pepper,
  freshly ground
2 t. honey
1 can (6 ounces) tomato paste
2 c. apples (tart), peeled and chopped
Hot cooked brown rice

Cut lamb into 1 inch cubes. Saute onion and garlic in olive oil until golden brown. Add curry powder, paprika, ginger, jalapeno pepper and honey. Blend well. Add lamb and brown all sides. Add tomato paste and enough boiling water to cover. Stir well. Cover and simmer for 3 minutes over low heat. Add apples and cook for 15 minutes longer. Serve with rice. Makes 4 Servings.

Hanley's Banana Soy Milk

Base:
  1 c. soaked soybeans   1½ c. water

Blend 1 minute...cook 1 hour in double boiler.

Milk:
  1 c. base   ⅛ t. sea salt
  3½ c. spring water   1-4 bananas
  1 t. vanilla

Add base (above) with milk ingredients. Blend well. Serve over cereal and 1-3 tablespoons carob for a creamy, non-sweet cereal topping.

CHAPTER 37

Circulation Blockage In Legs (Intermittent Claudication)

For a while I debated with myself the need to include this category of illness in Foods That Heal, because food alone cannot help to alleviate it.

Then I learned from alternative doctors that this is a common condition for which orthodox physicians have no satisfactory treatment and that many patients suffer amputations and often death, because they have little or nothing to go on—usually just a low fat-low cholesterol diet, something with limited effectiveness.

Alternative doctors use the Haeger treatment, which, at least offers some relief and minimizes the need for amputations.

Symptoms And Therapy

Exactly what is intermittent claudication? A partial blockage of blood circulation in the legs, resulting in increasing pain until the person can walk no farther. After a brief rest, he or she can again walk a short distance.

A prominent Swedish surgeon specializing in artery diseases, Knut Haeger, M.D., experimented to see if he could extend the walking range of intermittent claudication patients. He succeeded beyond expectations.[1]

Haeger gave 300 to 400 I.U. of vitamin E to numerous patients and had them become more active, walking each day. Invariably, this regime increased the amount of blood circulated in the leg and, therefore, permitted patients to walk farther before being stopped by pain.

Patients who exercised without taking the vitamin E extended their walking range only slightly, compared with those who took the vitamin.

Patience Brings Positive Results

Haeger states that there's no such thing as "instant improvement" with this regime. Improvement could take three months or more.

The most exciting result of the experiments was that in the group of 95 patients exercising and taking vitamin E there was the need for only one amputation. Among the 104 patients who were not on the vitamin, there was a requirement for 11 amputations — 11 times as many!

Exactly how did this regimen improve the walking range? Evan and Wilfrid Shute, the Canadian doctors whose landmark clinical work advanced the cause of vitamin E, indicated that this vitamin increased peripheral circulation.

However, the Haeger theory holds that vitamin E makes it possible for leg muscles to do more work. Then, as the patient can walk farther, he or she increases the blood circulation.

Whether or not Haeger's theory is correct, his regime gets desired results. As part of the 300 to 400 I.U. of vitamin E taken in daily, here are foods most rich in this vitamin in terms of International Units per less than four ounce portions:

Wheat germ, 160; safflower nuts, 35; sunflower seeds, 31; whole wheat, 30; sesame oil, 26; walnuts, 22; hazelnuts, 21; peanut and soy oil, 16; almonds, 15; olive oil, 14; cabbage, 7.8; brazil nuts and peanuts, 6.5; cod liver oil, 5.4; cashews, 5.1; soy lecithin, 4.8; spinach, 2.9; asparagus, 2.5; broccoli, 2.0; butter, 1.9; parsley, 1.8; oats, barley and corn, 1.7 and avocados and pecans, 1.5.

Lynda's Prune-Wheat Germ Bread

1½ c. Whole Wheat Flour	½ c. Butter
⅓ c. Honey	2 Eggs
½ c. Toasted Wheat Germ	½ c. Dairy Soup Cream
1¾ t. Apple Pie Spice	1 c. Diced Pitted Prunes
1½ t. Baking Soda	½ c. Walnuts, Chopped
¼ t. Sea Salt	¼ c. Unsweetened Applesauce

In large mixing bowl combine flour, wheat germ, apple spice, soda and salt. Add butter and cut in until mixture resembles coarse crumbs. Beat eggs, applesauce, honey and stir in sour cream. Blend into flour mixture along with prunes and nuts. Stir just until mixed. Spoon into greased 9 inch loaf pan and bake at 375 degrees for about 50 minutes, or until a wooden toothpick inserted in center comes out clean. Cool in pan or on rack for 10 minutes. Remove cake from pan and cool. Serve warm or cool with butter or cream cheese.

Wild Bill Goin's Banana-Nut Drink

1 t. fiber	½ c. brewers yeast
½ c. ground raw sunflower seeds	2 t. pure vanilla
2 very ripe bananas	2 c. spring water
½ c. non-instant milk powder	2 t. wheat germ

In blender or food processor combine all ingredients and mix well. This is thick and very rich. Serve for an on-the-run breakfast or for a nutritious snack. Serves four one-cup servings.

Maureen's Parsley Sauce

Mince a bunch of parsley and a clove or two of garlic, depending on how you feel about garlic. At our house we use two or three cloves, and mince it very fine. Add a bit of olive oil, sea salt and pepper to taste. Grate a little fresh Romano or fresh Parmesan cheese and mix it all together. We call it Parsley Sauce and it's absolutely fantastic on steak, fish or fowl and it's good on salads as a dressing.

Lesta's Date-Nut Spread

1 c. dates, pitted	¼ c. plain yogurt
½ c. pistachios	½ c. non-instant dry milk powder

Blend all together in blender. If too thin to spread, add more dry milk powder. Spread on celery stalks for appetizers.

The California Cooler

3 avocados, halved and peeled	Ice
3⅓ c. unsweetened grapefruit juice	Mint, for garnish
¾ c. honey	

Puree avocados with grapefruit juice and honey. Chill. Pour into ice filled glasses. Serve with straws. Makes 6 to 8 servings.

CHAPTER 38

Circulation Problems

If nutrient and oxygen-carrying blood can't efficiently pass through arteries to and from your trillions of cells — if your circulation is limited — you may soon be out of circulation with one or more serious, if not critical, medical disorders:

(1) obstruction of arteries to the heart and cramping with pain in the chest (angina pectoris);

(2) an area of heart tissue which has died because blood supply has been cut off (heart infarct);

(3) blockage of a blood vessel to the brain (cerebral thrombosis);

(4) impeded blood flow to the leg;

(5) diabetic complications;

(6) emphysema;

(7) kidney disorders;

(8) deterioration of the eye's retina;

(9) a disease characterized by rigid muscles, muscle weakness, slow movements and tremors (Parkinson's disease);

(10) senility;

(11) stroke;

(12) varicose veins.

How Circulatory Problems Happen

Many researchers believe that arteries start to narrow with degeneration of their walls. Fibrin, a blood component rushes to the scene to clot and seal the stress point. This irregularity seems to be the site at which a buildup begins.

Cholesterol is just one ingredient in the buildup on walls of the arteries, including fibrin, calcium, triglycerides, ceroids and, sometimes, blood platelets.

A study by Dr. William B. Kountz of 288 low thyroid patients with elevated blood cholesterol—his patients and those from the infirmary of Washington University, St. Louis — revealed advanced blood vessel disease in all patients averaging 67 years of age.[1]

Kountz gave thyroid supplements to half of this group and none to the other half, the controls. After five years, he found the fatality rate of controls twice as high as that of patients on thyroid hormone.

Although this study indicates that proper thyroid gland function or proper supplementation protects or regains a healthy circulatory system, other therapies also seem to work.

Of Vitamins And Arteries

Vitamins C, B-6 and E also make key contributions to keeping arteries clean and blood free-flowing. An article in the respected Lancet magazine states that 1000 mg of vitamin C a day prevented blockages in arteries that bring on heart attacks and strokes, and also lowered blood cholesterol levels.[2]

In rabbit experiments, Dr. Anthony Verlangieri, then at Rutgers University, discovered that a deficiency of vitamin C in the daily diet led to the loss of certain chemical compounds in artery linings, creating irregularities, ideal accumulation places for harmful plaques. A high intake of vitamin C assured that these chemicals would stay where they belong, making for smooth artery linings.[3]

Twenty-two years of experiments by Dr. M.L. Riccitelli, of Yale School of Medicine, produced results similar to those of Verlangieri.[4]

Various foods can keep cholesterol and triglycerides under control: dietary fibers such as oat bran, olive oil, and raw carrots. (See Section on Cholesterol and 20 natural ways of lowering blood cholesterol.)

Many natural foods or supplements help keep blood from clotting when it isn't supposed to—among them, garlic or liquid garlic (the odorless type); onions, cantaloupe, and olive oil and ginger.

The Villain Stress

Deficiencies of certain vitamins can cause biochemical stress. Stressors can come in any packages—physical exposure to extreme heat or cold or to gruelling labor; negative emotions (unhappiness, frustration or depression), unrelenting financial pressure, and among others, demanding daily deadlines.[5]

Whatever the form of stress, it makes blood pressure rise, adrenal glands engorge and the thymus and lymph glands shrink. Just as a buildup of biochemical gunk in arteries can restrict blood flow, so can stress, by constricting arteries.

Therefore, managing and reducing stress is just as important as eating properly. (See section on Stress.)

Exercise: Good Stuff!

Individuals who cannot manage stress properly often resort to vigorous physical exercise to relax. This is excellent, because physical activity helps release stress and, at the same time, keeps arteries and capillaries supple and youthful.[6]

Inactive capillaries often collapse and, then, cannot provide enough food and oxygen to muscles which they're supposed to service.[7]

A simple, no-cost-for-equipment exercise like brisk walking for a half hour or more daily can send the blood rushing to the farthest outposts of the body. More athletic individuals can go in for greater physical activity: bike-riding, jogging, running, or swimming.

Foods That Help Keep Arteries Clear

Earlier, we mentioned vitamins C, B-6 and E, which contribute to smooth and unimpaired arteries. Here are foods richest in vitamin C in milligrams per less than four ounce portions: acerola cherries, 1100; guavas, 240; black currants, 200; parsley, 170; green peppers, 110; watercress, 80; chives, 70; strawberries, 57: persimmons, 52; spinach, 51; oranges, 50; cabbage, 47; grapefruit, 38; papaya, 37; elderberries and kumquats, 36; dandelion greens and lemons, 35; cantaloupe, 33; green onions, 32; limes, 31; mangoes, 27; loganberries, 24; tangerines and tomatoes, 23; squash, 22 and raspberries and romaine lettuce, 18.

Best bets for foods high in vitamin B-6 in terms of milligrams per less than four ounce units are: brewer's yeast, 4.0; brown rice, 3.7; whole wheat, 2.9; royal jelly, 2.4; soybeans, 2; rye, 1.8; lentils, 1.7; sunflower seeds and hazelnuts, 1.1; alfalfa, 1; salmon, 0.98; wheat germ, 0.92; tuna, 0.90; bran, 0.85; walnuts, 0.73; peas and liver, 0.67; avocados, 0.60; beans, 0.57; cashews, peanuts, turkey, oats, chicken and beef, 0.40; halibut, 0.34 and lamb and banana, 0.32.

Food sources and supplements with the highest number of International Units of vitamin E per less than four ounce servings are: wheat germ, 160; safflower nuts, 35; sunflower seeds, 31; whole wheat, 30; sesame oil, 26; walnuts, 22; corn oil and hazel nuts, 21; soy and peanut oil, 16; almonds, 15; olive oil, 14; cabbage, 7.8; brazil nuts and peanuts, 6.5; cod liver oil, 5.4; cashews, 5.1; soy lecithin, 4.8; spinach, 2.9; asparagus, 2.5; broccoli, 2; butter, 1.9; parsley, 1.8 and oats, barley and corn, 1.7.

Thus far, we have talked mainly about preventing arteries from narrowing or blocking. However, what can be done about already existing reduction of circulation? Over and above earlier-mentioned thyroid therapy where indicated, there's chelation therapy.

Orthodox medicine often bad-mouths chelation, which uses a chemical called EDTA, dripped into the bloodstream intravenously. The orthodoxy, which insists on double-blind studies for everybody else's therapies, favors heart bypass surgery with all its risks—including that of death—a surgical technique never proved by a double-blind study. Would this be a double standard?

Heart bypass has had some successes. However, it usually costs twenty to thirty times what a 20-treatment chelation course would cost. Bypass patients often suffer a painful, long-term recovery, while chelation patients have no pain and no recovery period. Further chelation improves circulation in all parts of the body, not just the heart area.

There's one hitch. The Medical Monarchy — more accurately, dictatorship—has conned government authorities into approving heart bypass for Medicare reimbursement and not approving chelation therapy for such reimbursement. Even private insurance companies are under the thumb of the Medical Monarchy, which is answerable to no one. Maybe congress could rectify this condition.

Insurance company lemmings plunge over the financial brink, paying out astronomical sums that could be saved if chelation therapy were reimbursable, avoiding the emergencies that bring on money-squandering heart bypass surgery.

All right. How does chelation work? EDTA dripped into the veins slowly removes calcium, the cement which holds together the biochemical gunk narrowing or blocking arteries and weakens the structure so that this debris slowly enters the bloodstream, circulates to the kidneys and is thrown off.

In the infancy of chelation, some mishaps occurred due to too rapid removal of calcium and to the loss of vitally needed minerals. Now, however, the technique has been perfected and minerals are added by intravenous dripping. Many of the alternative doctors on the list in the back of the book do chelation or can make referrals. Otherwise, the American College of Advancement in Medicine, 23121 Verdugo Drive, Suite 204, Laguna Hills, CA 92653, can pinpoint a chelation expert in your area. The phone number is (714) 583-7666.

There you have it: preventive and therapeutic methods for encouraging the highest quality circulatory system.

CHAPTER 39

Colds

One thing nobody wants in common with anybody else is the common cold, the source of assorted human miseries.

So, do you protect yourself with vitamin C?

Alternative doctors say, "Yes." Orthodox doctors say, "No."

Who's right?

Mr. Vitamin C himself, Dr. Linus Pauling, two-time winner of the Nobel Prize, offers answers in his book, How To Live Longer And Feel Better. (W.H. Freeman and Company).[1]

Pauling, in the late 1960s started championing large doses of vitamin C, from 1000 mg on up into the stratosphere and refers to a dissenting article in Mademoiselle Magazine of November, 1969, written by Dr. Frederick Stare, then chairman of the department of nutrition at the Harvard School of Public Health—noted for his anti-supplement stance —and identified as "One of the country's Big Names in nutrition."[2]

The Numbers Game

Stare stated that this business about vitamin C being helpful in coping with colds had been disproved some 20 years before in a "careful study" at the University of Minnesota. Half of 5,000 students were given a large dose of vitamin C and the other half were given look-alike pills with no nutrient values (placebos).[3]

For two years, researchers checked on the medical histories of all students involved and discovered that there was no difference in how often, how severe and how long the colds lasted, asserted Stare.[4]

Dr. Pauling went back to the medical journal carrying the article on this particular study by Cowan, Diehl and Baker, and noted that what Stare called a "careful study" actually involved four hundred students, rather than 5,000.[5] But what's a little error of 4,600 among friends?

Scientific Inaccuracy

He also noted that the "careful study" was conducted for six months, rather than two years?[6] Who's going to quibble over a year and one-half error for mere scientific accuracy?

Further, Pauling discovered that Stare's "large dose of vitamin C" was just 200 mg. Despite this, Cowan, Diehl and Baker found that the vitamin C-taking students had 31 percent fewer days of illness than those who didn't take the vitamin.[7]

How could the researchers fail to realize that a 31 percent difference is statistically significant? And, beyond this, how could someone of Dr. Stare's stature overlook it, too? How could everyone but Dr. Pauling miss it?

One can only conclude that, before writing the Madamoiselle article, scientist Stare should have made a more careful study of the "careful study" to make sure it proved his point instead of Dr. Pauling's.

Convincing Studies

Dr. Pauling refers to a controlled study by biochemist G. Ritzel.[8] Schoolboys taking 1000 mg of vitamin C daily reported a decrease in number of colds by 45 percent and a decrease by 30 percent in number of days of illness per cold. Including the Ritzel study, Pauling summarized results of 16 controlled research projects to find the percentage of decrease in illness of test subjects taking varying amounts of vitamin C daily.[9]

Individuals taking 70 to 200 mg of vitamin C daily, averaged a decrease in illness per person of 31 percent in comparison with placebo subjects. Those taking larger amounts averaged 40 percent.[10]

Pauling quotes the American Medical Association statement released to the press in 1975 with the headline, "Vitamin C Will Not Prevent or Cure the Common Cold."[11] This announcement was based on two publications presented in the Journal of the American Medical Association

(JAMA), one by Karlowski and associates and another by Dykes and Meier—the latter a review of other studies.[12]

Results of these studies hardly justified the AMA headline — particularly, that of Dykes-Meier, which omitted numerous well-structured investigations which presented opposing findings, writes Pauling.[13] Even the Dykes-Meier study admitted that vitamin C reduces the amount of illness connected with the common cold.

No Room For Improvement!

So that readers of the Journal of the American Medical Association would have a thorough analysis of all existing evidence, Dr. Pauling prepared a short but thorough coverage of 13 controlled studies and submitted it to the editor of JAMA.[14]

Twice the editor returned the paper to Pauling for small revisions, which he made. Six months later, the editor rejected the paper as "not wholly convincing."[15]

Apparently, the Dykes-Meier publication, omitting key studies was more convincing than a more comprehensive one prepared by a two-time Nobel prize winner!

Pauling declares that it was improper for the JAMA editor to publish only one side of a scientific or medical question and also to block the proper discussion of a question by sitting on a paper for six months, preventing its timely submission to another publication.[16] Eventually, the Pauling paper found a home in Medical Tribune.

High C Levels, Low Infection

Over and above the Pauling findings are several solid studies which show that taking supplementary vitamin C offers various kinds of protection against colds.

In an experiment by the Naval Medical Research Institute, vitamin C plasma levels of 28 men on a 68-day submarine patrol were noted frequently. Those with the lowest plasma levels of vitamin C manifested twice as many cold symptoms as the men with highest vitamin C plasma levels.[17]

An Australian study demonstrated that individuals who had contracted colds reduced the duration of their infection by 19 percent, simply by taking 1000 mg of vitamin C daily.[18]

A carefully controlled, double-blind study by Terence W. Anderson, Ph.D, of the University of Toronto School of Hygiene, produced results which surprised Dr. Anderson, who, some years before, had determined to prove Linus Puling wrong in saying that vitamin C could reduce duration of the common cold.[19]

Five hundred test subjects received 1000 mg of vitamin C daily. This was upped to 4000 mg on the first three days of an illness. Five hundred others received a look-alike nothing pill (a placebo). As in all double-blind studies, neither participants, nor the researcher knew who was getting what.[20]

Test results showed that those on the vitamin C supplement were confined indoors with colds 30 percent fewer days than the others. Here's the most dramatic fact: 40 percent more of the vitamin-takers stayed entirely free of all types of illness, including colds, than the placebo-takers.[21]

More Cold-Fighters

Although vitamin C is the foremost cold-fighter, there are other nutrients that also battle for you: vitamins A, B-complex, E and the mineral zinc. Immune system strength against the 80 to 100 cold-causing viruses is built by eating foods rich in these nutrients and, in certain instances, by taking vitamin and mineral supplements.

Studies of human beings and animals revealed that a deficiency of vitamin A weakened the ability of the immune system to defend against colds and other physical ailments, and the addition of vitamin A reversed the condition.[22]

The full range of B vitamins also bolsters the immune function. Research shows that a lack of vitamin E shuts down part of the immune function, the making of antibodies and the multiplication of white blood cells which destroy virus and other invaders. Even moderate amounts such as 200 I.U. daily help to reverse the damage.[23]

Zinc: Mineral Marvel

As a contributor to controlling colds, zinc, like vitamin C among vitamins, is a superstar among minerals for strengthening the immune function, particularly in reviving function of the thymus gland, the key gland of the immune system.

Even the most senior of senior citizens have experienced a revival of thymus function with zinc added to their diet. Research shows that as little as 15 mg of zinc can recharge the thymus and, consequently, the immune function. [24]

Zinc lozenges allowed to melt in the throat have helped relieve soreness and drive away other cold symptoms. They sell in health foods stores at potencies of 25 to 50 mg.

In one study, 11 percent of the zinc lozenge users got rid of all cold symptoms within 12 hours. Twenty-two percent conquered their colds in 24 hours. Fifty percent were free of all cold symptoms in four days, and 88 percent had no colds within seven days. [25]

In sharp contrast, all takers of placebos showed cold symptoms after four days. Just 49 percent of them had defeated their colds by the seventh day.

Folk Remedies

One of the most powerful anti-cold weapons in the Jewish mother's arsenal is chicken soup, which has been found to loosen phlegm in nose and throat and speed the end of the cold. Modern science is finally learning by experimentation what Jewish mothers knew all along.

Jean Carper in The Food Pharmacy (Bantam) states that George Washington, our first president, treated a cold by eating a hot roasted onion before going to bed.

Another folk remedy for colds and sore throat is sliced onions cooked slowly — not browned — in water until almost a syrup. Add a spurt of lemon and a tablespoon of honey and mix well. Some persons strain the onion out. Others drink it down with the syrup.

Garlic is a renowned folk remedy for colds. Two cloves eaten raw daily are said to help relieve you of colds and friends. Odorless garlic fluid, capsules or tablets are helpful, too. I rarely get a cold, but if I do, I take eight spurts of garlic fluid from the squeeze bottle into half a glass of water and drink it down three times daily. And soon, I'm back to normal.

Vitamin-Rich Foods For Colds

Foods richest in vitamin A—or its precursor—in International Units per less than four ounce portions are: cod liver oil, 200,000; sheep liver, 45,000, beef liver, 44,000; calf's liver, 22,000; dandelion greens, 14,000; carrots, 11,000; yams, 9,000; kale, 8,900; parsley and turnip greens, 8,500; spinach, 8,100; collard greens and chard, 6,500; watercress, 5,000; red peppers, 4,400; winter squash, 4,000; egg yolk and cantaloupe, 3,400; endive, 3,300; persimmons and apricots, 2,700; broccoli, 2,500; pimentos, 2,300; swordfish, 2,100; whitefish, 2,000; romaine, 1,900; mangoes, 1,800; papayas, 1,700; nectarines and pumpkin, 1,600; peaches and cheese, 1,300; eggs, 1,200; cherries, lettuce and cream, 1,000; tomatoes and asparagus, 900; and halibut, 850.

Inasmuch as vitamin B-complex is difficult to obtain in food form, preventive medicine specialist Gary Gordon, M.D. recommends that his patients take a vitamin B-complex tablet or capsule in a potency of 50 mg for the major fractions. (Gordon and his name and address are included on the list of alternative physicians in the back of the book.

Among the best food sources of vitamin C in milligrams per less than four ounce servings are: rose hips, 3,000; acerola cherries, 1,100; guavas, 240; black currants, 200; parsley, 170; green peppers, 110; watercress, 80; chives, 70; strawberries, 57; persimmons, 52; spinach, 51; oranges, 50; cabbage, 47; grapefruit, 38; papaya, 37; elderberries and kumquats, 36; dandelion greens and lemons, 35; cantaloupe, 33; green onions, 32; limes, 31; mangoes, 27; loganberries, 24; tangerines and tomatoes, 23; squash, 22; raspberries and romaine lettuce, 18 and pineapple, 17.

Richest food sources of vitamin E in international units for less than four ounce servings are: wheat germ, 160; safflower nuts, 35; sunflower seeds, 31; whole wheat, 30; sesame oil, 26; walnuts, 22; hazelnuts, 21; peanut oil, 16; almonds, 15; olive oil, 14; cabbage, 7.8; brazil nuts and peanuts, 6.5; cod liver oil, 5.4; cashews, 5.1; soy lecithin, 4.8; spinach, 2.9; asparagus, 2.5; broccoli, 2.0; butter, 1.9; parsley, 1.8; oats, barley

2.5; broccoli, 2.0; butter, 1.9; parsley, 1.8; oats, barley and corn, 1.7; avocados and pecans, 1.5; salmon, 1.4; bee pollen, 1.3; rye, 1.2 and cheese, eggs, leeks and coconut, 1.00.

Excellent foods for zinc content in milligrams per less than four ounce servings are: herring, 110; wheat germ, 14; sesame seeds, 10; torula yeast, 9.9; blackstrap molasses, 8.3; maple syrup, 7.5; liver, 7; soybeans, 6.7; sunflower seeds, 6.6; egg yolk, 5.5; lamb, 5.4; chicken, 4.8; molasses, 4.6; brewer's yeast, 3.9; oats, 3.7; rye, 3.4; whole wheat, 3.2; corn, 3.1; coconut and beef, 3.0; beets, turkey and walnuts, 2.8; barley, 2.7; beans and avocados, 2.4; peas, 2.3; bleu cheese, 2.2; eggs, 2.1 and buckwheat, 2.0.

Caroline's Wheat Germ Liver

⅔ c. plain wheat germ, toasted
½ t. sea salt
1 t. oregano, dried
Freshly ground black pepper to taste
4 t. fresh lemon juice

4 t. sesame oil
1½ lbs. calf's liver
  (cut into ½ inch slices)
½ c. unsalted butter
4 lemon wedges

Combine wheat germ, sea salt, oregano and pepper on a large plate and toss gently to mix. Blend lemon juice and sesame oil and brush or rub liver. Lay oiled liver onto seasoned wheat germ, turn to coat both sides. Set dredged liver onto a fine-meshed rack and allow to sit for 10 minutes. Heat oil (or butter) over a low-medium heat in a large skillet. Add slices of liver and saute for approximately 4 minutes, turning once, until liver is medium-rare. Transfer to a plate and serve immediately with lemon wedges. Serve with baked yams and fresh green salad. Makes 4 servings.

Chrissy's Fruit Salad

2 c. fresh pineapple, cubed
2-3 bananas, sliced
1-2 papayas, peeled, seeded and
  cut into bite size
2 T. lemon juice
  (to prevent discoloration of fruits)
½ grapefruit, peeled and chopped

2 c. apple, cut in bite size
½ c. pitted dates, sliced
½ c. walnuts or pecans
½ c. unsweetened coconut
½ c. orange, peeled and cut in bite size
2 T. wheat germ

Mix all ingredients together. Fruit salad is delicious dressed only in its own juice, but you may want to make it in an ambrosia. To do this, add

AMBROSIA DRESSING. Serve in lettuce cups or in pineapple boats. Serves 6.

Ambrosia Dressing

1 c. home-made mayonnaise
½ c. raw certified skim milk

1 T. vanilla
2 T. honey or to taste

Blend in blender. Add a pinch of nutmeg to taste.

CHAPTER 40

Colon Complications (Diverticular Diseases)

A subtle sickness, diverticulosis, one of the diverticular diseases, can exist for a long time without warning symptoms.

Then it can deteriorate into diverticulitis — inflammation of the lower intestine lining and — wham! — the pain can be knifing.

All right. How does this sequence of events start?

With extreme constipation, with fecal matter hardening and compacting in the lower bowel, which is a tube in segments and surrounded by muscles. When waste matter is long, moist and thick, these muscles easily squeeze it downwards from one segment to the next, eventually expelling it through the rectum. This action is called peristalsis.

Hardened fecal matter breaks into fragments, and the hard fragments press on the tender bowel lining and cause it to balloon outward. These small bulges are also formed by pressure of intestinal gas, claim some authorities.

Diverticulosis Becomes Something Worse

Fecal matter collects in these thin-walled balloons and invites bacteria, which make the mass putrefy. Eventually the putrefaction causes the delicate membrane to become irritated, then inflamed, uncomfortable and, suddenly, painful.

This condition spells the end of diverticulosis and the start of diverticulitis. And that spells trouble, right here in Intestine City.

A skilled surgeon can remove the inflamed balloons, but his scalpel cannot cut away the underlying causes for diverticular disease. So, more diverticula soon appear.

Complications Of Diverticulosis

A grim fact rarely mentioned in medical literature is that the putrefactive bacteria in the balloons can actually bring on a form of anemia caused by a deficiency of folic acid, even when the diet provides enough of this nutrient.[1] (See the section on Anemia.) The enemy bacteria intercept folic acid before the victim of diverticular disease has a chance to benefit from it.

Remember that a single enemy bacterium fissions and fissions, becoming a menacing and undermining military force of two million within seven hours.[2] To beat them, you bring in your own military force, friendly bacteria such as lactobacillus acidophilus in a high quality yogurt, in acidophilus milk, and/or in cultures of these organisms from health food stores.

Just three capsules of such cultures can supply as many as 100 million living lactobacillus acidophilus and lactobacillus bifidus microorganisms —a welcome army. This is like calling out the biochemical marines!

Nutrition-oriented medical doctors usually recommend the intake of a pint to a quart of yogurt daily or an equal amount of acidophilus milk or a capsule containing more than 33 million lactobacillus acidophilus organisms. (See the Section on Milk Intolerance.) Sometimes even milk-intolerants can take yogurt without problems. For milk intolerants, there are also lactobacillus acidophilus products based on carrots.

If the patient stays on this regime for months and keeps reinforcing his friendly army, the good guys eventually win. Then it is necessary to make sure the Recommended Daily Allowance (RDA) for folic acid—between 400 and 800 mcg—is met to correct the anemia, because now that the enemy bacteria are overwhelmed, this vitamin will no longer be intercepted.

Following are the richest food sources of folic acid per milligram in units of just less than four ounces: torula yeast, 3; brewer's yeast, 2; alfalfa, 0.80; soybeans, 0.69; endive, 0.47; chickpeas, 0.41; oats, 0.39; lentils, 0.34; beans and wheat germ, 0.31; liver, 0.29; split peas, 0.23; whole wheat, 0.22; barley, 0.21; brown rice, 0.17; sprouts, 0.14; asparagus, 0.12; green peas, 0.11; sunflower seeds and collard greens, 0.10; spinach, 0.080; hazelnuts and kale, 0.070; peanuts, soy lecithin, and walnuts, 0.060; corn,

0.059 and brussel sprouts, broccoli, brazil nuts and almonds, 0.050.

The Disease Can Be Controlled

How can the problem of diverticular disease be solved? With a higher fiber diet, say numerous authorities. People of underdeveloped nations who subsist on corn, beans and peas and wheat, often get our sympathy. However, in one respect they are better off than people in our developed nation. They have only 1/50th the diverticular disease that we have, thanks to their high fiber diet.[3]

Dr. Denis Burkitt, a world authority on fiber and its relation to colon health, points an accusing finger at the typical American diet: low in fiber and high in refined carbohydrates, protein and fats.

The value of a high fiber diet was demonstrated not long ago in an in-depth study of 100 diverticular disease patients at the Royal Liverpool Hospital (England). Researchers found that of patients who religiously followed a high-fiber diet, 91 percent showed no return of symptoms for from five to seven years.[4]

Other studies have revealed similar benefits of the high fiber diet. The fact that many British and American hospitals are putting diverticular disease patients on a high fiber diet has reduced the number of patients needing surgery for this condition by 90 percent, says Dr. Burkitt.[5]

Dangers Of Overdoing

Some patients become overzealous in trying to control their colon condition, taking too much fiber at once without enough extra water, and have developed a bowel obstruction requiring surgery. The British Medical Journal warns against this practice and describes the painful consequences to a man who ate 16 tablespoons of fiber at a sitting.[6]

Richard Kunin, M.D. advises no more than two tablespoons of bran a day at only one meal.

An 80-day study at Cornell University revealed that the type of bran eaten makes a difference in correcting diverticular problems.[6] Coarse bran proved to be superior to fine bran in holding more water in waste material and in moving fecal matter through the bowels more quickly.

One of the best grain fibers is oat bran. Some individuals are so hung up on wheat bran that they are not aware that many foods can offer effective fiber—among them: apples, carrots, potatoes, root vegetables, (like turnips) spinach, beans—actually, all legumes—all whole grains, and nuts such as walnuts, peanuts and almonds.

Whatever choices we make may be able to help in controlling diverticular disease.

A Whole Salad

¼ c. yogurt
¼ c. bleu cheese dressing
½ T. brewers yeast
Alfalfa sprouts
¼ c. oats
Red cabbage, chopped

¼ head romaine lettuce
½ c. brown rice (cooked in water containing cube of chicken bouillon)
Bean sprouts
Sun flower seeds

Mix all ingredients together and serve.

CHAPTER 41

Constipation

A doctor friend calls constipation—too few and usually difficult bowel movements—the most widespread and least necessary physical ailment.

"Laxatives would not be the hottest best-sellers in over-the-counter medicines if people knew the many natural ways of correcting constipation," he often says. "They cost Americans $200 million annually."

All right, so how does a victim of constipation become a regular guy or gal? By the following, says a doctor friend:

1. Making sure there's enough fiber in the diet.

2. Discovering and eliminating food allergens.

3. Eating at least a cup of lactobacillus acidophilus-containing yogurt daily.

4. Taking in at least 60 mcg of folic acid each day.

5. Making certain of not being hypothyroid (having a low thyroid function), and, if hypothyroid, correcting the condition.

BONUS: Exercising daily, particularly doing bends at the mid-section.

Hazards Of Constipation

When food wastes idle through the intestines, mild to frightening physical ailments can result—hemorrhoids and varicose veins, appendicitis or cancer.

The longer waste matter is pressed against the tender tissues of the colon, the longer bowel bacteria have to change normal substances in the stool into cancer-causing chemicals, sometimes bringing about intestinal cancer.

Chronic constipation can cause colon disorders such as diverticulosis—pouches in the bowel wall where fecal matter can lodge and putrify—and diverticulitis, swelling and inflammation of these pouches.

Beating The "Civilized Diseases"

Often a tablespoon or two of bran daily is all that separates a person from ability to resist what Dr. Denis Burkitt, an authority on the colon and waste matter, calls the "civilized diseases" or to become a victim of them.

Burkitt offers a rather unique bathroom test for telling whether or not the diet contains enough fiber and whether or not a person is in danger of developing the civilized diseases.

Floaters are stools containing enough fiber to make them float. Sinkers are heavy and hard and indicate that the person may be headed for problems. Let's talk more about the numbered causes of constipation above:

1. So far as fiber is concerned, seven tablespoons of oat bran have been found to keep bowel movements regular and to guard against diseases of Western society—intestinal tract ailments, heart and artery disorders and degenerative diseases such as cancer. Whole grain breads and cereals are key fiber contributors.

Fiber in vegetables and fruit is helpful but, aside from that in carrots, is not quite as effective as fiber in bran.

2. Of great importance is discovering and dealing with food allergies. The section on food sensitivities and allergies offers a list of the foods to which many of us are allergic, guidance in taking the Coca test and also in how to use challenges to reveal which foods contribute to constipation.

3. Eating yogurt containing lactobacillus acidophilus (LA) implants friendly bacteria to colonize the intestines and outnumber the unfriendly bacteria which may contribute to constipation and to the possible start of cancer. So does taking a lactobacillus acidophilus supplement, which hurries the process of colonizing.

4. Sometimes a deficiency of folic acid may cause constipation. No one fully understands why.

5. Low thyroid function slows down all body functions, including bowel

contractions necessary to move wastes out efficiently. In first generation hypothyroids, sometimes a 225 microgram kelp tablet daily—this contains iodine, the most important food for the thyroid gland—helps to correct this condition. Hypothyroids of the second generation and beyond may require prescribed thyroid tablets.

Bonus: Exercise brings more blood, oxygen and nutrients to the intestines to keep them in health and tones up the tissues for more efficient moving out of waste matter.

Research Results

FIBER: In an experimental controlled study, the eating of bran upped the number of bowel movements and reduced intestinal transit time. Corn bran proved superior to wheat bran.[1]

In another experimental controlled study, 10 grams (less than a tablespoon) of wheat bran two times daily proved markedly superior to a bulk laxative in 10 constipated geriatric patients. The bran reduced bowel transit time from 126 hours to 89 hours.[2]

When wholegrains are mentioned, the backers of white flour and bread always bring up the point that whole grain products contain phytic acid which supposedly makes calcium, iron, magnesium, manganese and zinc impossible for the intestine to absorb.

A recent comparative study by Eugene Morris, of the U.S. Department of Agriculture's Human Nutrition Research Center, destroys this idea.[3] Ten men ate two bran muffins with each meal for thirty days. For fifteen days, they ate muffins with phytic acid stripped from the bran. Then they ate muffins made from whole grain flour.

For the first five days on the muffins with phytic acid, the men did lose more of the needed minerals than when on the other muffins. However, after that they absorbed almost the same amount of minerals as when on the muffins without phytic acid.

LACTOBACILLUS ACIDOPHILUS: This friendly bacteria corrected constipation in 305 of 356 patients. In another experiment, lactobacillus acidophilus relieved symptoms of many constipation-causing conditions: idiopathic ulcerative colitis. irritable colon and, among others, mucous colitis.[4]

NUTRIENTS: In an experiment with three women who were proved to be deficient in folic acid and suffered from chronic constipation, along with other symptoms—among the major ones: depression, fatigue and restless legs—all patients recovered when given 60 mg of folic acid daily.[5]

It is almost impossible to obtain this amount of folic acid from food without eating forty or fifty pounds of produce. Human requirements for this vitamin vary, so the needs of some surpass their ability to obtain it from food.

I rarely need a fiber product, because I eat fresh vegetables and fruits, as well as whole grain products. However, when I do, I favor a product made from whole fruits, vegetables and grains, plus acidophilus.

Natural ways of winning the war against constipation cited here offer alternatives to spending $200 million plus annually for laxatives!

Rice-Garbanzo Casserole

Cooking rice in Apple Juice instead of water:

1½ c. brown rice	¾ c. garbanzos
3 c. pure apple juice	½ lb. peas, with buds left on
½ c. chives, finely chopped	4 medium carrots
1 red bell pepper, chopped	2 ears of corn

Place rice, apple juice, chives and bell pepper in crockpot and cook for 3 hours. Meanwhile, steam garbanzos (which have soaked overnight in water) for 1 hour. Add peas, carrots and corn to steamer and continue steaming for another 10 to 15 minutes. Remove vegetables, along with garbanzos, to rice in crockpot. Serve when ready. Crockpot will keep warm without cooking any further.

Pineapple Health Shake

¼ c. powdered skim milk	2 T. fiber
1 t. honey	1 t. brewers yeast
1 glass unsweetened apple juice	

Put in blender and mix until frothy.

Sprout Salad

1 c. alfalfa sprouts
1 c. wheat sprouts
1 c. mung bean sprouts
1 c. sunflower seed sprouts

¼ c. green pepper, finely chopped
¼ c. green onions, chopped
1 large avocado, chopped
Poppy seed dressing (below)

Mix all ingredients together in large bowl. Toss lightly with dressing and serve immediately.

Poppy Seed Dressing

¼ c. poppy seed
¼ c. unsweetened pineapple juice
1 t. kelp

2 t. lime juice
2 t. honey
¼ c. olive oil

Blend together all ingredients, except oil. Turning blender on low speed, add oil very slowly in a steady stream. Stir in a few extra seeds. Chill until ready to serve.

CHAPTER 42

Cramps

No respecter of persons, cramps work their exquisite torture on anyone and everyone now and then: individuals who exercise themselves to exhaustion and those whose only exercise is avoiding exercise.

Subtle to obvious physical and biochemical events can bring on cramps —improperly used or fed muscles, tight and binding shoes, four-inch high heels, standing longer than usual, bending in an unaccustomed manner, walking with longer, more vigorous strides than usual, exercising without a warmup, stretching beyond normal range in bed at night, sleeping with a leg twisted or resting in an unaccustomed position or malnourishment: a junk food diet, a crash diet or not following a nutrient-rich regime in pregnancy.

Physical conditioners, coaches, athletes and long-time joggers tell me that the best way to get rid of cramps is to prevent them.

Warmups And Proper Nutrition

Death and taxes are inevitable, but cramps are not, if you use your muscles sensibly and eat nutritionally as well as recreationally.

Warmups raise body temperature gradually, making muscles work faster, more efficiently, and with less proneness to cramping. Athletes ease into physical activity—first, by gentle stretching, then by more strenuous stretching.

Easy does it. Joggers often start by walking. Fast walkers usually start slowly and gradually shift into longer strides and greater speed. Their bodies tell them when they are ready.

Outdoor winter sports—skiing or ice-skating—particularly dictate a slow warmup. After all, cold air and wind-chill direct blood from the skin and outer parts of the body to the center, cutting down circulation in toes, feet and legs, fingers, hands and arms. This makes muscles stiff and slow-reacting.

Cramps Made To Order

Weekend or vacation athletes are prime candidates for cramps—as are middle-age persons who forget that fifty year old muscles are no longer twenty.

Even if you treat your muscles the way you want them to treat you, you can still suffer from cramps, if you don't eat properly.

A medical doctor told me about a patient who did just that. Often during the night, she turned over and stretched. Instant agony! A cramp gripped the calf of a leg. She screamed in pain, massaging a knot of muscle with both hands.

After examining her diet sheet, the physician had her drink two glasses of milk daily, eat a cup of plain yogurt, take three calcium-magnesium tablets — 1,000 mg of calcium and 500 mg of magnesium — and also a tablespoon of cod liver oil to supply vitamin D to assure absorption of calcium and its deposition in teeth and bones and also at least 30 I.U. of vitamin E to prevent cramping.

Only three days after starting on this regime, she lost her cramps.

A calcium shortage brings out the worst in muscles. Calcium makes them contract and is the key mineral in transmitting signals throughout the nervous system and, significantly, in areas where nerves are attached to muscles and help to control them. A deficiency causes the sending of erratic signals and the abnormal contracting of muscles.[1]

More To The Story Than Calcium

If lack of calcium isn't the problem, it could be a deficiency of potassium or magnesium. Potassium is a stellar performer in muscle health and function — as well as an aid in transmission of impulses through nerves. A lack of potassium causes explosions of electrical charges to muscles, rather than a smooth transmission, bringing on abnormal responses — muscle twitches, tremors and cramps.[2]

Richard Kunin, M.D. explains that excessive sugar in the diet can create a shortage of potassium, bringing with it cramps and other neuromuscular ailments.[3]

Richest food sources of potassium per milligram in less than four-ounce units are: kelp, 12,000; torula yeast, 2,000; brewer's yeast, 1,900; soybeans, 1,700; beans, 1,200; parsley, peas and sprouts; pistachios, 970; wheat germ, 950; sunflower seeds, 920; chickpeas, 800; almonds, 770; sesame seeds and brazil nuts, 720; peanuts, 670; pecans and avocados, 600; lentils, 590; veal, 580; halibut, 530; salmon, 510; rye, 470; walnuts and cashews, 460; buckwheat, 450; turkey, 440; millet and chicken, 430; potatoes, 410; wheat, 390; liver, 380; beef and bananas, 370 and oats, 350.

In a potassium deficiency, it is conceivable that a banana, a dish of wheat germ cereal or a handful of sunflower seeds could stand between you and muscle cramps.

Magnesium: Another Mighty Mineral

Sometimes additional magnesium-containing foods can foil the muscle mutiny: cramps, tremors and tics.

When a vitamin B-6 supplement alone could not relieve foot and leg cramps or spasms in his pregnant patients, John Ellis, M.D. added magnesium, and most of his patients returned to normal.[4]

Richest food sources of magnesium in milligrams per less than four ounce serving are: kelp, 740; blackstrap molasses, 410; sunflower seeds, 350; wheat germ, 320; almonds, 270; soybeans, 240; brazil nuts, 220; bone meal, 170; pistachios and soy lecithin, 160; hazelnuts, 150; pecans and oats, 140; walnuts, 130; brown rice, 120; chard, 65; spinach, 57; barley, 55; coconut, 44; salmon, 40; corn, 38; avocados, 37; bananas, 31: cheeses, 30; tuna, 29; potatoes and cashews, 27 and turkey, 25.

Vitamins Get Into The Act

Aside from vitamin B-6, mentioned earlier, a few other nutrients keep muscles from cramping: vitamin C and vitamin E.

Two groups of soldiers were put through arduous maneuvers, struggling up steep mountain paths carrying heavy packs and equipment. One group took vitamin C until their tissues were saturated. The second group received no vitamins.

The first group suffered no cramps, little fatigue and recovered quickly from the ordeal. The second endured severe cramps and fatigue, feeling exhausted for days.[5]

Best supplement and food sources of vitamin C in milligrams per less than four ounce servings are: rose hips, 3,000; acerola cherries, 1,100; guavas, 240; black currants, 200; parsley, 170; green peppers, 110; watercress, 80; chives, 70; strawberries, 57, persimmons, 52; spinach, 51; oranges, 50; cabbage, 47; grapefruit, 38; papaya, 37; elderberries and kumquats, 36; dandelion greens and lemons, 35; cantaloupe, 33; green onions, 32; limes, 31: mangoes, 27; loganberries, 24; tangerines and tomatoes, 23; squash, 22; raspberries and romaine lettuce, 18 and pineapple, 17.

Convincing Evidence For Vitamin E

Numerous alternative medical doctors I know have had amazing success in using vitamin E against every kind of cramp: night time leg and foot cramps—some of them persisting for years—abdominal, rectal and even menstrual cramps.

Two Los Angeles medical doctors, Samuel Ayres, Jr. and Richard Mihan, tackled some of the most difficult and longest-enduring cases of leg cramps with vitamin E — and, in most instances, won.[6]

Slightly more than half of the patients had suffered from leg cramps for longer than five years — many for twenty to thirty years and more. About one quarter of the patients had severe leg cramps every night or several times nightly.

Three hundred international units of vitamin E daily—sometimes less — relieved 103 of 125 patients completely or almost completely. Four hundred international units eliminated cramps of the remainder.[7]

When the vitamin E was discontinued, the cramps came back, but again ended — usually within a week — when the supplement was resumed. Response was so dramatic that the two researchers went so far as to refer to vitamin E as the cramp medicine.

Without eating giant servings, it is virtually impossible to combat cramps with the amounts of vitamin E in natural foods. However, the following richest food sources of this vitamin — listed according to International Units per less than four ounce portions — serve as an excellent accompaniment to vitamin E supplementation:

Wheat germ, 160; safflower nuts, 35; sunflower seeds, 31; wheat, 30; sesame oil, 26; walnuts, 22, hazelnuts, 21; peanut oil, 16; almonds, 15; olive oil, 14; cabbage, 7.8; brazil nuts and peanuts, 6.5; cod liver oil, 5.4; cashews, 5.1; soy lecithin, 4.8; spinach, 2.9; asparagus, 2.5; broccoli, 2.0; butter 1.9; parsley, 1.8; oats, barley and corn, 1.7; avocados and pecans, 1.5; salmon,, 1.4 bee pollen, 1.3 and rye, 1.2.

Lamb And Beans

1½ c. lima beans, dried	Sea salt to taste or kelp
(washed and drained in water)	Pepper
3 lbs. lamb steaks, cut into pieces	5 cloves of garlic, chopped
¼ c. olive oil	¼ t. season salt
1 onion, sliced	

Cover beans with 4 cups of water. Bring to a boil (for 2 minutes). Cover pan and let stand for 1 hour. Brown lamb in olive oil and put in a 3-quart size casserole dish. Add onion and 1 cup of hot water. Cover and bake in preheated moderate oven at 350 degrees for 1 hour. Pour off fat and liquid. Add beans with bean liquid. Season meat and beans. Cover and bake for 1½ hours longer,adding more water if necessary. Add parsley for garnish. Makes 4 servings.

Maureen's Parsley Sauce

Mince a bunch of parsley and a clove or two of garlic, depending on how you feel about garlic. At my house I use two or three cloves, and mince it very fine. Add a bit of olive oil, sea salt and pepper to taste. Grate a little fresh Romano or fresh Parmesan cheese and mix it all together. I call it Parsley Sauce and it's absolutely fantastic on steak, fish or fowl and its good on salads as a dressing.

CHAPTER 43

Cravings (For Food)

Would you believe it, a huge bowl of thick and steaming lentil soup for breakfast?

Neither did I, but there was portly Joe, the husband of my new friend Donna, putting it away with obvious pleasure. When he came up for air, I asked, "How come lentil soup for breakfast?"

"It keeps me filled up for hours, and I don't crave snacks all morning. This means I lose two pounds a week."

Joe had read a study that lentils are a stick-with-you food that kills cravings, ideal for breakfast.

Why not? Several other friends who encompass too many calories tried it, and were able to resist those wicked, sugar-laden, coffee-break delights. And, sure enough, they, lost weight, too.

Beware Of Skipping Breakfast!

Some individuals think that skipping breakfast is a good way to lose weight. If there's a worse way, I can't remember what it is. Low blood sugar from fasting all night sinks even lower when the person tries to resist eating until noon. In this half-starved, weakened condition, he or she is easily overwhelmed by cravings and subject to binge eating.[1]

A high blood sugar level is an excellent first-line of defense against cravings. However, sometimes a person needs even more: the ability to avoid temptation. Knowing the location of bakeries, cookie shops, and candy stores can help one detour away from appetite-alluring aromas and sights.

Lead Us Not Into Temptation

The same goes for supermarkets and restaurants. We all know where the sugary and chocolaty temptations beckon to us. So it's easy to avoid them — even at the checkout counter. You just look over and beyond them.

A similar technique works in restaurants where a tempting pastry display — plump cream puffs, napoleons, chocolate eclairs — greets you as you enter. Ignore it! Otherwise, a second exposure, when the waitress wheels up the seductive pastries, can beat down your weakening resistance. Better yet, avoid restaurants which display these bad goodies.

It is not always possible to avoid temptation. So then you take a scripture from the Bible and "Flee from temptation." Walk or run to high ground.

One of my well-rounded friends complains about tempting cakes, cookies or candies in the cupboard. It is my unpleasant duty to remind her that they "did not grow there. Someone had to stash them there, and I think I know who it is."

My system for avoiding such tempters is easy. I don't permit them in the house. If I did, it would be inviting in Trojan horses — or chocolate rabbits — that could undo me and add to me.

The Full Feeling Helps

A feeling of fullness helps to control cravings. I use a health food powder mixed with water, nonfat or low-fat milk that offers that full feeling, plus power-packed nutrition: balanced amino acids, fiber, key vitamins and minerals and, best of all, carnitine, the substance shown by many studies to strengthen heart and liver function and to help in burning, rather than storing, body fat.

Besides curbing cravings, this formula tastes great!

There you have it: my system for controlling cravings, instead of letting them control me. To a large extent, this method has kept me in the same size clothing I wore in college. And, to beat temptation, I don't necessarily have to eat lentil soup for breakfast.

However, lentil soup is a tasty filler. Below is my recipe for it. Be my guest!

Maureen's Cravings-Killing Lentil Soup

4 c. stock or water	1 t. nutmeg
1 c. dried lentils	1 t. cayenne pepper (optional)
1 large white onion, diced	1 t. celery seed
2 stalks celery w/tops, chopped	1 t. thyme
½ green bell pepper, diced	1 bay leaf (remove before serving)
2 medium carrots, cut in rounds	3 sprigs parsley
1 t. cumin	1 t. sweet basil

Soak lentils for 2 hrs. (or overnight) to retain maximum vitamins, minerals & enzymes. Cook in soaking water. To avoid gas, drain soaking water & cook in fresh water. Bring liquid to a boil and add lentils. Reduce heat and simmer for 30 minutes, partially covered. Add remaining ingredients and simmer for 20 minutes. Add 1 tablespoon of tamari last to preserve its nutritional content. Remove half of soup from pan to blender and whiz for a few seconds to obtain a thick lentil puree. Mix back into remaining soup in pot. Stir to desired consistency. Top with minced parsley.

CHAPTER 44

Depression

Once the late Dr. Carlton Fredericks gave me his candid opinion on mood-elevating drugs as opposed to vitamins and minerals in coping with emotional disorders such as depression.

"Drugs hide the symptoms, and nutrients usually remove the cause."

Anyone who suffers from depression may, at first, lean on a crutch and fill a doctor's prescription for a mood-elevating drug, but he or she would much rather get down to the basic cause and eliminate it than make drug-taking a way of life.

Fortunately, psychiatrists now realize that all depression is not caused by emotional conflicts and that such over-simplifications are only for the over-simple. In fact, many psychiatrists now add nutrition to their therapy.

And why not? Sigmund Freud, the father of psychoanalysis, predicted that a biologic or physiologic therapy would someday prove to be more effective in coping with emotional illness than psychotherapy. Carl Jung agreed.[1]

Over-Simplifying The Complex

My friend Richard Kunin, M.D. of San Francisco, in Mega-Nutrition (McGraw-Hill), one of the new breed of physicians, says it better than I can:

"Depression is actually one of the early signs of nutritional depletion." Dr. K. cites the classic Kinsman-Hood study, showing that a vitamin C-deprived diet for two to six weeks sent every one of the test subjects into depression.[2]

Studying deficiency disease in depth led Dr. Kunin to a lightning flash of understanding as to why orthodox doctors often miss the diagnosis for depression. Deficiency of calories — starvation or crash diets — and of nutrients brings on depression way before it creates observable symptoms of physical illness.[3] So how can anybody but an alternative doctor who takes a thorough dietary history make a correct diagnosis?

The biochemical bottom line for certain types of depression experienced by women is depletion of nutrients, states Kunin, particularly related to menstrual periods, to the time right after childbirth and to use of the Pill.[4]

A complex depletion in menstruation — loss of blood and cells of the uterus — must be made up with folic acid, vitamins B-12 and B-6, protein and the minerals iron and zinc.[5]

Yet these crying needs go unmet, largely because of the gross over-simplification of the problem, reducing it to the need for iron for "tired blood". Dieting to lose weight aggravates already existing depletions. Depression can't be far behind.[6]

Post-Partum Blues And More

The same sort of thing happens to women who have delivered babies — but with far more serious complications which could even lead to death. Kunin cites the fact that psychiatric wards are filled with young mothers so depressed that many want to commit suicide. Again, nutritional depletion has driven them this far.[7]

Creating a new life — the double nutrient burden — then having to produce a quart of milk daily to nurse the infant, the tremendous stress of feeding the baby around the clock, and the strain of adjusting to a different family relationship and lifestyle are drains on energy, hormones, nutrients. Is it any wonder that depression results? The answer to nutrient depletion is not the psychiatric ward, but super-nutrition, he says.[8]

A third kind of depression exclusive to women — again invited by nutrient depletion — is oral contraceptive-induced depression, particularly before the menstrual period. The Pill steps up the need for the vitamins folic acid and B-6 and for zinc.

Biochemist Dr. Jeffrey Bland suggests a maintenance level of 800 micrograms of folic acid, 25 mg of vitamin B-6 and 20 mg of zinc for takers of oral contraceptives.[9]

Many alternative doctors recommend drinking extra water and taking a tablespoon of a vegetable oil daily, because the latter contains essential fatty acids (EFAs). After all, the brain is made up mainly of water, fat and some cholesterol. (If insufficient cholesterol is derived from food, the liver produces it.)

Natural Causes

Now it would certainly be wrong to say that all depression originates from nutrient depletion. Some comes from emotional conflicts resulting from phases of living and life-shaking daily events.

The person who aimed at becoming chairman of the board and, in his early fifties, finds himself supervisor of the mailroom may have a feeling of futility and depression. The same goes for the local beauty contest winner with Hollywood star aspirations, whose beauty has faded as her mid-section has expanded and she serves as an extra. Depression often dogs the home-oriented woman whose whole reason for being has been her now-departed children, leaving her an empty-nester.

However, even in such instances, the depth of despair probably could be lessened with super-nutrition, because, in these days of depleted soils and depleted and processed foods, few people fill every nutritional need.

Underlying Nutritional Stresses

Earlier we touched on vitamin B-6 deficiency depression created by the oral contraceptive pill. Alternative doctors usually advise 50 mg daily for a month, then 10 to 20 mg a day for maintenence and then back to the higher dosage just prior to the menstrual period to prevent menstrual depression.

A McGill University study found folic acid levels of depressed patients far lower than those of psychiatrically ill and medically ill patients.[10] It is possible to get sufficient folate from foods to exceed the RDA. (See list of folic-acid rich foods below.)

A deficiency of certain amino acids that are precursors to neurotransmitters, chemicals that relay signals from one nerve cell to another, can contribute to depression: L-phenylalinine and tyrosine. These two nutrients at 500 to 1000 mg a day for a two week period have been shown to lift deprssion in many patients.[11] Let me sound a warning. Phenylalinine in large doses can cause blood pressure to rise, sometimes appreciably, and is best used with guidance of an alternative medical doctor.

Large amounts of B vitamins, including choline, and much lecithin, when combined with pantothenic acid, serve as precursors to the neurotransmitter acetylcholine. In high potencies, this, too, is best used with a qualified physician's guidance, because, if taken by a manic-depressive in the depressed state, it could plunge the person into a profound depression.[12]

On the other hand, the amino acid tryptophan, also a neuro-transmitter precursor, has been shown to combat depression with no side effects, as demonstrated when test subjects in a controlled, double-blind study took a large amount daily, six grams—more than can be obtained from a pound of soybeans.[13]

Low Thyroid, Low Mood

Another important cause of depression is low thyroid function. (See section on Thyroid Function, Low.) Mark Gold, M.D. examined depressed individuals—350 inpatients and 44 outpatients—at Fair Oaks Hospital in Summit, New Jersey and discovered a significant amount of low-level hypothyroidism, which made him believe that depression can be the first symptom of early thyroid gland failure, which the usual thyroid function tests are not sensitive enough to pick up.[14]

The conventional thyroid function lab tests among depressed patients detected only 10 percent of hypothyroids. Ninety percent of depressed individuals who proved to be hypothyroid clinically had normal blood tests. Dr. Gold's study convinced him that all psychiatric patients should be checked for hypothyroidism, because if thyroid function is reduced by just 10 percent, brain function is reduced by the same amount, resulting in depression and other negative emotional conditions.[15]

Broda O. Barnes, M.D., Ph.D, a well-known thyroid authority, states that first generation hypothyroids usually can correct their condition by taking a kelp tablet daily. Kelp is rich in iodine, the thyroid's major nutrient. However, hypothyroids of the second generation or beyond can overcome depression and many other symptoms of low thyroid function by taking natural, desiccated thyroid prescribed by a physician.

Allergies And Hypoglycemia: Depressors

Depression, among other negative emotions, has been brought out in test subjects by having them eat foods to which they were allergic or by permitting their blood sugar level to drop low. (See Section on Allergies and Low Blood Sugar.)

Allergies can worsen low blood sugar, and low blood sugar can worsen effects of allergies.

Many simple, folksy ways of reducing depression really work. One of them is regular, vigorous exercise, such as walking in the sunlight. Letting the sunlight into your home does, too. As an Italian proverb puts it, "When the sun does not enter, the doctor does."

Another depression chaser is establishing and keeping a network of close relatives and friends to discuss problems and offer and receive social support. Still another is adopting a pet, a satisfying therapy for many individuals.

Following are lists of foods and supplements which are highest in vitamin B-12, protein, iron and zinc and, then, folic acid, vitamin B-6, and in iodine.

First, let's look at the foods which have the highest content of vitamin B-12 in milligrams per units of less than four ounces: liver, 0.086; sardines, 0.034; mackerel, 0.0100; red snapper, 0.0088; salmon, 0.0047; lamb, 0.0031; swiss cheese, 0.0021; eggs, 0.0020; haddock, 0.0017; muenster cheese, 0.0016; swordfish and beef, 0.0015 and bleu cheese, 0.0014.

So far as protein is concerned, the best sources are meat, poultry and fish, eggs, milk, nuts, beans and peas.

Best sources of iron in supplements and foods in milligrams in units of less than four ounces are: kelp, 370; bone meal, 82; torula yeast, 18; brewer's yeast, 17; kidney, 13; soy lecithin and caviar, 12; pumpkin seeds, 11; sesame seeds, 10; wheat germ, 9.4; blackstrap molasses, 9.1; liver,

8.8; pistachios and egg yolk, 7.2; sunflower seeds, 7.1; chickpeas, 6.9; millet, 6.8; lentils, 6.7, walnuts, 6.0, parsley, 5.0; almonds, 4.7 and oats, 4.5.

These are foods and supplements with the highest ratings in zinc in milligrams per units of less than four ounces: herring, 110; sesame seeds, 10; torula yeast, 9.9; blackstrap molasses, 8.3; maple syrup, 7.5; liver, 7.0; soybeans, 6.7; sunflower seeds, 6.6; egg yolk, 5.5; lamb, 5.4; chicken, 4.8; regular molasses, 4.6; brewer's yeast, 3.9; oats, 3,7; bone meal, 3.6; rye, 3.4; whole wheat, 3.2; corn, 3.1; coconut and beef, 3.0; beets, turkey and walnuts; barley. 2.7 and beans and avocados, 2.4.

Here are supplements and foods richest in folic acid in terms of milligrams per unit of less than four ounces: torula yeast, 3.0; brewer's yeast, 2.0; alfalfa, 0.80; endive, 0,47; chickpeas, 0.41; oats, 0.39; lentils, 0.34; beans and wheat germ 0.31; liver, 0.29; split peas, 0,23; whole wheat, 0.22; barley, 0,21; brown rice, 0.17; asparagus, 0.12; green peas, 0.12; sunflower seeds and collard greens, 0.100, spinach, 0.080; hazelnuts and kale, 0.070; peanuts, soy lecithin and walnuts, 0.060 and corn, 0.059.

These supplements and foods are the best sources of vitamin B-6 in milligrams per units of less than four ounces: brewer's yeast, 4.0; brown rice, 3.6; whole wheat, 2.9; royal jelly, 2.4; soybeans, 2.0; rye, 1.8; lentils, 1.7; sunflower seed and hazelnuts, 1.1; alfalfa, 1.00; salmon, 0.98; wheat germ, 0.92; tuna, 0.90; bran, 0.85; walnuts, 0,73; peas and liver, 0.67; avocados, 0.60; beans, 0.57; cashews, peanuts, turkey, oats, chicken, and beef, 0.40; halibut, 0.34 and lamb and banana.

Foods and supplements richest in iodine in terms of milligrams per less than four ounce units are: kelp, 180, cod liver oil, 0.84; haddock, 0.31; cod, 0.14; chard and beans, 0.10; perch, 0.074; sunflower seeds, 0.070; herring, 0.052; turnip greens, 0.047; halibut, 0.046; peanuts and cantaloupe, 0.020; liver, 0.019 and soybeans, 0.017.

(WARNING. Only very small amounts of iodine are needed: just 35 micrograms for an infant, ranging slightly upward from 45 mcg for the six month to the year old, to 60 mcg for the one to three years old, 80 mcg for the four to six year old; 110 mcg for the seven to ten year old on up from 115 mcg for teen-agers to 150 mcg for lactating women. Three foods on the above list could well supply the daily requirement of most adults.)

Special Cocktail

4 large T. fresh brewers yeast	1 t. honey
1 glass papaya juice	1 t. rose hips powder

Mix all ingredients in papaya juice. This nutritious drink will greatly help digestion. Drink 30 minutes before meal.

Shoulder Lamb Steaks

6 shoulder lamb steaks	¼ c. spring water
3 T. sesame oil	3 T. blackstrap molasses
1 onion, minced	1 T. worchestershire sauce
1½ c. tomato sauce	2 t. kelp
½ c. vinegar	6 fresh peaches, peeled and sliced

In large skillet, brown steaks on both sides in oil. Remove. Add onion and cook until soft. Add tomato sauce, vinegar, water, molasses, worchestershire and kelp. Stir to blend. Return steaks to skillet; spoon some sauce over top. Cover pan and simmer over low heat, turning occasionally (about 1 hour, or until steaks are tender). Add peaches and simmer covered for 5 minutes longer. Serve at once with cooked rice. Makes 6 servings.

CHAPTER 45

Diabetes

Elevated blood sugar in diabetes is due to a breakdown of the body's energy-use system. Glucose, a simple sugar taken from foods, serves as our fuel to produce heat and energy.

Glucose circulates in the blood to body cells but cannot penetrate the cell wall receptors unless attached to molecules of insulin, a hormone produced by the pancreas. When there's not enough insulin, sugar accumulates in the blood and circulates helplessly, eventually entering the kidneys and then the bladder for excretion in the urine.

How does diabetes develop? In several ways. Alpha and beta cells in an area of the pancreas called the Islets of Langerhans are out of balance.

Checks And Balances Are Imbalanced

Beta cells secrete insulin, which by escorting glucose into cells, lowers blood sugar levels. Alpha cells secrete a hormone called glucagon, which, when blood sugar becomes too low, triggers the turning of glycogen, sugar stored in the liver, into glucose for release into the bloodstream.

Hormones of the beta and alpha cells are supposed to check and balance one another. However, in the diabetic, blood sugar manages to rise too high for several reasons.

Repeated assaults on the pancreas with large amounts of refined and quickly absorbed sugar force this gland to work overtime in producing insulin. Eventually, it becomes exhausted and produces too little insulin.

A Chromium Crisis

A shortage of insulin is not always the problem. Sometimes it's a shortage of the trace mineral chromium. Insulin needs tiny amounts of chromium to be able to escort glucose through cell walls. Studies by Dr. Walter Merz, chief of the U.S. Department of Agriculture's Vitamin and Mineral Research Division, show that a deficiency of chromium can bring on diabetes.[1]

Most diabetes which comes on in the middle or later years (maturity onset diabetes), results from a diet of highly processed, chromium-impoverished foods. A list of chromium-rich foods will be offered later.

Some authorities feel that a little-appreciated cause of diabetes is the fact that the beta cells—for whatever reasons—produce a fore-runner of insulin that really doesn't do the full job, instead of a biologically active form.[2]

Many Theories

Still other experts suggest that diabetes is a two-hormone disorder triggered by a shortage of insulin production and a surplus of blood sugar-raising glucagon, as indicated by experiments conducted at the University of Texas Southwestern Medical School.[3]

All of these theories and still more indicate that there can be many reasons why diabetes develops. Heredity makes us more likely to be diabetic. Several studies show that children born of at least one diabetic parent are more prone to be diabetic than those from non-diabetic parents. Children of at least one diabetic parent tend to develop diabetes because they have inherited a pancreas that operates poorly or cell receptors which fail to take in glucose efficiently.[4]

Negative environmental factors, too, have been blamed: poor food selection, preparation, use and repetition from one generation to another.

The Stresses Of Life

Stress also must be counted in. One of the adrenal gland hormones, epinephrine, spurted into the bloodstream when we are threatened in a fight-or-flight situation increases free fatty acids in the bloodstream and shuts off the release of insulin. Continued and intense stress could upset the checks and balance system of the pancreas hormones and invite diabetes.[5]

Another form of stress, gross overweight (obesity) can cause diabetes, says Dr. W. John Butterfield, Professor of Medicine at Guys Hospital in London. An amazing similarity exists in how the body handles sugars and starches in diabetes and in obesity.[6]

Dr. Butterfield reveals results of his testing, comparing how well three groups were able to take glucose into their cells. Juvenile diabetics could absorb no sugar into their cells, indicating that they lacked ability to produce insulin. Older diabetics and obese normal subjects took up glucose in about the same manner. Lean control subjects took up more sugar than did the heavyweights.[7]

Obesity Encourages Diabetes

Here's how Dr. Butterfield explains the way in which progressive weight gain encourages diabetes. With the continuation of obesity, less and less insulin is able to reach insulin-responsive muscles. So less and less glucose uptake occurs there, making it necessary for an increasing amount of insulin to be formed.[8]

When obesity reaches vast proportions, there is too much tissue area for the pancreas to service. Frequently, not enough supply of insulin can be made to meet demand.

Dr. Butterfield offers another significant observation about why obese people are prone to diabetes. When body fat competes with muscle for insulin, the fat wins. This means that then carbohydrates are changed into still more fat.[9]

First-Aid From High Fiber

A high-fiber diet helps both obese and lean diabetics, says James Anderson, M.D., noted biochemist at the University of Kentucky, who has researched high-fiber diets for many years. Both groups reduced blood fats and the need for insulin.[10]

Many obese patients lost weight on the Anderson diet of raw foods: fruits, vegetables, bran, nuts, seeds and whole grains. Patients who showed the most improvement in their diabetes were those who lost the most weight.

Outstanding fiber foods are almonds, apples, blackberries, broccoli, corn, fresh peas, kidney beans, plums, potatoes, prunes, raisins, spinach, sweet potatoes, wholewheat bread and zucchini.

Advice From An Ex-Diabetic

By avoiding the typical high fat, high sugar and low fiber diet, it is possible to prevent and manage diabetes, writes Associate Professor Somasundaram Addanki, a biochemist and nutritionist at Ohio State University College of Medicine.[11]

A diabetic who married a diabetic, Professor Addanki says that he and his wife did not develop diabetes until they had left their native India and had begun eating the typical western diet.[12]

In a *United Press International* news story, Professor Addanki admitted to six years of diabetes and diabetic impotency before he stopped eating sugar, white flour products and fatty foods and got rid of this ailment.[13]

By Its Symptoms Shall Ye Know It

One medical disorder whose symptoms reveal it clearly is diabetes: excessive thirst, frequent urinating of large amounts of fluid, constant hunger, systemic hyperacidity, high sugar level in both blood and urine; rapid weight loss, severe itching, fatigue and marked weakness.[14]

How can diabetes best be prevented and managed?

1. By junking junk foods — sugar, white flour and fatty foods, a la Professor Addanki.

2. By adding fresh fruits, vegetables and whole grains to the diet for live enzymes and fiber.

3. By making certain our intake of chromium is adequate.

Junk foods are processed foods—canned, boxed, packaged—rather than live, uncooked and enzyme-rich foods. Excellent fiber foods were listed earlier in this section.

Best Food Bets For Chromium

Foods which contain chromium have only tiny amounts of this trace mineral. However, that's all right, because we need only very small quantities. We can be assured of getting enough chromium by selecting and eating the right foods. Here they are in milligrams per less than four ounce portions:

Thyme, 1.00; black pepper, 0.37; whole wheat, 0.18; cloves, 0.15; seaweeds, 0.130; brewer's yeast, 0.063; corn oil, 0.047; vegetables, 0.040; fruits, 0.030; honey, 0.029; chicken, 0.026; blackstrap molasses. 0.022; parsley, 0.021; butter, 0.021; nuts and grains, 0.020; maple syrup, 0.018; eggs, 0.017, and brown rice, 0.016.

When I have told my TV program listeners about the foods which contain the most chromium, they seem to prefer taking a chromium food supplement based in yeast. This has a potency of 200 micrograms per tablet. One tablet per day has proved effective for many diabetics, my alternative doctor friends tell me.

Dr. Jonathan Wright says that diabetes can often be controlled by what you don't eat as much as by what you do eat. "Eliminate refined sugar. Sugared fare—so-called civilized foods—brought a marked rise in diabetes among diverse people throughout the world: New Zealand Maori, North Canadian Eskinmos, South African blacks and Yemenite Jews."

Folk Remedies Sometimes Help

All sorts of foods and plants have a reputation for helping to prevent or control diabetes.

Broiled stems of a Mexican variety of cactus, Opuntia streptacantha Lemaire, help to control non-insulin dependent diabetes by lowering blood glucose and insulin levels, say Mexican scientists.[15]

Researcher Alberto C. Frati-Munari and associates at the Hospital de Especialidades in Colonia La Raza, compared two groups after a 12 hour fast—one fed broiled stems of the cactus and the other given only water. Blood glucose levels and insulin decreased in the cactus-fed group, but not in the group given water.

Although they have no conclusive answer, the researchers feel that the cactus improves the effectiveness of available insulin.

This cactus, whose broiled stems serve as a common food in various arid parts of Mexico, can also be found in the deserts of the southwestern United States.

Legumes To Stand On

Through the years in folk medicine, legumes—beans, peas and lentils—have had a reputation for controlling diabetes. Research by Dr. James Anderson shows why.[16]

A cup of cooked navy or pinto beans daily slashed the need for insulin injections by some thirty-eight percent in one group of test patients. Individuals with adult onset diabetes — those whose ability to secrete insulin has slowed down — have eliminated the need for insulin shots through the Anderson bean diet.

Dr. Anderson theorizes that this fare works because beans make for such a slow rise in blood sugar that less insulin is needed and, further, contributes to the production of more insulin-receptors on cells. This gives insulin more escape hatches and. therefore, the means of ushering additional sugar out of the blood.

In a study to determine soybeans' influence on lowering cholesterol — they worked well — biochemist Andrew P. Goldberg, of Washington University, found that soybeans also kept insulin levels under control, a strong recommendation for diabetics to eat them.[17]

A Bonus For Diabetics: Physical Exercise

So much is said about diet for prevention and control of diabetes, but so little is said about one of the best non-food methods of accomplishing this: regular physical exercise.

Lionel H. Opie, M.D., of the Ischemic Heart Disease Laboratory of the University of Capetown, South Africa, writes in the "American Heart Journal" that regular exercise may prevent diabetes.[18]

Opie has found that cycling, running or vigorous walking help in prevention and control of diabetes by:[19]

1. improving the ability to use blood sugar properly and lessening the amount of insulin secreted.

2. helping body cells to get the most out of available glucose.

3. decreasing the negative influence of an occasional heavy intake of carbohydrates.

Something that Dr. Opie didn't say that should be said is that daily, vigorous exercise often contributes to loss of weight and, consequently, a better chance to prevent diabetes and control it.

Not long ago a study showed that persons with a pot belly were more prone to develop diabetes, as well as heart disease—something which should be seriously considered.[20]

Zucchini Cake

2½ c. whole wheat flour	1 c. honey
2 c. zucchini squash, grated	½ c. black strap molasses
1 c. slivered almonds	2 eggs
1 c. apricots, chopped	2 t. baking powder
1 lime or lemon	1 c. spring water
1 c. safflower oil (cold press)	

Beat eggs. Add honey and molasses while beating. Grate rind of lime and add with lime juice. Mix flour and baking powder. Add water and oil alternately. Add zucchini and apricots. Place in 9 x 13 baking dish. Sprinkle top with slivered almonds. Bake in 350 degree oven for 40 to 45 minutes.

Happy Cat's Liver And Onions

2 Large Yellow Onions, Diced	½ lb. Beef Liver
4 Cloves of Garlic, Minced	1 t. Basil
¼ t. Thyme	½ t. Marjoram

The secret is in the herbs and not cooking the liver to the point where it is brown in the middle. Combine onions with garlic and Thyme in a skillet. Steam-stir in a small amount of spring water until tender and browned slightly (approximately 20 minutes) over medium heat. Add liver and herbs to onion mixture and cook covered until liver is pink inside and has clear juices. Serve hot with lightly steamed carrots and broccoli seasoned to taste with season salt. Makes two servings.

CHAPTER 46

Diarrhea

Webster's New World Dictionary has a few choice words to describe diarrhea: "Excessive frequency and looseness of bowel movements."

This doesn't begin to describe the discomfiture—often, the pain—and inconvenience of diarrhea, which exists as a disease entity and also as the symptom of some other ailments. (The danger of diarrhea is that, along with waste matter, nutrients hurry through too fast to be absorbed. Death can result from excessive diarrhea in infants who become dehydrated.)

A list of causes for diarrhea could stretch from horizon to horizon. So we'll deal only with the majors:

1. Antibiotics intended to kill off harmful bacteria to clear up an infection also kill off friendly bacteria, causing too rapid transit of wastes.

2. Food poisoning. The body throws off toxic bacteria as fast as it can.

3. Stress and anxiety. The mind can't rid itself of concerns and worries, so the bowel acts sympathetically.

4. Food allergy. The bowel discharges what it can't tolerate.

5. Difficulty in digesting gluten, a protein substance found in wheat, barley, oats and rye. Again, the body hurries to get rid of something it cannot tolerate. Patients with celiac disease — a disorder rising from difficulty in digesting gluten — often are deficient in vitamin B-6 and magnesium. The latter is necessary to utilize vitamin B-6.

6. Pellagra, caused by lack of niacin, invites the three "D"s: Diarrhea, Dermatitis and Dementia. Although pellagra is no longer a widely prevalent cause of diarrhea, lack of sufficient niacin still is.

7. Sorbitol, an artificial sweetener in many food products and beverages: processed foods, baked foods, ice cream, gum, jelly and carbonated drinks. Natural sorbitol is found in certain fruits, mainly prunes, noted

for their laxative effect.

8. Super high intakes of vitamin C. All of us have different levels of bowel tolerance for vitamin C.

9. Colitis (inflammation of intestinal walls) and other major diseases of the colon, including cancer.

10. Eating and drinking food in underdeveloped countries with poor sanitation: fresh fruits, vegetables and salads, foods bought from street vendors, drinking of water from local sources. This form of diarrhea from bacteria known as Escheria coli was labeled "Montezuma's Revenge" by Americans who picked it up in Mexico. The term is now used worldwide in undeveloped countries where Americans travel.

Coping With Diarrhea Naturally

1. A regime to re-colonize depleted friendly bacteria is liberal daily amounts of a high quality yogurt with lactobacillus acidophilus, six to 12 tablets of lactobacillus acidophilus, and a diet high in fiber and unrefined carbohydrates. (This regimen won't work if the patient is still being given antibiotics.)

2. Bananas may be a golden solution to diarrhea, because they contain pectin, which can tighten up loose bowels. On top of this, they provide key minerals often lost in diarrhea: magnesium and potassium.

3. Carob, also rich in pectin, normalizes bowel movements, as demonstrated in numerous well-structured experiments.

4. Managing stress properly helps to cope with diarrhea: seeking and finding solutions to what makes us anxious; exercising vigorously and regularly to release tensions and developing faith in being able to handle crises.

5. Finding and eliminating food allergens. (This process is elaborated under the section on Allergies.)

6. Eliminating gluten-containing grains, if a medical doctor's diagnosis reveals a gluten-intolerance.

7. Adding niacin to the daily vitamin supplement regime.

8. Being alert to note and eliminate sorbitol-containing foods.

9. Learning the bowel tolerance for vitamin C.

10. Providing sufficient fiber-rich foods to cope with colitis and other

intestinal disorders.

11. Taking proper precautions while traveling in underdeveloped countries: boiling local water before drinking it or acquiring pure bottled spring water. At this writing, Dr. Carol Tacket, of the University of Maryland School of Medicine, has developed a powdered cow's milk which stops traveler's diarrhea. Cows are exposed to the Escheria coli bacteria, causing them to make antibodies in blood and milk to kill the bacteria. The milk is dehydrated in easy-to-carry form.[1]

Tacket and associates gave one group of ten healthy men and women the special antibody-containing powdered milk and another group of ten a look-alike placebo, then exposed all twenty to the bacteria. Not one of the ten on the antibody-rich powdered milk developed diarrhea. Nine out of ten of the others came down with it.[2]

The Stopper

1 pint plain yogurt	1 T. fiber
3 bananas	

Chop bananas and mix with yogurt and fiber.

CHAPTER 47

Ears, Ringing (Tinnitus)

Ringing in the ears doesn't begin to describe the variety of noises that bedevils victims of tinnitus: the buzz of a horsefly; the hiss of steam, the throb of a car engine, the rasp of a handsaw, or the roar of a waterfall.

The satanic sounds persist loud and clear, so that the victim can't ignore them.

One tinnitus patient confided to me: "Sleep? What's that? All I hear day and night is that infernal, torturing noise. It never lets up. It annoys me if I try to sleep, talk, read, work, watch TV or listen to musical tapes."

Some sufferers get relief by turning up the sound of a radio, tape player or TV a notch above the tinnitus noise.

Major Causes

Authorities on tinnitus generally agree that victims are tuned into various noises of their body at work. The most common is the rush of blood through arteries or capillaries, particularly those in a snailshell-shaped organ (the cochlea) which is a crucial part of the inner ear for hearing.[1]

Others are static caused by the unceasing minute movement of body cells, the constant contraction of ear muscles, alternating action of the tongue's soft palate; continual hollow sounds from inflammation of the mucous membrane; a clicking noise from jawbone movement; a throbbing sound from impaired blood circulation in the carotid artery or capillaries near the ear and last, but no less irritating, a whirring racket from the jugular vein of individuals suffering from pernicious anemia or iron deficiency anemia. (See Section on Anemia).[2]

Various medicines and drugs bring toxins which can contribute to tinnitus: quinine and salicylates in many aspirins, antibiotics such as aureomycin and streptomycin; relaxants or sleeping pills (barbiturates), cocaine, heroin, opium and marijuana and opium. If these drugs are stopped in time, the tinnitus often stops, too.

Exposure to chemicals and gasses used in industry and business can sometimes invite tinnitus: poisonous fluids (anilines) used for making dyes, resins, varnishes and, among others, rocket fuel; arsenic, benzene, lead, mercury, phosphorus and carbon monoxide, fumes from cleaning solvents, and illuminating gas.

If a job exposes you to these toxins, the obvious course is to request a departmental transfer, or to find a job in another industry or business. A new, clean environment often helps to correct tinnitus.

Corrective Action

Orthodox doctors usually advise tinnitus patients "to learn to live with it."

Of course, it is far better to learn to live without it — to take some positive action. Stopping drinking and smoking sometimes reverses the condition, doctors tell me.

A deficiency of the trace mineral manganese and the B vitamin choline can cause tinnitus, say some research reports. Choline is a biochemical forerunner of the nerve messenger acetylcholine.

Best food sources of manganese by milligram in less than four ounce units are: cloves, 26; ginger, 8.7; buckwheat, 5.1; oats, 4.9; hazelnuts, 4.2; chestnuts, 3.7; wheat, 3.6; pecans, 3.5; barley, 3.2; brazil nuts, 2.8; sunflower seeds, 2.5; ginseng, watercress, peas and beans, 2.0; almonds, 1.9; turnip greens and walnuts, 1.8; brown rice, 1.7; peanuts, 1.5; honey, 1.4; coconut, 1.3 and pineapple, 1.1.

Best food sources of choline by milligrams in less than four ounces are: soy lecithin, 2,900; egg yolk, 1,700; chickpeas, 780; lentils, 710; split peas, 700; brown rice, 650; liver, 550; caviar, 540; eggs, 500; wheat germ, 400; soybeans and green beans, 340; green peas, 270; cabbage and torula yeast, 250; spinach, peanuts and brewer's yeast, 240; sunflower seeds, 220; sprouts, 210; blackstrap molasses, 150; alfalfa, bran and barley, 140;

asparagus, 130; lamb, flax seed and potatoes, 110 and veal.

Pernicious anemia, caused by an acute deficiency of vitamin B-12, and iron deficiency anemia, have been found to bring on tinnitus. If deterioration has not gone too far, then correction of these disorders should remove the basic problems and tinnitus.

My friend Jonathan Wright, M.D., in fact, has reversed tinnitus caused by these two anemias, simply by bolstering patients' diets with vitamin B-12 and iron.

Best food sources of vitamin B-12 in milligrams in units of less than four ounces are: liver, 0.086; sardines, 0.034; mackerel and herring, 0.0100; snapper, 0.0088; flounder, 0.0064; salmon, 0.0047; lamb, 0.0031; Swiss cheese, 0.0021; eggs, 0.0020; haddock, 0.0017; muenster cheese, 0.0016; swordfish and beef, 0.0015, and halibut and bass, 0.0013.

Richest food sources of iron in milligrams per less than four ounces are: kelp, 370; bone meal, 82; torula yeast, 18; brewer's yeast, 17; kidney, 13; soy lecithin and caviar, 12; pumpkin seeds, 11; sesame seeds, 10; wheat germ, 9.4; blackstrap molasses, 9.1; liver, 8.8; pistachios and egg yolk, 7.2; sunflower seeds, 7.1; chickpeas, 6.9; millet, 6.8; lentils, 6.7; molasses and walnuts, 6; parsley, 5; almonds, 4.7; oats, 4.5; cashews, 3.8; rye, 3.7 and wheat, 3.5.

Cornish Game Hens

2 cornish game hens	1 T. apple juice concentrate
2 garlic cloves	1 egg white (yolk discarded)
1 t. chives	¼ t. ginger powder
½ c. dates, pitted and chopped	Pinch of ground cloves

Wash hens thoroughly and dry. Stuff with wild rice to simmer in cavity of hens. Mix all other ingredients, with the exception of honey, and boil 5 minutes. Fill cavities with hot liquid, tying hen at neck. Secure opening so liquid will remain within cavity. Blend honey with ginger and rub over skin of hen to glaze. Roast in covered baking pan in hot oven until tender, basting frequently with liquid from bottom of pan. Serves 4.

Shirley Foreman Fruit Salad

1 fresh pineapple
1 c. fresh raspberries or
strawberries

1 c. blueberries
1 c. melon balls
Ginger lime dressing

Cut pineapple in half through crown. Remove core and chunk fruit. Toss lightly with raspberries, blueberries and melon balls. Spoon into pineapple shells. Drizzle with Ginger Lime Dressing (below). Makes 4 to 6 servings.

Ginger Lime Dressing

¼ c. honey
¼ c. orange juice
2 T. lime juice

1 T. crystallized ginger, chopped
1 t. lime peel, grated

Combine all ingredients well.

CHAPTER 48

Eczema

Some individuals pronounce eczema "EK-z-ma" (correct). Others pronounce it ek-ZEE-ma (wrong). However you pronounce it, eczema is a real trial, a stubborn disorder characterized by a permanent inflammation, a rash that itches and burns, crusted and scaly skin which often has cracks and breaks and weeps.

Eczema appears to be a hereditary allergic reaction to some outside irritant which manifests itself in the upper layer of the skin. Many of its victims have previously experienced asthma or hay fever.

What To Do About It?

Several nutritional approaches mentioned in medical literature have brought relief to eczema sufferers. A Yale University researcher injected 24 to 50 mg of vitamin B-6 into the vein or under the skin of eczema patients and reported improvement of the condition.[1] (No mention was made as to whether this vitamin, taken by mouth, would bring about similar results.)

Essential Fatty Acids To The Rescue

Without sufficient essential fatty acids (EFA), it is impossible to have healthy and beautiful skin, hair and nails. An essential fatty acid is a substance such as linoleic acid that the body can't synthesize. Therefore, it has to be a regular part of the daily diet.

In a deficiency of EFAs, or if EFAs can't be translated into gamma-linoleic acid (GLA) — and this is a difficult biochemical hurdle — skin lesions like those in eczema and fish skin (ichthyosis) occur, along with hair loss and brittle, cracking nails.[2]

Zinc deficiency blocks this translation. Various experiments have shown that children with eczema present low levels of EFA. Other experiments reveal that depriving children of EFAs invites eczema.

The Promise Of Evening Primrose Oil

Infants fed mother's milk derive preformed GLA, eliminating the need for forming this compound from linoleic acid.[3] Very few food supplements offer preformed GLA—among them evening primrose oil, black currant seed oil, and borage seed oil. Evening primrose oil has been the most thoroughly researched.

Just three capsules of evening primrose oil offer the amount of GLA in a day's supply of mother's milk.[4] Although EFAs have been of some help for eczema, their benefits seem to be limited by their content of linoleic acid convertible to GLA.

And, speaking of GLA, a double-blind, placebo-controlled experiment at the University of Bristol (England) demonstrated a modest yet significant improvement in eczema of adults as well as children.[5]

One of the most severe forms of eczema, atopic eczema, was significantly improved on high dosages of evening primrose oil, as exhibited by a double-blind, controlled, cross-over study of varying doses of evening primrose oil on ninety-nine patients.[6] There were no side effects.

Atopic eczema, endured by multi-millions of individuals, is only one of many dissimilar diseases which are biochemical relatives—allergies, asthma and hay fever, to name several.

Here's what atopic ailments have in common: they run in families; they are based on deficiencies of certain essential blood ingredients—including elements for making prostaglandins, controllers of numerous body processes; they are also founded on immune system deficiencies, which reduce a defense system's effectiveness in coping with threatening invaders.[7]

An Unusual Approach

A foreign medical journal mentions experiments with eczema patients done in the Soviet Union.[8] Researchers extracted carotene—a vitamin A precursor—from pumpkins and treated eczema patients with it in two ways: orally, 20 to 40 drops twice daily as a food supplement and as an ointment rubbed on eczematic areas.

Sixteen of nineteen patients — including some infants — were considerably improved or apparently cured. Twenty-four of 33 patients with microbial eczema and six of seven individuals with hyperkeratosis (skin scaliness) were markedly improved or cured.[9]

These research projects give new hope to individuals tormented by the trying manifestations of eczema.

CHAPTER 49

Epstein-Barr Syndrome (Viral Exhaustion Syndrome)

Another one of those diseases that orthodox medicine feels is "all in the mind," but is all too evident in the body, is Epstein-Barr syndrome, whose worst symptom is devastating exhaustion.

The first major outbreak in recent history of what alternative doctors call "the chronic viral fatigue syndrome," occurred in the tiny mountain community of Incline Village, Nevada.

A guest on my television interview program, Robert Cathcart, M.D., who was practicing in Incline Village during the initial outbreak, observed:

"Many people go to their doctors with this profound fatigue. Exhausted women are especially moody before their periods and experience many menstrual problems.

"One day they are feeling fine. Then they catch something like the flu or, maybe, mononucleosis and never seem to recover from it. (See the section on Mononucleosis.) Some are so fatigued they feel they will never be normal again. They develop food sensitivities, or, maybe, even arthritis.

"All the doctor's lab tests turn out normal. The patient is told, 'You're okay. Perhaps you should see a psychiatrist,' " says Dr. Cathcart.

Better advice is to see a doctor who realizes that the patient and symptoms are sometimes more important than laboratory tests, that physical ailments exist which are sometimes beyond detection by present tests.

Getting The Upper Hand

I remember reading newspaper accounts of the Epstein-Barr epidemic at Incline Village. People were so exhausted they had to quit school or work. One man closed his barbershop, because he was too overwhelmed with fatigue to function.

"When conventional medical doctors recognize this condition, they generally use a drug called acyclovir given intravenously." says Dr. Cathcart. "My experience is that this doesn't work very well."

Dr. Cathcart, a pioneer in using massive doses of vitamin C (which he calls ascorbate) to combat difficult-to-manage diseases, has his patients take 30 to 100 grams of vitamin C daily. This adds up to 30,000 to 100,000 milligrams. Inasmuch as it is impractical to swallow 60 to 200 500 mg tablets of vitamin C each day, Dr. Cathcart recommends that his patients use ascorbate in powder or granulated form. One level teaspoonful contains four grams (4,000 mg). The freshest supply of this form of vitamin C can be obtained at health food stores.

Some patients are intimidated by such high dosages. but Dr. Cathcart explains that they are necessary to reinforce the white blood cells which "eat up bad viruses and bad bacteria." He adds that, "When patients are deeply ill with Epstein-Barr virus, they feel so bad, because they have toxins throughout their body. These toxins are technically called 'free radicals'."

Neutralizing Free Radicals

What's a free radical? An oddball molecule with one electron missing. It is out of harmony with nature, and figuratively runs amuck, trying to pick up another electron, damaging or destroying healthy body cells. Free radicals form from oxidation that goes on continuously in our trillions of cells, from radiation, from chemicals in air, food and water, and even from exercise.

"Let me explain this," says Dr. Cathcart. "When we exercise, we generate free radicals—particularly the sick person. However, exercise in the healthy person generates more free radical scavengers."

Diseases such as Epstein-Barr and mononucleosis bring on free radicals in hordes.

Free radicals almost overwhelm the tissues, so super-high doses of vitamin C, supplied on a regular basis, act as free radical scavengers, and neutralize and mop them up. Gigantic doses of ascorbates can cause diarrhea, but the sicker a person is, the more counteracting vitamin C is necessary and the less chance there is of diarrhea, because the body needs this ascorbate ammunition to combat the virus, states Dr. Cathcart.

Of All Things, Exercise?

Now the last thing in the world that the exhausted victim of Epstein-Barr syndrome would appear to need is exercise. Yet that is exactly what Dr. Cathcart says is a necessity, but only after the patient's tissues have been well saturated with ascorbate.

"Normally, exercise would cause remission for Epstein-Barr sufferers. However, if we first absolutely saturate them with vitamin C and then, exercise them, they tend to get relief from their symptoms," he informs.

"Exercise steps up blood circulation and drives ascorbates into the deepest tissues of the body," states Dr. Cathcart. "By taking large doses of vitamin C by mouth and intravenously and then, after a few days, exercising, you drive it into the tissues."

You don't cure persistent viruses such as chronic hepatitis, herpes, or Epstein-Barr, informs Dr. C, but saturating people with ascorbates reactivates them and puts them back to school or work.

More Nutrients Needed

In addition to enormous amounts of acorbates, Dr. Cathcart advises his patients to take other nutrients to strengthen the immune system to fight the good fight: vitamin A, chromium, manganese, selenium and zinc.

Supplements and foods richest in vitamin A in International Units per less than four-ounce units are: cod liver oil, 200,000; sheep liver, 45,000; beef liver, 44,000; calf's liver, 22,000; dandelion greens, 14,000; carrots, 11,000; yams, 9,000; kale, 8,900; parsley and turnip greens, 8,500; spinach, 8,100; collard greens and chard, 6,550; watercress, 5,000; red peppers, 4,400; squash, 4,000; egg yolk and cantaloupe, 3,400; endive, 3,330; persimmons, and apricots, 2,700; broccoli, 2,500; pimentos, 2,300; swordfish, 2,100; whitefish, 2,000; romaine lettuce, 1,900; mangoes, 1,800; papayas, 1,700; nectarines and pumpkin 1,600; peaches and cheeses, 1,300; eggs, 1,200 and cherries, lettuce and cream, 1,000.

Best food and supplement sources of chromium in milligrams per less than four ounce units are: thyme, 1.00; black pepper, 0.37; whole wheat, 0.18; cloves, 0.15; brewer's yeast, 0.063; corn oil, 0.047; vegetables, 0.040; fruits, 0.030; honey, 0.029; chicken, 0.026; blackstrap molasses, 0.022; parsley and butter, 0.021; nuts and whole grains, 0.020; maple syrup, 0.018; eggs, 0.017; brown rice, 0.016; corn syrup, 0.015 and meats and tomatoes, 0.014.

Foods and supplements with the highest values of manganese in terms of milligrams per less than four ounce units are: tea leaves, 28; cloves, 26; ginger, 8.7; buckwheat, 5.1; oats, 4.9; hazelnuts, 4.2; chestnuts, 3.7; whole wheat, 3.6; pecans, 3.5; barley, 3.2; brazil nuts, 2.8; sunflower seeds, 2.5; ginseng, watercress, peas and beans, 2.0; almonds, 1.9; turnip greens and walnuts, 1.8; brown rice, 1.7; peanuts, 1.5; honey, 1.4; coconut, 1.3; pineapple, 1.1; parsley, 0.94; spinach, 0.82; grapefruit and lettuce, 0.80; tea, 0.69, bananas, 0.64; carrots, 0.60; berries, 0.55, brewer's yeast, 0.53 and yams, 0.52.

Richest food and supplement sources of selenium in milligrams per less than four ounce units are: corn, 0.40; cabbage, 0.25; whole wheat, 0.13; beans, 0.12; vegetable oils, 0.100; onions, 0.080; chicken, 0.070; beets, 0.065; barley, 0.062; tomatoes, 0.060; soybeans, 0.054; saltwater fish, 0.053; liver, 0.050; brown rice, 0.039; alfalfa and peanuts, 0.038 and meat, 0.022.

Best food and supplement sources of zinc in milligrams per less than four ounce units are: herring, 110; wheat germ, 14; sesame seeds, 10; torula yeast, 9.9; blackstrap molasses, 8.3; maple syrup, 7.5; liver, 7.0; soybeans, 6.7; sunflower seeds, 6.6; egg yolk, 5.5; lamb, 5.4; chicken, 4.8; brewer's yeast, 3.9; oats, 3.7; bone meal, 3.6; rye and whole wheat, 3.4; corn, 3.1; coconut and beef, 3.0; beets, turkey and walnuts, 2.8; barley, 2.7; beans and avocados, 2.4; peas, 2.3; bleu cheese, 2.2; eggs, 2.1 and buckwheat, 2.0.

Salaman Salmon
(Stuffed Peppers)

4 green peppers, split and seeded	Sea salt and pepper to taste
1 t. minced onion	1 t. fresh lemon juice
1 c. whole wheat bread crumbs	1 can salmon, flaked
1 egg	2 T. butter
½ c. whole milk	⅛ T. thyme

Boil peppers in salted water for 5 minutes and drain. Mix remaining ingredients, except butter. Fill peppers with mixture. Melt butter and mix with remaining crumbs. Sprinkle on top of peppers. Bake in preheated oven at 300 degrees for approximately 30 minutes. Makes 4 servings.

Connie Haus's Lentil Recipe

½ onion, quartered	¼ t. oregano
1 garlic clove, minced	¼ t. nutmeg
1 t. olive oil	⅓ t. basil
1 15 ounce can tomato sauce	¼ t. sea salt
½ c. spring water	¼ t. thyme
¼ c. lentils, washed	Dash tabasco sauce

Saute onion and garlic in oil. When tender, add other ingredients. Simmer 45 minutes over low heat. Serve over hot cooked vegetable pasta. Serves 4.

Peggy's Super C-Caeser Salad

½ c. parsley, chopped	1 garlic clove, finely chopped
¼ c. lemon juice	1 T. anchovy paste
¼ c. spring water	1 T. honey
¼ c. cider vinegar	2 T. Romano Cheese, grated
¼ to ½ t. vegetable salt	¾ c. olive oil
¼ t. fresh cayenne pepper	

Put all ingredients, except oil, in blender. Blend until smooth. While blending, add oil gradually in medium speed until mixture thickens. Chill well. Serve on romaine lettuce.

CHAPTER 50

Eye
(Macular
Degeneration)

Many individuals handicapped with the serious eye condition called macular degeneration don't seem to understand the nature of their problem.

This is probably because little has been written on the subject in the popular press. There's no better time than now or place than here to talk about it.

First, the macula is a part of the retina, the light-sensitive membrane at the back of the eye that registers images. The retina is like the film in a motion picture camera. As individuals age, some of them experience the narrowing or hardening of the tiny arteries in the macula, as well as in other parts of the head and body.

Then the macula does not get enough blood and, with it, nutrients and oxygen, and slowly begins to starve. As the macula deteriorates, central vision gradually becomes blurred. This often leads to blindness. High blood pressure sometimes ruptures the small arteries in the macula, causing leakage and eventual blindness.

Positive Action May Help

Orthodox medicine offers little to a patient with macular degeneration. Alternative medicine holds out more than a degree of hope, however. Sometimes, chelation treatment is used to remove cholesterol, calcium and other debris that clogs arteries. A leading alternative physician, James Julian, M.D., of Hollywood, California, refers to chelation and use of the chemical EDTA as a "Roto-rooter for the arteries."

With circulation restored in the macula, deterioration can be halted.

In rare instances, the deterioration has even been reversed and central vision improved. The proper nutritional approach often puts the brakes on macular degeneration in time to preserve sight.

Several studies indicate that macular degeneration may be prevented by taking a zinc supplement.

Minerals That Guard The Macula

Zinc is a vital part of eye tissues, especially those in the macula, which have a high degree of protein turnover. Zinc deficiencies often mimic those of vitamin A, as in night blindness.

Dr. Jeffrey Bland, in his monthly audio tape series, Preventive Medicine Update (HealthComm, Inc. of Gig Harbor, Washington), finds that abnormal zinc and copper metabolism is responsible for many disorders of the retina.[1]

Another mineral which has proved helpful in preventing macular degeneration is the trace element selenium. Selenium promotes a certain enzyme (glutathione peroxidase), which protects eye tissues from damage from oxidation and free radical attack.[2]

(Oxidation continues on a 24-hour basis in our cells, creating free radicals. A free radical is an atom, highly charged with energy. It has one electron of a pair missing, and runs amuck in search of another electron, damaging or destroying healthy cells in the macula and elsewhere. There can be millions of them.)

How Selenium Works

A deficiency of selenium reduces the activity of this enzyme, which, then, is limited in ability to quench free radicals. So tissues of the macula are attacked and damaged. Selenium appears to be instrumental in protecting the eyes from senile macular degeneration and too little selenium in the diet may lead to macular degeneration.[3]

Like zinc and selenium, vitamin C, shown by studies at Stanford University Medical School, protects against damage of various eye tissues, including the macula and the lens.[4]

In the 1984-85 Yearbook of Nutritional Medicine (Keats Publishing,

Inc.), eye authority Ben C. Lane, O.D., mentions the need for supplementation of vitamin C and vitamin B-6 — the latter particularly in wet senile macular degeneration.[5] In wet maculopathy, the eye tissues leak fluids.

Dr. Lane recommends 250 mg of vitamin C three times daily and vitamin B-6 in a potency of 50 mg twice daily. He also points out that most patients with macular degeneration eat their flesh proteins well done, destroying much of the vitamin B-6 in foods which are rich in this nutrient.

Foods That Fight Macular Degeneration

It is possible to get enough of the mineral zinc in foods to reach the level of 50 mg daily, which Dr. John Trowbridge of Houston, Texas usually recommends for patients with macular degeneration.

This is also true of selenium. Foods can offer enough of this trace mineral to satisfy the daily requirement of 200 micrograms (not milligrams). One can easily take in as much as 250 mg of vitamin C in foods and/or supplements three times daily. However, it is impossible to ingest 50 mg of vitamin B-6 twice daily in foods alone, although foods and supplements serve as a foundation for taking B-6 pills or capsules.

Following are the foods and supplements richest in zinc in terms of milligrams per unit of less than four ounces: herring, 110; wheat germ, 14; sesame seeds, 10; torula yeast. 9.9; blackstrap molasses, 8.3; maple syrup, 7.5; liver, 7.0; soybeans, 6.7; sunflower seeds, 6.6; egg yolk, 5.5; lamb, 5.4; chicken, 4.8; regular molasses, 4.6; brewer's yeast, 3.9; oats, 3.7; bone meal, 3.6; rye, 3.4; whole wheat, 3.2; corn, 3.1; coconut, and beef, 3.0; beets, turkey and walnuts, 2.8; barley, 2,7; beans and avocados, 2.4; peas, 2.3; bleu cheese, 2.2; eggs, 2.1; buckwheat, 2.0; mangoes, 1.9 and millet, brown rice and almonds, 1.5.

Here are the best food sources of selenium in milligrams per less than a four ounce unit: corn, 0.40; cabbage, 0.25; whole wheat, 0.13; beans and peas, 0.12; onions, 0.080; chicken, 0.070; beets, 0.065; barley, 0.062; tomatoes, 0.060; soybeans, 0.054; saltwater fish, 0.053; freshwater fish and liver, 0.050; brown rice, 0.039; alfalfa and peanuts, 0.038; meat, 0.022; garlic and rye, 0.020; egg yolk, 0.018; oats, 0.012; lentils and brewer's yeast, 0.011 and eggs, 0.0100; cheeses, 0.0080, torula yeast, 0.0040; beans, 0.0030 and carrots, 0.0022.

Food supplements and foods which have the highest amounts of vitamin C are the following in milligrams per units of less than four ounces: rose hips, 3,000; acerola cherries, 1,100; guavas, 240; black currants, 200; parsley, 170; green peppers, 110; watercress, 80; chives. 70; strawberries, 57; persimmons, 52; spinach. 51; oranges, 50; cabbage, 47; grapefruit, 38; papaya. 37; elderberries and kumquats, 36; dandelion greens and lemons, 35; cantaloupe, 33; green onions, 32; limes, 31; mangoes, 27; loganberries, 24; tangerines and tomatoes, 23; squash, 22; raspberries and romaine lettuce, 18 and pineapple, 17.

Richest supplement and food sources of vitamin B-6 in milligrams per units of less than four ounces are: brewer's yeast, 4.0; brown rice, 3.6; whole wheat, 2.9; royal jelly, 2.4; soybeans, 2.0; rye, 1.8; lentils, 1.7; sunflower seeds and hazelnuts, 1.1; alfalfa, 1.00; salmon, 0.98; wheat germ, 0.92; tuna, 0.90; bran, 0.85; walnuts, 0.73; peas and liver, 0.67; avocados, 0.60; beans, 0.57; cashews, peanuts, turkey, oats, chicken and beef, 0.40; halibut, 0.34; lamb and bananas, 0.32; blackstrap molasses, 0.31 and corn and egg yolk, 0.30.

CHAPTER 51

Eye Problems

Inability to see well in the black of night after leaving a brightly lighted building, a condition called night blindness, has been charged to a vitamin A deficiency, as long as I can remember.

A shortage of this vitamin may still be a cause, but it is no longer the only cause, says clinical biochemist Daniel Bankson at the University of North Carolina in Chapel Hill.[1]

Experiments with rats spotlight the fact that previous researchers in night blindness have been in the dark about an even more critical deficiency: that of protein.

When fed a third to a fifth of their normal protein requirement as well as four times their daily ration of vitamin A, the rats became acutely night-blind, even though they had ample vitamin A in their eye tissues.

Then these animals were fed a balanced diet—just enough calories to maintain their size and weight—with one exception: not enough protein. Again, they showed normal levels of vitamin A in their eyes. However, now the night-blindness was even worse.

Before the Bankson experiment, researchers thought that protein deficiency limited delivery of the proper amount of vitamin A stored in the liver. However, the fact that the eyes showed adequate levels of vitamin A shatters this theory.

Undoubtedly, a shortage of protein in the diet is a major reason for night-blindness, although Bankson cannot, as yet, explain why.

Vitamin A: Not To Be Ignored

Even though vitamin A deficiency is no longer the sole reason for this eye condition, it still can be shown by solid studies to cause sensitivity to bright headlights and other glare, to quickly tiring eyes, inadequate daytime vision and to an unpleasant package of eye disorders: conjunctivitis (inflammation of the mucous membrane covering the front of the eyeball); corneal ulcer (an open sore on the window of the eye); inflammation of the iris, the colored portion of the eye that encircles the black pupil, and sties, tiny abscesses that form in follicles of eyelashes.[2]

Night blindness should never be treated lightly for two reasons: it is one of the major causes of auto accidents and it signals a dietary deficiency which should be corrected to prevent a far more serious eye disease. Some alternative doctors recommend taking both protein and vitamin A, because a long-term deficiency of vitamin A could lead to retinitis pigmentosa, a gradual deterioration of the retina and total blindness.[3]

Studies have revealed that victims of this disease—thousands each year in the United States—show an alarmingly low blood level of vitamin A, due mainly to inability to absorb this vitamin from food or supplements. Injected water-based vitamin A brought about a dramatic improvement in some patients.

Retinitis pigmentosa is best treated by a nutrition-oriented ophthalmologist.

Another serious eye disorder which can lead to irreversible blindness is xerophthalmia, often caused by a vitamin A shortage, too.[4] The eye loses internal lubrication, and the mucous membrane covering the front of the eyeball and the cornea become dry and thickened.

B-2 Deficiency And Its Consequences

Deficiency of vitamin B-2 can contribute to itching, burning and crying when there's really nothing to cry about. Like the rest of the trillions of cells that add up to become you and me, cells of the cornea must take in oxygen. A shortage of this vitamin forces nearby tissues to form many tiny blood vessels, enabling blood to deliver oxygen closer to the cornea.[5] Result? Bloodshot eyes.

Serious eye conditions, over and above what have been covered here—cancer of the eye, cataracts, glaucoma and macular degeneration—are dealt with in their own sections of this book.

So much for the more serious eye ailments. Can anything be done nutritionwise for eye deficiencies such as near-sightedness and strabismus (cross-eyes to you and me)?

Adelle Davis offers the answers in Let's Get Well (Harcourt, Brace & World), her fine meaty book. (Vegetarians, no offense intended.) Near-sightedness is associated with stress and too little calcium intake or its faulty absorption, contributory to tension and or spasms of small muscles holding eye lenses.

Both calcium and "large amounts" of vitamin E have corrected near-sightedness and cross-eyes in children, she writes.[6] Bearing out her idea of stress as a major cause of near-sightedness, she cites statistics in days of national prosperity and, then, in depression times.[7]

In a survey, nearsightedness of school children in carefree, prosperous times (1925) skyrocketed from 25 percent to 72 percent at the stressful height of the Great Depression (1935).[8]

Still another nutrient showed the ability to stop the progress of near-sightedness in children in an experiment at Guy's Hospital in London: protein. When added to the diet of part of the children, protein arrested the development of this condition. Children on the usual hospital fare showed continued deterioration of sight.

Putting Lazy Eyes To Work

Nutrition is not the only course to follow to improve eyesight. How about exercise? Does that sound ridiculous? That's what I thought, too, until I tried it. I read the literature of a company which has the farsightedness (no pun intended) to begin to teach about eyeglasses and contact lenses being crutches and of the need for exercising eyes, like any other part of the body.

Eyeglasses are optical crutches to which the eyes adapt. They never get better from wearing glasses. They become invalids. This company offers an alternative, constructive exercises to reeducate eye muscles, based on those in the perennial best-selling book, The Bates Method for Better Eyesight Without Glasses.

I really didn't want to read the company's literature, because I had just been fitted for glasses to correct my far-sightedness. Then I noted that the firm's kit could help various eye conditions: astigmatism, farsightedness, nearsightedness, presbyopia (old age sight) and hypersensitivity to light.

One of the company's methods was familiar to me, palming, placing the palms of the hands over the eyes to rest them, relax them and to stimulate circulation to them. So I tried a vision kit and, within a month, my eyes were so improved by what is called "aerobic" exercises that I threw away my glasses.

I am happy to know that there is an exercise approach to correct eye problems, just as there are nutritional methods. Now I know how to exercise my eyes for better vision. I also know the proper foods to eat to keep them well. To me, that's out of sight!

In this section, I offered research on various nutrients which appear to help the eyes: protein, vitamins A, B-2, E and the mineral calcium. Foods with the most protein are meat, poultry, fish, eggs, legumes, nuts ands grains.

Supplements and foods richest in vitamin A and its precursor, beta-carotene, in international units per less than a four ounce serving are: cod liver oil, 200,000; sheep liver, 45,000; beef liver, 44,000; calf's liver, 22.000; dandelion greens, 14,000; carrots, 11,000; yams, 9,000; kale, 8,900; parsley and turnip greens, 8,500; spinach, 8,100; collard green and chard, 6,500; watercress, 5,000; red peppers, 4,400; squash, 4,000; egg yolk and cantaloupe, 3,400; endive, 3,300; persimmons and apricots; broccoli, 2,500; pimentos, 2,300; swordfish, 2,100; whitefish, 2000; romaine, 1,900; mangoes, 1,800; papayas, 1,700; nectrines and pumpkin, 1,600; peaches and cheeses, 1,300; eggs, 1,200 and cherries, lettuce and cream, 1,000.

Best bets for supplements and foods high in vitamin B-2 in milligrams per units of less than four ounces are: torula yeast, 16; brewer's yeast, 4.2; liver, 4.1; royal jelly, 1.9; alfalfa, 1.8; bee pollen, 1.7; almonds, 0.92; wheat germ, 0.68; mustard greens, 0.64; egg yolk, 0.52; cheeses, 0.46; human milk, 0.40; millet, 0.038; chicken, 0.36; soybeans and veal, 0.31; eggs and sunflower seeds, 0.28; lamb, 0.27; peas, blackstrap molasses, parsley and cottage cheese, 0.25; sesame seeds, 0.24; egg white, lentils, rye and beans, 0.22; spinach, turkey, broccoli and beef, 0.22.

Supplements and foods richest in calcium in milligrams for units of less than four ounces are the following: bone meal, 40,000; dolomite, 21,000;

sesame seeds, 1,200; kelp, 1,100; cheeses, 700; brewer's yeast, 420; sardines and carob, 350; molasses, 290; caviar, 280; soybeans and almonds, 230; torula yeast, 220; parsley, 200; brazil nuts, 190; watercress, salmon and chickpeas, 150; egg yolks, beans, pistachios, lentils and kale, 130; sunflower seeds and milk, 120; buckwheat, 110; maple syrup, cream and chard, 100; walnuts, 99; spinach, 93; endive, 81; pecans, 73; wheat germ, 72; peas, 70; peanuts, 69; eggs, 54 and oats, 53.

Here are supplements and foods with the largest amounts of vitamin E in international units per servings of less than four ounce; wheat germ, 160; safflower nuts, 35; sunflower seeds, 31; whole wheat, 30; sesame seed oil, 26; walnuts, 22; corn oil and hazelnuts, 21; soy oil and peanuts oil, 16; almonds, 15; olive oil, 14; cabbage, 7.8; brazil nuts and peanuts, 6.5; cod liver oil, 5.4; cashews, 5.1; soy lecithin, 4.8; spinach, 2.9; asparagus, 2.5; broccoli, 2.0; butter, 1.9; parsley, 1.8; oats, barley and corn, 1.7 and avocados and pecans, 1.5.

CHAPTER 52

Fatigue

Recently I read a news story stating that a diagnosis doctors aren't keen about making is one for fatigue. First, there are so many ailments which can cause fatigue that it's sometimes difficult and time-consuming to get the right answer and, second, because there are so many patients with this complaint.

However, most frustrating for doctor and patient is that tests sometimes fail to offer even a clue. So the diagnosis is "nothing organically wrong," making the patient seem like a neurotic or hypochondriac, although he or she knows something is organically wrong. Then comes more frustration: endless doctor-hopping and money wasted for no satisfaction.

Most common causes of fatigue are low thyroid function (hypothyroidism), low blood sugar (hypoglycemia), Candida albicans, allergies and various forms of physical and emotional stress, including deficient intake of nutrients.

Unmasking The Culprits

On several occasions when he spoke at National Health Federation meetings, Broda O. Barnes, M.D. and Ph.D, an authority on thyroid function, told me, "In my 40-plus years as a medical doctor, four out of five of my thousands of patients with the complaint of fatigue turned out to be hypothyroid."

In his numerous published papers and at physicians' coventions and meetings, he advised doctors to rule out hypothyroidism before considering any other diagnosis for extreme fatigue. He also advised them to request that their patients take the Barnes Basal Temperature Test, the armpit test described in the Section on Thyroid Function (Low).

Yet, most doctors still use conventional laboratory tests which are not sensitive enough to catch many subtle cases of hypothyroidism.

As stated in the section Thyroid Function (Low), first generation hypothyroids can usually correct this condition with a daily kelp tablet containing 225 mcg of iodine or a diet which contains foods rich in iodine. (See list at the end of this section.) Second generation hypothyroids or beyond usually need prescribed thyroid supplement. Alternative doctors are familiar with the Barnes Basal Temperature Test, which, for many years, was mentioned in the Physicians Desk Reference (PDR).

The files of Dr. Barnes, who practiced for many years in Fort Collins, Colorado, bulged with cases of super-fatigue which were turned around within weeks by kelp or thyroid hormone supplementation—mainly the latter.

Low Blood Sugar Can Sap Your Strength.

Like low thyroid function, low blood sugar (hypoglycemia) can reduce you to lowest terms physically and emotionally. On a lengthy list of most common symptoms of this disorder, compiled by hypoglycemia authority, Dr. Stephen Gyland, of Jacksonville, Florida, exhaustion ranks third, a complaint of 87 percent of the patients. [1]

Before I came of age nutritionally, I was an airline stewardess in the days when Pontius was a pilot. The work was so exhausting I practically lived on coffee. It was almost as if I were on a coffee I.V.

After a gruelling, long flight, I was drained, practically collapsing, and felt like the "Totalled Woman." A wiser mind than mine directed me away from coffee and junk food to higher protein content small meals, spaced to keep my blood sugar level stable. Those small changes in diet worked big changes in me. The gal who thought she couldn't live without regular coffee fixes really began to live when she divorced herself from the coffee pot.

Many years later, I learned that alternative doctors use the very method I followed for correcting low blood sugar. And it works! (See the Section on Low Blood Sugar.)

Breakfast-Skipping Means Energy-Dipping

One of the cardinal sins of many who complain of fatigue is trying to lose or control weight by skipping breakfast, an open invitation to hypoglycemia. First, this won't melt off poundage, so it's a useless exercise. (The right meal to skip for weight loss is dinner. See the Section on Overweight (How to Be a Good Loser).

Not eating breakfast means that you've already had 12 or more hours without food. Tacking on another four hour fast until lunchtime, means some 16 hours without food and, therefore, a low, low blood sugar level and depressing fatigue, if not exhaustion.

Numerous experiments underscore that, in most instances, no breakfast means no energy — particularly the classical U.S. Department of Agriculture study by Elsa Orent-Keiles and Lois F. Hallman.[2]

Blood sugar levels after various types of breakfasts were compared: (1) unsweetened black coffee; (2) unsweetened black coffee and a donut; (3) citrus fruit, toast with butter and jam, bacon, and coffee with sugar and cream and (4) the remaining breakfasts were like number three, but with the addition of milk and breakfast cereal or milk and eggs.

Those who drank their breakfast—black coffee only—experienced a steadily falling blood sugar, intense hunger, headache, and weakness. Those who ate breakfast two and three experienced a rapid rise in blood sugar, then an off-the-cliff drop to the fasting level within three hours. Test subjects were unhappy, and looking forward to lunch.

The remaining breakfasts, with much more protein, boosted the blood sugar—but not as high as that of the others—and it stayed high far longer, then declined more slowly.

All groups were given the identical lunch: a sandwich and coffee. Those who had had black coffee and the high carbohydrate breakfast, showed hypoglycemia not long after the meal. However, the beneficial effects of the higher protein breakfast—sustained good energy and well-being—continued through the entire afternoon without low blood sugar symptoms.

A sometimes disastrous result of breakfast-skipping is such ravenous hunger that the person may devour more calories at lunch than his or her usual breakfast and lunch would have provided. An even worse consequence could be binge-eating on junk foods.

The Yeast Crisis And Fatigue

Although based on a different biological premise, Candida Albicans (fungus overgrowth) has this in common with hypoglycemia: it is best managed by a no-sugar diet. (This eliminates almost all fruit. As elaborated in the Section on Candida Albicans, this benign yeast in the colon spreads to various parts of the body. Fatigue overwhelms the patient.)

Since the world began, people have lived with Candida in their colons, but only in the past generation has this organism become a take-over guy. Antibiotics kill harmful bacteria but also annihilate friendly organisms that keep Candida albicans in check. Cortisone and hormones in the birth control pill also cause the yeast to thrive, as does the diet of refined sugar and flour which so many Americans follow.

Once friendly bacteria are implanted by means of good quality yogurt or supplements of lactobacillus acidophilus and they have time to colonize the colon, the Candida albicans retreats, and energy slowly returns.

Allergy Route To Low Energy

One of the little-suspected causes of fatigue is allergy from environmental sources and food. Many hard-to-diagnose cases of exhaustion turn out to be allergies. In a sense, an allergy is a metabolic rejection of one or more substances to which most individuals don't react. The immune system makes a special type of antibody to attack the offending substance.

Eventually the allergen-bearing blood bathes the entire system. One theory is that we are attacked at our point or points of weakness. We suffer fatigue, because the energy-use system is particularly vulnerable. Another theory is that an allergy is a form of stress. A certain allergen may keep the adrenal glands working continuously and, in this way, wear them down, producing exhaustion.

A young woman who owned a novelty manufacturing company came to me for a referral to a doctor. Her complaint was fatigue beyond fatigue. She had to lock her office door to take frequent naps, morning, noon and afternoon in order to survive. If she had a business appointment at night, she made it fairly late, so that she could nap for an hour before going out.

"Maureen, I've got everything I need business-wise, financially, and socially, but I can't continue living a fractional life. Do you suppose I have sleeping sickness?" she asked.

"Not likely," I replied. "I'll set up an appointment for you with one of the best alternative physicians I know."

We went on talking. Inasmuch as her fatigue was a continuing thing, I reasoned it was caused by hypothyroidism, hypoglycemia, or possibly Candida albicans. However, the Barnes Basal Temperature Test had shown her to be normal, as had the six-hour glucose tolerance test taken for low blood sugar.

None of her medical history indicated Candida albicans, so I questioned her about allergies. "Do you ever experience any symptom other than fatigue — no matter how mild?"

It turned out her eyes watered when she came into the office in the morning. However, the fatigue was no worse then. After more discussion, she suddenly showed a light of recognition. It seemed that, early each day, the cleaning woman freshened up her private bathroom with a strong-smelling disinfectant.

"Come to think of it, my eyes water a little when I enter the office," she admitted. "But could something as innocent as a disinfectant cause the eye-watering and my fatigue?"

I directed her to a special kind of medical doctor, a clinical ecologist. Sure enough, when he challenged her with the disinfectant, tears welled up in her eyes, and, in a short time, she felt weighed down with fatigue. He advised her to have the cleaning woman stop using the chemical. And, good news, my friend stopped developing tears in her eyes, and her energy level slowly but markedly increased by the week's end.

"It's incredible," she gushed several weeks later. "My energy level is almost up to normal now."

Although allergy is not a prime suspect in fatigue, anemia usually is — especially iron-deficiency anemia. In fact all types of anemia — iron-deficiency, pernicious and megaloblastic — have one thing in common: they limit the oxygen which can be delivered to body cells. Without enough oxygen, we can't have efficient metabolism, and, therefore, cannot generate enough energy or warmth. (See the section on Anemia.)

Iron-deficiency anemia, of course, is corrected by iron-rich foods and pernicious anemia by foods which contain large amounts of vitamin B-12. Vegetarians are particularly susceptible to this kind of anemia. Megaloblastic anemia occurs when the diet is deficient in the B vitamin folic acid.

All Kinds Of Stress

Stress can come in various forms, shapes and intensities. It can be physical or emotional. However, if persistent, such as anxiety or worry, it can cause adrenal deficiency, draining these glands' hormone resources, like the grinding away of a car starter can drain a battery.

Adrenal exhaustion can produce overwhelming fatigue which studies show is correctible in time with the nutrients pantothenic acid and vitamin A.[3] (Lists of foods rich in these vitamins will be offered at chapter's end.)

In an experiment, prisoner volunteers deprived of pantothenic acid for 25 days became so exhausted and seriously ill that the test had to be called off. Even on a regime of 4,000 milligrams of pantothenic acid daily, the volunteers recovered slowly.[4]

Although a deficiency of pantothenic acid is especially critical in adrenal exhaustion, a shortage of virtually any vitamin or mineral can cause fatigue or exhaustion, if the deficiency persists for long enough.

All of which tells us to keep our diet balanced with meat, poultry, fish, eggs, fresh vegetables and fruit (none of the latter with Candida albicans, however), whole grains, nuts and seeds.

The disorders named above are the major causes of fatigue. Yet there are still other reasons: inability to sleep —See the Section called Sleeplessness— smoking, drinking, failing to exercise, skipping meals, too rigid a weight-loss diet; carrying around much excess weight, and being bored with life with its emotional overtones of unhappiness.

Now let's look at foods needed to correct hypothyroidism and adrenal and physical exhaustion, too: iodine and pantothenic acid and vitamin A.

Iodine can be found in most liberal amounts in terms of milligrams per less than four ounce units in these supplements and foods: kelp, 180; cod liver oil, 0.84; haddock, 0,31; codfish, 0.14; chard and beans, 0.10; perch,

0.074; sunflower seeds, 0.070; herring, 0.052; turnip greens, 0.047; halibut, 0.046; vegetable oils, 0.024; peanuts and cantaloupe, 0.020; liver, 0.019; soybeans, 0.017; pineapple, 0.016, potatoes, 0.015; cheeses, 0.011 and lettuce, 0.010.

Here are the supplements and foods richest in pantothenic acid in terms of milligrams per less than a four ounce unit: royal jelly, 35; brewer's yeast, 11; torula yeast, 10; brown rice, 8.9; sunflower seeds, 5.5; soybeans, 5.2; corn, 5.0; lentils, 4.8; egg yolk, 4.2; peas, 3.6; alfafa , 3.3; whole wheat, 3.2; peanuts, 2.8; rye, 2.6; eggs, 2.3; bee pollen and wheat germ, 2.2; bleu cheese, 1.8; cashews, 1.3; chickpeas, 1.2; avocado, 1.1 and chicken, turkey and walnuts, 0.90.

Sources with the highest amounts of vitamin A or its precursor in terms of International Units per less than four ounce units are: cod liver oil, 200,000, sheep liver, 45,000; beef liver, 44,000; calf's liver, 22,000; dandelion greens, 14,000; carrots, 11,000; yams, 9,000; kale, 8,900; parsley and turnip greens, 8,500; spinach, 8,100; collard greens and chard, watercress, 5,000; red pepper, 4,400; squash, 4,000; egg yolk and cantaloupe, 3,400; endive, 3,300; persimmons and apricots, 2,700; broccoli, 2,500; pimentos, 2.300; swordfish, 2,100; whitefish, 2,000; romaine lettuce, 1,900, mangoes, 1,800; papayas, 1,700 and nectarines and pumpkin. 1,600.

Mary Archer's Pepper Liver

2 onions, sliced in rings	1 t. jalapeno pepper, chopped
1 green pepper, thinly sliced	1 t. cumin
2 tomatoes, chopped	½ t. tamari
1 lb. beef liver, cut in thin strips	

Place onion rings, green pepper and jalapeno pepper slices in large skillet and steam-stir in enough spring water to prevent sticking until onion begins to turn transparent. Add tomatoes and stir over medium heat until onion and pepper are tender. Place liver strips over onion mixture. Add spices and cover. Steam liver until tender. Pink juices should remain in slices. Add tamari, stirring liver and vegetables to combine. Serve with brown rie or boiled potatoes. Serves 4.

Bean Salad

2 apples, peeled
¼ c. lemon juice
½ c. cider vinegar
1 T. red wine vinegar
½ c. oil
1 T. frozen apple juice concentrate,
   unsweetened
¼ c. pickle juice
2 garlic cloves, minced
1 t. brewer's yeast

½ t. oregano
½ t. onion powder
¼ t. dill weed
1 t. spike
6 c. total of beans - made up of cooked
   garbanzo, kidney, green beans and
   yellow wax beans
1 medium onion, sliced into rings
1 c. celery, diced

Blend apples in blender with lemon juice. Add vinegars, oil, apple concentrate, pickle juice and seasonings. Place beans, onion and celery in large bowl and pour dressing over top. Let stand in refrigerator overnight. The longer it stand, the better the flavor. Makes 10 to 12 servings.

CHAPTER 53

Frost-Bite

What can foods possibly have to do with being or not being frostbitten? More than you can imagine.

Individuals with arteries narrowed by deposits of cholesterol, calcium, and other byproducts of foods are the most frequent victims of frostbite, because they have a decreased volume of blood circulating to the skin.

(See the Section on Cholesterol, 20 Ways To Lower It Naturally.)

Beta blockers and smoking also reduce blood flow to exposed skin and elsewhere.

For the benefit of you who have come no closer to experiencing frostbite than opening your refrigerator's freezer door, frostbite is the freezing of the skin and tissues underlying it.

Long exposure to the frigid air—this is no commercial—or icy winds stops the blood circulation to the face, ears, nose, fingers and hands, toes and feet. As a cross-country skier, I, along with other enthusiastic skiers, sometimes ignore temperature and experience frostbite—hard, pale, cold skin that has no feeling. However, most of the time, I powder the inside of my ski socks with cayenne pepper, which keeps me snuggly warm.

The Folklore Treatment: A "No-No"

Once frost-bitten, you make a mistake if you rub the frozen parts with snow. Expose them to warmth—not heat, inasmuch as your numbed skin can't sense the degree of temperature. If no convenient shelter is near, it is best to warm the affected area with other body parts. Tuck frozen hands in the armpit or hold frozen toes in the hands. Another alternative is wrapping a blanket or towel around the frostbitten body part.

251

Usually frozen fingers or toes will thaw out normally in warm surroundings, becoming red and painful. If you fail to recover in a short time, see an emergency doctor quickly for treatment to avoid the possibility of dry gangrene, which may necessitate having a finger or toe removed.

Dear friends of mine, Ronn and Connie Haus, the chief executive officers of Family Christian Broadcasting, Channel 42, in Concord, California had an unusual problem that led to frostbite.

Ronn, playing basketball with his son, managed to get jammed in the ribs. To lessen the pain, he lay down with an ice pack over the sore area and, due to a hectic, exhausting work schedule, fell asleep. When he woke up, he was frostbitten. Connie called me for some sisterly advice.

I suggested peeling several bananas and laying the soothing inner part of the peel on the frost-bitten area. At first, Ronn laughed at this old folk remedy. However, to his credit, he tried it and got instant relief. The next day, the frostbitten portion looked and felt almost normal. In the Section on Skin Irritations, Abrasions and Insect Bites, you will read more about the wonderful banana peel.

So much for what to do after the damage is done. How about preventing frost-bite by diet? Several of my Canadian doctor friends tell me that much experimentation has been done in Canada with guinea pigs, rats, monkeys, and human beings to prevent frostbite by a high intake of vitamin C.

And every experiment (reported in reputable journals) showed that a liberal intake of vitamin C, indeed, stimulates the body to generate greater body-heat and made animal and man more cold-resistant.

Reported in the Canadian Journal of Biochemical Physiology, research by Dr. J.M. Leblanc and associates, revealed that a daily intake of 425 mg of vitamin C was a far better protection against discomfort from cold and frostbite than a daily intake of 25 mg.[1]

Is it possible to derive as much as 425 mg of vitamin C from food each day? Yes, but it is sometimes difficult to obtain fresh vegetables and fruit in cold climates. However, food supplements such as rose hips are usually available and can supply even more than that. So can vitamin C pills or capsules.

Winter sports participants often live in warmer climates, have access to fresh fruits and vegetables the year around, and can fortify themselves before flying to winter resorts, and taking vitamins while there.

That is what I do before driving up to the great snow slopes near Lake Tahoe.

Here are supplements and foods richest in vitamin C in milligrams per less than four ounce units:

Rose hips, 3,000; acerola cherries, 1,100; guavas, 240; black currants, 200; parsley, 170; green peppers, 110; watercress, 80; chives, 70; strawberries, 57; persimmons, 52; spinach, 51; oranges, 50; cabbage, 47; grapefruit, 38; papaya, 37; elderberries and kumquats, 36; dandelion greens and lemons, 35; cantaloupe, 33; green onions, 32; limes, 31; mangoes, 27; loganberries, 24; tangerines and tomatoes, 23; squash, 22 and raspberries and romaine lettuce, 18.

CHAPTER 54

Gall Bladder Disorders

Nobody pays much attention to the gall bladder. After all, hardly anybody knows what it does. And as long as it performs the job, why bother with it?

There's only one problem with this line of thought. Neglect and failure to do the right things to keep the gall bladder healthy could bring on inflammation or gallstones and such pain that you couldn't pay attention to anything else.

A homely, four-inch long, pear-shaped organ tucked between the liver lobes, the gall bladder has the unspectacular job of storing and concentrating bile, which the liver produces, and releasing some into the small intestine when signalled that some fat has arrived for digestion.

When gallstones form, they move out with the bile and choke off the narrow neck of the gall bladder or the even smaller bile duct below, intense pain strikes on the upper right side of the abdomen or between the shoulder blades. The knifing pain gets worse for several hours, then subsides, replaced by a sick feeling with the possibility of vomiting.

Underlying Cause

Occasionally the blockage—several small stones or a medium-sized one—breaks when the stones fall back into the gall bladder or move through the bile duct into the intestines.

The American Medical Association Family Medical Guide (Random House) says that a million new cases of gallstones occur each year. Autopsies reveal that 2½ times more women have gallstones than men. Seventy percent of American Indian women older than thirty have them for an unexplained reason. About 20 percent of senior citizens develop gallstones.

If blockage of bile flow persists for long, many complications can occur: obstructive jaundice, infection of the gall bladder and inflammation when the trapped bile stagnates.

Certain preventive measures can be taken to keep the gall bladder happy, without a gallstone to its name, and cooperative to you and your health. However, to help the cause, you should know bile and your gall bladder better.

Getting To Know You

Bile is a green blend of acids, cholesterol, lecithin, minerals, pigments and water, whose job it is to work on digested fats, carotene and fat soluble vitamins A, D, E, and K so that they can pass through the intestinal wall into the blood. Lecithin dissolves fat into droplets so small that enzymes can encompass and process them for absorption. B-complex vitamins influence the gall bladder to empty its content on command.

Troubles start when the diet is to high in refined sugar and starches and too low in protein, when too little bile is formed by the liver, and the gall bladder is too lazy to empty its content when the right hormone issues its command.

In too large particles for enzymes to process, fat can't be readily absorbed, unites with calcium and iron from food, frustrates these minerals from entering the blood where they can do some good, forms a hard soap, then hard-packed fecal matter and causes constipation.

Frightening Consequences

Persistent stealing of essential iron and calcium can bring on iron-deficiency anemia, osteoporosis (honeycombed bones) or osteomalacia (weak and caving-in bones). (See Sections on Osteoporosis and Osteomalacia.)

Without enough bile, fats melted at body temperature cover carbohydrates and protein, making it hard for enzymes to continue the digestion process. So bacteria attack this partially digested mess, bringing on gas and uncomfortable and often painful inflation, contributing to an odoriferous bowel movement and an equally foul breath.

Even with an adequate intake of protein and carbohydrates, insufficient bile can cause malnutrition—just as it can by limiting absorption of the fat-soluble vitamins A, D, E and K and carotene. Inability of enough vitamin A to get into the bloodstream is one of the causes of night blindness and other serious consequences, if this condition persists. (See the Section on Eye Problems).

Adelle Davis, in her monumental work, Let's Get Well (Harecourt, Brace and World) mentions the perils of a low-fat or no-fat diet recommended by some individuals for gall bladder diseases, gallstones and blockage of the bile duct, referring to an American Medical Association suggestion that the diet contain at least 25 percent fat. A low-fat diet would prevent absorption of nutrients mentioned in the above paragraph, invite deficiency, and bring on medical ailments more devastating than gall bladder disorders.

What Causes Gallstones?

Supposedly, a high fat-high cholesterol diet causes gallstones. This popular belief may be far less popular and far less believable when evidence of animal experiments is presented.

One group of hamsters was purposely fed a diet deficient in vitamin E. A second group received ample vitamin E. The first group developed gallstones. The second did not.[1]

Experimental animals purposely fed much cholesterol and fats — saturated or unsaturated—along with sufficient vitamin E, showed no sign of gall stones. On the same regime without enough vitamin E, they developed them.[2]

Other researchers put hamsters on a vitamin E-deficient diet with no fat or cholesterol, and they, too, formed gallstones.[3]

Vitamin E: Opponent Of Gallstones

One theory about gallstone formation holds that dead cells from the gall bladder's inner membrane act as the nucleus around which stones form. But why doesn't this happen when vitamin E is plentiful? Vitamin A protects integrity of skin and internal membranes. However, without enough vitamin E to guard it, vitamin A is attacked by oxidation, permitting membrane cells to die and drop into the bile.

A second theory is that stones are less likely to form from cholesterol when the diet has a high content of lecithin, which homogenizes cholesterol — also fat — and holds it in this condition.

Royal Gall Bladder Flush

Many people have gallstones without knowing it, because they may be small enough to pass cleanly and painlessly. Once in a while, I go on what I call the Royal Gall Bladder Flush, because it gets rid of cholesterol stones and makes one feel like a queen or king.

It works on a seven-day plan. From Monday to Saturday, I drink all the apple juice I can contain, along with my regular diet.

On Saturday, I eat my usual lunch. Three hours later, I dissolve two teaspoons full of di-sodium phosphate or Epsom salts in a small amount of hot water. Ugh! It tastes that bad. So I wash it away with a glass of fresh grapefruit juice. I repeat this routine in two hours.

For dinner, I eat half a grapefruit and drink a glass of freshly squeezed grapefruit juice.

Just before going to bed, I blend a half cup of warm and unrefined olive oil with half cup of grapefruit juice and drink it. The combination is not that bad. Or you can take half cup of unrefined olive oil blended with a half cup of freshly squeezed lemon juice.

Then I go to bed, lying on my right side with my right knee pulled as close to my chest as I can for a half hour.

On Sunday morning, I take two more teaspoonsful of di-sodium phosphate or Epsom salts in a small amount of hot water at least an hour before I eat.

That morning's bowel movement contains small, green, irregularly-shaped cholesterol stones the size of kiwi fruit seeds to grape seeds and a few just smaller than cherries.

I use the Royal Flush every three to six months.

Now, in summary, the ideal diet to keep the gall bladder normal appears to be moderately high in protein and low in refined carbohydrates, with B-complex, and lecithin supplemented by a liberal amount of vitamin E.

Best protein sources are meat, poultry, fish, eggs, milk and milk products, nuts, legumes and whole grains.

Only two food sources contain liberal amounts of lecithin: soy beans and eggs. Therefore, some individuals prefer to take a lecithin supplement. B-complex vitamins to stimulate the gall bladder to empty its content with vigor can be found in a combination of brewer's yeast, torula yeast, and desiccated liver tablets or in a B-complex tablet.

Richest supplement and food sources of vitamin E in International Units per less than four ounce portions are: wheat germ, 160; safflower nuts, 35; sunflower seeds, 31; whole wheat, 30; sesame oil, 26; walnuts, 22; corn oil and hazelnuts, 21; soy oil and peanut oil, 16; almonds, 15; olive oil, 14; cabbage, 7.8; brazil nuts and peanuts, 6.5; cod liver oil, 5.4; cashews, 5.1; soy lecithin, 4.8; spinach, 2.9; asparagus, 2.5; broccoli, 2.3; butter, 1.9; parsley, 1.8; oats, corn and barley, 1.7 and avocados and pecans, 1.5.

CHAPTER 55

Gas (Intestinal)

A subject little discussed and much-suffered is intestinal gas.

Uncomfortableness and bloating come from three major sources: (1) eating too fast or too nervously; (2) overeating and (3) digesting food inefficiently and, therefore, incompletely.

In the first instance, a person bolts foods or gulps fluids and swallows air. If not released through the mouth, this air moves downward.

Overeating, especially as a way of life, overwhelms available digestive enzymes, leaving some food undigested. Putrefactive bacteria break it down and, in the process, produce foul gas.

Inefficient digestion caused by insufficient hydrochloric acid, bile and digestive enzymes leads to the same end.

Some years ago, the Reader's Digest published a classic article, Mealtime Madness, showing that the dining table is not only the place for eating, but also for carrying on family arguments and rehashing the day's frustrations — negative factors which make individuals eat under stress — too nervously and too fast. Result? Intestinal gas. Bloating and odor tell a person immediately that his or her digestion needs a tuneup.

Some Solutions

In all three causes of intestinal gas, the solutions are visible in the problems: merely reverse them. Trade in mealtime madness for mealtime peace and peace of mind. This is within your control.

Similarly, substitute moderate eating for over-eating. The opportunity to get rid of bloating, painful and, sometimes, embarrassing flatulence, can work as an incentive for reduced intake.

So far as digestive deficiencies are concerned, you can get guidance from a nutrition-oriented doctor after he or she draws a focus on specific causes. (See the list of alternative doctors in the back of the book.) Sometimes, something as simple as several hydrochloric acid tablets or capsules right after meals can solve the problem.

Some digestive aids in health food stores contain hydrochloric acid, bile and several digestive enzymes.

Certain Problem Foods

One food is notorious for producing intestinal gas: beans. Sulfur-containing foods—broccoli, brussels sprouts, cabbage, cauliflower, eggs and dried appricots—can produce that rotten egg odor (hydrogen sulfide) so familiar to chemistry students.

Fiber from grains is indigestible to us, but certain intestinal micro-organisms don't find it so. Individuals who increase their fiber intake too fast run the risk of producing intestinal gas.

Milk can promote gas in lactose-intolerant persons. (See Section on Milk Intolerance) This is because they lack an enzyme called lactase, necessary for the breaking down of the milk sugar lactose.

How To Cope With Problem Foods

Straight out of folk medicine, I got the formula which works for making beans less bean-like. Boil beans for a few minutes, shut off the heat, let them stand for an hour or two. Drain out the water, and add new water. The thrown-away water supposedly removes objectionable substances. This method also works with lentils and peas.

People who are milk-intolerant can often tolerate yogurt with no negative results. If that doesn't work, they can buy lactase products at any health food store. These will help them digest undigestible milk and other dairy products and reduce—possibly eliminate—dairy products-caused flatulence.

A product which proves helpful to millions of people in conquering gas comes right out of folk medicine: charcoal. Several studies reveal that activated charcoal, a heath food store item, can cut the production of gas by 75 percent.

Another wonder-worker is garlic, which decimates the army of putre-factive bacteria.

The simple suggestions mentioned here have helped millions to solve an important problem.

Jean Martin's Cranberry Relish

10 sweet apples	1 lb. cranberries
7 sweet oranges	Pinch sea salt

Chop apples fine. Peel 6 of the oranges, leaving the peel on one orange. Wash it well, scrubbing with a brush. Quarter all oranges to remove seed. Blend all oranges until fine in blender with sea salt. Put cranberries through coarse food chopper, or whirl lightly in blender with enough of the blended oranges to turn over in blender. Mix all ingredients. Chill and serve. May need to add honey if fruit is not sweet. Serves 8.

CHAPTER 56

Glaucoma

Glaucoma, a build-up of sight-destroying eye pressure, can be so subtle that many persons may not even be aware of it—at least in the early stages.

Glaucoma is caused by excessive fluid (aqueous humor) between the window of the eye (cornea) and its lens. This liquid continues to be secreted and drained off. A blockage of the drain causes tremendous pressure on, and progressive damage to the optic nerve, usually leading to blindness. Conventional therapy is oral drugs, eye drops and/or surgery.

Telltale Symptoms

Without fail and without delay, see an opththalmologist, a medical doctor who deals with eye diseases, when any of the following symptoms appear: decreased or blurring vision; colored halos around artifical lights; pain in or near the eye; an enlarged pupil (the circular opening in the iris); unusual watering or discharge from the eyes; change of eye color; a clouded cornea and or hardness of the eyeball; nausea or outright vomiting present with these symptoms; tiredness and moderate discomfort in the eye — especially following TV or motion pictures in a dark room; deteriorating sight in poor light and gradual loss of side vision.

See An Optometrist Or Ophthalmologist Regularly

The best insurance for the only set of eyes you will ever have is to take them to an optometrist or to an alternative ophthalmologist for examination at least twice a year, whether or not you need glasses. A standard part of both the optometrist and the ophthalmologist's examination is testing for glaucoma. If the pressure is abnormal, the optometrist recommends that you see an ophthalmologist, who can take action to control the condition.

Normal And Dangerous Eye Pressure

The normal reading for eye pressure ranges between 15 and 20. Any measurement over 20 is suspect. Extreme readings can surpass the fifties and sixties.

If you have glaucoma, follow guidelines established by an ophthalmologist. Second, carry an identification card which your ophthalmologist has or can obtain from the National Foundation for Eye Care. This will prove useful for two purposes: (1) so that your family practitioner won't prescribe a medicine or drug which could worsen the glaucoma, and (2) to forewarn emergency doctors of your condition in the event that you have an accident which renders you unconscious.

Nutritional Control

Authorities who know glaucoma best say that it cannot be cured, "only controlled". One of the newer methods of establishing control, as revealed in Italy by Michele Virno, M.D. and associates before the Roman Ophthalmological Society, is by means of high potency vitamin C: a half gram for every 2.2 pounds of body weight five times daily (35 grams) for a person weighing 150 pounds.[1]

Internal eye pressure plunged to its lowest point within four to five hours after patients ingested their first installment of vitamin C. Numerous individuals reduced their eye-pressure to the safe range within 45 days—something the usual oral drugs and eye drops could not always accomplish.

Is This High Intake Really Safe?

Commenting on results, Dr. Linus Pauling agrees with experimenters that this regime is safe, although it caused some stomach upset and diarrhea, ending in three or four days.[2]

The biochemists do not clearly understand how vitamin C controls glaucoma. However, professor G.B. Bietti, director of the Eye Clinic of the University of Rome, the scene of the experiment, made these significant observations:[3]

1. Vitamin C is effective taken orally or by intravenous injection—the latter in the form of sodium ascorbate in daily installments of .4 grams to 1 gram per every 2.2 pounds of body weight.

2. Benefits of this regime can be prolonged indefinitely—at least for the seven months duration of the experiment—by means of divided daily dosages of 125 mg per 2.2 pounds of body weight taken two, three, or four times.

3. Vitamin C can also be taken along with conventional glaucoma medications when the latter cannot control the condition.

Make Your Ophthalmologist Aware!

Most ophthalmologists know about vitamin C therapy for glaucoma. However, if your ophthalmologist is not familiar with this regime, let him or her read this section.

Other Key Considerations

Many precautions must be exercised during treatment:

1. Let your ophthalmologist know immediately if you have any marked and unexpected physical reactions to his or her medications.

2. Try to stay calm and peaceful, not permitting the day's stressful events to provoke you to anger, fear or worry.

3. Avoid heavy lifting or pushing, because these actions put undue stress upon the eyes and can often nullify the benefits of your doctor's treatment.

4. Refrain from stimulants such as coffee and tea, which act upon the eyes like emotional stress.

5. Promote easy bowel regularity as recommended in the section called Constipation, because straining could build up pressure in the eyes. (Very likely, the high amounts of vitamin C will assure that constipation won't exist.)

6. Avoid protracted periods using the eyes in darkness, such as in a

motion picture theater, and stay out of very bright sun whenever possible. Glaucoma can be controlled and your vision protected.

Grandmother's Baked Apple

1 fresh medium apple	⅛ t. cloves, ground
⅛ t. cinnamon	1 T. spring water

Wash and core apple. Place in shallow baking dish. Mix spices and water together. Pour over apple. Bake moderate in 350 degree oven until done, about 35 minutes.

Stuffed Leg Of Lamb

1 T. wheat germ	2 t. walnuts, finely chopped
1 t. brewers yeast	2 t. lemon rind, finely chopped
½ lb. spinach	¼ c. pine nuts
1 T. olive oil	½ c. soft whole grain bread crumbs
½ c. scallions, chopped	1 egg, beaten
2 large garlic cloves, chopped	7½ to 9 lbs. leg of lamb,
¼ c. fresh parsley	boned and butter fried
3 T. fresh mint	(your butcher can do this for you)

STUFFING:

Steam spinach for 3 minutes. Drain and squeeze out water, and chop (this should equal ½ cup). Heat oil in a small pan. Saute scallions and garlic for 2 to 3 minutes. Combine spinach, scallion mixture, parsley, wheat germ, brewers yeast, mint, lemon rind, walnuts, pine nuts, bread crumbs and egg. Blend well.

LAMB:

Place lamb on work surface and skin—side down. Make gashes in thick meaty parts to flatten if necessary. Grind pepper over lamb. Squeeze lemon half over top and rub juice in. Spoon nut-herb stuffing over lamb. Using your hands, work stuffing into folds (or pockets) of meat and spread evenly. Roll meat up and fasten with trussing needle, and kitchen string. Tie lamb roll 2 or 3 times with string to make a compact, oblong roast. Remove skewers. Rub outside with oil and rosemary and place on a rack set in a roasting pan. Cover and set aside to marinate at room temperature for 1 hour. Preheat oven to 325 degrees. Roast lamb, uncovered, for 12 to 15 minutes per pound for medium, or 20 minutes per pound for well done. Baste often with pan juices during roasting. Allow roast to rest 10 minutes on a heated platter before slicing. Makes 8 servings.

Marinated Bean Salad

4 c. garbanzos

4 c. green beans

1 green pepper, finely chopped

1 onion, finely chopped

1 t. honey

1 T. olive oil

3 T. lemon juice

Place garbanzos and green beans in bowl. Add pepper and onion. Mix honey, oil and lemon juice. Pour over mixture. Let stand several hours before serving. Serves 4.

CHAPTER 57

Gout

Almost exclusive to males, gout is a hereditary condition in which harmful chemicals gather in and around joints—particularly that of the big toe—and cause acute inflammation. This disorder has often been managed by eating cherries or drinking cherry juice.

We owe the cherry treatment to an inflamed, gouty big toe that was part of a Texan named Ludwig W. Blau, Ph.D.[1]

Crippled, confined to a wheelchair, Blau wheeled himself to the cupboard, but couldn't eat most of what he saw there: foods high in the amino acid purine, a no-no for gout-sufferers: anchovies, bouillon, herring, meat extracts and sardines. (Organ meats are also high in purines.)

Accidental Discovery

Discouraged, he tried the refrigerator, saw a bowl of plump, red cherries, sampled them, and, hooked, ate the bowlful. Next morning, wonder of wonders, the pain and inflammation in his foot were almost gone, so he decided to eat at least six cherries daily. Soon he was delivered from the wheelchair, pain, and gout and able to resume business actively.

Forgetting to take his cherry supply with him on a business trip, Blau soon found his big toe throbbing and excruciating. A few days after he resumed eating six to eight cherries a day, his gout diminished.

Instead of pooh-poohing the cherry story, Blau's family physician tried the therapy on 12 patients, all of whose gout or arthritis were improved by eating cherries or drinking cherry juice. Dr. Blau described the results in Texas Reports on Biology and Medicine.

More About The Cherry Cure

While cherries didn't seem to help rheumatoid arthritis, cherry juice contributed to reduced pain in some patients.

A high concentration of uric acid in the blood causes gout. Nutrients in cherries seem to keep uric acid from crystallizing and becoming deposited in joints.

Dr. Blau discovered that cherries of any kind appear to work: fresh or canned, sweet or sour or a mixture of the two. How soon does relief from gout usually occur? In 10 days or less. However, one patient just under 60 years of age ate her six to eight cherries for a month before her pain diminished.

What nutrients make cherries gout-effective? Their calcium-phosphorus ratio is excellent. They contain about 191 mg of potassium to every 100 grams and two mg. of sodium to 100 grams — a negligible amount of sodium—a good portion of vitamin A precursor: 100 International Units per 100 grams for sweet cherries—and, remarkably, 1,000 I.U. per 100 grams for the sour cherries —as well as traces of vitamins B-1, B-2, niacin and vitamin C.

A fruit other than cherries supposedly cured the gout of famous Swedish botanist Linnaeus: fresh strawberries, which he ate in large amounts every morning and evening.[2]

Other Approaches

Two other therapies are said to work—one from folk medicine and the other from the pages of the respected Merck Manual. Through the ages, the flowers of the broom plant brewed into a tea were supposed to cure gout.

Copious amounts of water — three or more quarts daily — have been recommended by the Merck Manual for gout and for preventing formation of kidney stones.

Millet Cereal

1 bottle cherry juice   1 c. millet
2 bananas

Try replacing the milk and sugar you normally put in your cereal with natural cherry juice…"tastes great!"

Cherry Salad

1 fresh pineapple
1 c. strawberries
2 large peaches (2 cups, sliced)
2 c. fresh cherries, pitted

½ c. honey
¼ c. lime juice
1 t. lime peel, grated

Cut pineapple in half lengthwise. Remove fruit; core and cut into bite-size pieces. In a 2½ quart glass container or bowl, layer half the pineapple, peaches and cherries and remaining pineapple. Blend orange juice, honey and lime juice. Pour over fruit. Top with lime peel. Makes six to eight servings.

CHAPTER 58

Gums And Tooth Socket Problems

"Be true to your teeth, or they will be false to you."

Whoever first made this statement really said a mouthful.

Dental neglect pays off in caries — a more respectable name for unrespectable cavities — gum ailments in periodontal disease — a fancy name for unfancy pyorrhea (infection and loosening of teeth in their sockets) — and, often, in false teeth.

Today "proper dental care" means more than just brushing and flossing teeth regularly and having a checkup and teeth cleaning semi-annually. It means proper nutrition to keep teeth, gums, and tooth sockets healthy. Although both aspects are important, some authorities feel that the latter is more important than the former.

One bit of evidence in favor of the nutritional approach is that, centuries ago, before toothbrushes, many people who worked under the sun and ate lots of fresh, raw, whole foods, took sound and healthy teeth to the grave. (Oh, to have had the breath mint concession!)

Opposite Viewpoint

Tooth socket deterioration starts with diseased gums, through which harmful bacteria invade and cause inflammation which then attacks the bone. This is today's popular belief.

It may not be popular tomorrow, thanks to findings by two Cornell University researchers: that bone loss through poor nutrition starts the deterioration process and that it all begins on the inside and works outward, not the other way around.

Well-based information holds that only one percent of the body's calcium circulates in the blood and in fluids between cells, but that this amount must be maintained at all cost. Therefore, when too little calcium is ingested, the shortage must be made up by drawing this mineral out of bone structures.

Some years ago, Cornell's Lennart Krook, D.V.M., Ph.D and Leo Lutwak, M.D., Ph.D and associates carefully examined jaw and bone structures of periodontal disease patients who had just died of other causes and discovered the priority order for withdrawal.[2]

First calcium is withdrawn from the jawbones (as shown by shrunken jawbones), then from the ribs and vertebrae and, finally, from arm and leg bones. As the jawbone and its tooth sockets shrink, bone pulls away from the teeth, causing them to loosen, irritating, then inflaming gums, and often bringing on bleeding.[3]

Jawbone degeneration — gum recession or a partially or fully visible tooth socket — is either. a sign that general osteoporosis, weakening honeycombed bones, is on the way or already happening in ribs and backbone.[4]

What To Do About It?

Krook and Lutwak concluded that most periodontal patients were taking in too little calcium. Checking into the diet of 10 volunteers—five women and five men of ages from 29 to 45—the researchers found that nine of ten were ingesting 400 mg or less calcium daily and had the deficiency symptoms to show for it: bleeding and inflamed gums (gingivitis) and loose teeth.[5] This is about half of the Recommended Daily Allowance (RDA). Many authorities feel that the RDA of 800 mg is too low, as did Krook and Lutwak, who gave 1,000 mg a day of calcium gluconolactate and calcium carbonate to the test subjects.

Results after six months of calcium supplementation were dramatic. Gum inflammation improved in every person and disappeared in three. Loose teeth tightened up in all but one case and, in one, returned to normal.[6]

The researchers who, at the start, had taken x-rays of volunteers' mouths, made comparative x-rays at study's end. Seven of the volunteers showed an increase of jawbone and a filling in of some bone which had parted from the tooth roots.[7]

All patients scored with two unexpected health improvements: a significant drop in blood pressure and cholesterol levels.[8]

A consensus of alternative medical doctors with whom I discussed the Krook-Lutwak supplementation recommended what they considered improvements: 1,200 mg of calcium, at least 400 I.U. of vitamin D, 10,000 I.U. of vitamin A, 600 mg of magnesium and at least 30 mg of zinc daily, as well as 500 mg of vitamin C or more. Best food and supplement sources for these minerals and vitamins will come later.

A Better Program

If working from the inside out with calcium alone proves effective, my doctor group felt the additional vitamins and minerals—all important to new bone formation — could speed and make more effective the bone rebuilding process.

The Journal Oral Surgery ran an article by Asger M. Frandsen, D.M.D., disclosing that vitamin A powerfully influences a process that goes on all the time: the tearing down of old bone cells and disposing of them and the forming of new ones to replace them. In a deficiency of vitamin A, the balance between the making of new bone tissue and the dissolving and disposing of the old bone cells may go out of balance, with new cells being created faster than old ones are being evacuated, causing abnormal bone formations which can bring on pain and other periodontal problems.[9]

Vitamin C also exerts a powerful influence on dental health. You get double duty out of this vitamin—in bone-building and gum-healing. All required minerals need a framework for laying down perfect bone. With too little vitamin C, that framework, made of a protein named collagen, can't be properly formed, and, therefore, neither can bone.

Just as vitamin C helps in forming collagen, so does it assist in the forming of connective tissue, a weblike fiber that binds cells together. Connective tissue in gums assists in the firming up of flesh to keep bacteria from penetrating to the tooth sockets and contributing to periodontal disease.

Vitamin C also helps to correct soggy, sore and bleeding gums. Longtime deficiencies of vitamin C make the collagen watery and weak.

Puffy gums which sometimes swell so much that they overlap part of the teeth, a condition called Vincent's disease or Trench Mouth, improves with the alternative dentist's treatment of vitamin C (500 mg or more), 200 mg of niacin and a 50 mg B-complex backup.

Today's dentists kill the infection with a local antiseptic — sometimes hydrogen peroxide — added to the nutritional regime above.

Stress Can Make You Dentally Ill!

While poor oral hygiene and diet plainly relate to tooth decay and periodontal problems, the relation of stress to these dental disorders is rarely considered. Yet the stresses of life can bring on cavities and gum diseases.

Researchers at Temple University School of Dentistry and the University of Alabama found that keeping calm, thinking soothing thoughts and learning to relax can help prevent tooth cavities and gum disorders.[10]

The Temple University group analyzed saliva of dental students prior to and after a 20 minute relaxation session. After the relaxation, the students' saliva became more watery, translucent and lower in content of harmful bacteria.

When a person is under stress — especially stress that never lets up — the saliva thickens, is less translucent and contains a far higher content of harmful bacteria.

Stress Attack: Beware Teeth And Gums!

Then salivary secretions are more capable of attacking tooth enamel.

University of Alabama researchers discovered that gum ailments, also, can often be attributed to stress.[11] Vincent's disease or trench mouth was once believed to be caused only by unsanitary living conditions in a combat environment such as the trenches of World War I.

Bacteria are not the only explanation, claim these investigators. Battle stress aggravates this ailment. Vincent's disease sufferers were found to have a high level of cortisol (an adrenal gland hormone) in their urine.[12]

The secretion of large amounts of cortisol lowers immune system response, allowing harmful bacteria to multiply more readily and rapidly.[13] Continued stress and emotional disorders cause even greater cortisol secretion and diminished immune response. More numerous enemy bacteria then attack tooth enamel and gums.

These researchers found that patients who have experienced negative, life-upsetting events often have deeper and more persistent anxiety and depression. Consequently, they seem to have more dental caries and gum disorders.[14]

Unsuspected Health Hazard

In cooperating with the dentist to preserve our teeth and gums through semi-annual checkups and cleanings, we may be bringing on a devastating condition through exposure to dental X-rays: cancer of the salivary (parotid) glands.[15]

So says researcher Susan Preston-Martin, Ph.D, associate professor of preventive medicine at the University of Southern California Cancer Center, who headed a team investigating this problem.

"Individuals who have had frequent dental X-rays — particularly in earlier decades when the amount of radiation necessary to achieve an X-ray image was many times higher than current technology requires, were found to be at highest risk," she states.[16]

Investigation of 408 patients with malignant and benign tumors was done through the USC Cancer Surveillance program, a registry of all new cancer cases diagnosed among Los Angeles County residents since 1972. Each case was carefully matched with a control in the same age and economic group.

Both cases and controls were interviewed regarding their histories of dental care.[17] Recall of dental history was validated for 25 percent of the pairs of cases and controls by checking dental records, which indicated comparable accuracy of information in two groups.

Cases with benign tumors and cases with malignant tumors had more cumulative radiation exposure of their parotid glands from dental X-rays than did controls.[18]

The study was undertaken when an earlier investigation related full-mouth dental X-rays before 1955 to cancer of the membrane covering the brain. Before the USC researchers started this project, it was known from studies of atomic blast survivors that salivary gland tumors could be caused by radiation. It was also known that 90 percent of exposure to radiation from man-made sources is from diagnostic X-rays.[19]

Even though radiation dosage used in dental X-rays is much lower than in the past, this source of radiation still contributes to an individual's chance of developing this rare cancer, states Dr. Preston-Martin, who indicates that the American Dental Association recommends X-rays only when clinically indicated.[20]

Seven Protective Nutrients

Of the seven nutrients mentioned above which help protect against tooth, gum and tooth socket deterioration — calcium, vitamin D, magnesium, vitamin A, niacin, vitamin B-complex, zinc and vitamin C — calcium deserves first mention.

Foods and supplements richest in calcium in milligrams per less than four ounce units are: sesame seeds, 1,200; kelp, 1,100; cheese, 700; brewer's yeast, 420; sardines and carob, 350; caviar, 280; soybeans and almonds, 230; torula yeast, 220; parsley, 200; brazil nuts, 190; watercress, salmon, and chickpeas, 150; egg yolk, beans, pistachios, lentils and kale, 130; sunflower seeds and cow's milk, 120; buckwheat, 110; maple syrup, cream and chard, 100; walnuts, 99; spinach, 93; endive, 81; pecans, 73; wheat germ, 72; peas, 70; peanuts, 69; eggs, 54 and oats, 53.

Best supplement and food sources of vitamin D in International Units per less than four ounce units are: cod liver oil, 20,000; sardines, 500; salmon, 400; tuna, 250; egg yolk, 160; sunflower seeds, 92; liver, 50; eggs, 48; butter, 40; cheese, 30; cream, 15; corn oil, 9.0; human milk, 6.0; cottage cheese and cow's milk, 4.0, bee pollen, 1.6 and bass, 1.0.

Many supplement and food sources are high in vitamin A content or its precursor. Here they are in International units per less than four ounce servings: cod liver oil, 200,000; sheep liver, 45,000; cow's liver, 44,000; calves' liver, 22.000; dandelion greens, 14,000; carrots, 11,000; yams, 9,000; kale, 8,900; parsley and turnip greens, 8,500; spinach, 8,100;

collard green and chard, 6,500; watercress, 5,000; red peppers, 4,400; squash, 4,000; egg yolk and cantaloupe, 3,400; endive, 3,300; persimmons and apricots, 2,700; broccoli, 2,500; pimentos, 22,300; swordfish, 2,100; romaine, 1.900; mangos, 1,800; papayas, 1,700; nectarines and pumpkin, 1,600; peaches and cheese, 1,300; eggs, 1,200; cherries, lettuce and cream, 1,000 and tomatoes and asparagus, 900.

Richest supplement and food sources of magnesium in milligrams per less than four ounce units are: dolomite, 13,000; kelp, 740; blackstrap molasses, 410; sunflower seeds. 350; wheat germ, 320; almonds, 270; soybeans, 240; brazil nuts, 220; bone meal, 170; pistachios and soy lecithin, 160; hazelnuts, 150; pecans and oats, 140; walnuts, 130; brown rice, 120; regular molasses, 81; chard, 65; spinch, 57; barley, 55; coconut, 44; salmon, 40; corn, 38; avocados, 37; bananas, 31, cheese, 30; tuna, 29 and potatoes and cashews, 27.

Best foods and supplements for zinc are the following in terms of milligrams per less than four ounce units: herring, 110; wheat germ, 14; sesame seeds, 10; torula yeast, 9.9; blackstrap molasses, 8.3; maple syrup, 7.5; liver, 7.0; soybeans, 6.7; sunflower seeds, 6.6; egg yolk, 5.5; lamb, 5.4; chicken, 4.8; regular molasses, 4.6; brewer's yeast, 3.9; oats, 3.7; bone meal, 3.6; rye, 3.4; whole wheat, 3.2; corn, 3.1; coconut and beef, 3.0; beets, turkey and walnuts, 2.8; barley, 2.7; beans and avocados, 2.4; peas, 2.3; bleu cheese, 2.2; eggs, 2.1 and buckwheat, 2.0.

Here are supplements and foods with the highest ratings for vitamin C content in milligrams per less than four ounce units: rose hips, 3,000; acerola cherries, 1,100; guavas, 240; black currants, 200; parsley, 170; green peppers, 110; watercress, 80; chives, 70; strawberries, 57; persimmons, 52; spinach, 51; oranges, 50; cabbage, 47; grapefruit, 38; papaya, 37; elderberries and kumquats, 36; dandelion greens and lemons, 35; cantaloupe, 33; green onions, 32; limes, 31; mangos, 27; loganberries, 24; tangerines and tomatoes, 23; squash, 22 and raspberries, romaine lettuce and pineapple, 17.

Richest supplement and food sources of niacin in milligrams per units of less than four ounces are: torula yeast, 100; brewer's yeast, 38; bee pollen, 19; peanuts, 17; liver, 16; salmon, 13; chicken and tuna, 12; swordfish and turkey, 11; halibut, 9.2; royal jelly, 8.2; veal, 7.8; sunflower seeds, 5.6; sardines and sesame seeds, 5.4; beef and alfalfa, 5.0; potatoes,

4.8; brown rice and wheat bran, 4.7; pinon nuts, 4.5; buckwheat and whole wheat, 4.3; wheat germ, 4.2; barley, 3.7; almonds, 3.5; peas, 2.6; beans, 2.4; millet, 2.3; soybeans and corn, 2.2; blackstrap molasses, 2.1 and lentils and chickpeas, 2.0.

Deviled Sardines

1 can (4 ounces) sardines in oil	½ t. sea salt
3 garlic cloves, Crushed	½ t. paprika
1 T. onion, minced	½ t. pepper
1 T. green pepper, minced	⅛ t. cayennetart,
1 T. prepared mustard	peeled and chopped
1 t. prepared horseradish	Juice of ½ lemon
1 T. spring water	Lemon and tomato wedges,
2 T. olive oil	pickles (optional)

Drain sardines and arrange on serving plate. Mix garlic, onion and green pepper. Add mustard, horseradish mixed with water and olive oil. Mix thoroughly. Add seasonings and lemon juice. Mix well and pour over sardines. Garnish with lemon and tomato wedges, and pickles (optional). Serve as appetizer with crackers, celery hearts. Serves 4.

Hot Stuffed Celery

Select stalks of celery having a deep curve. Fill with a mixture made from any of the following:

Peanut butter and sesame seeds	⅛ t. jalapeno pepper, minced
Cream cheese and grated carrots	Cheddar cheese and walnuts
or nuts and raisins	Cottage cheese and chopped cucumbers
Plain yogurt, fruit juice, wheat germ	

Use the stuffings for dates, prunes and apple halves.

CHAPTER 59

Hands,
Painful, Tingling
(Carpal Tunnel Syndrome)

By increasing their intake of vitamin B-6, some individuals have been able to avoid surgery for carpal tunnel syndrome, a disorder characterized by numbness, tingling and, often, pain in the hands or wrists.

Most prone to this ailment are individuals who eat much processed food, which is low in vitamin B-6, persons taking oral contraceptives, pregnant women, those with rheumatoid arthritis or diabetes, and the aged.

In order to understand the carpal tunnel syndrome drama, it is necessary to visualize the stage setting. The carpus is composed of eight small bones of the wrist, forming a tunnel around the median nerve.

A deficiency of vitamin B-6 is thought to bring about the above symptoms by putting pressure on the sensitive median nerve in one of two ways: (1) swelling fluid-containing membranes within the carpal tunnel or (2) thickening the ligament joining the two forearm bones at their ends, one or two inches from the start of the palm of the hand.

Intake of vitamin B-6 (pyridoxine) far above the required daily allowance (RDA) of two milligrams often corrects this ailment.

Right Foods Can Sometimes Right The Condition!

Can natural foods supply enough pyridoxine to manage carpal tunnel syndrome? Yes, in some instances, say nutrition-oriented physicians. But it could take a little more time and a lot more patience than if higher potencies of pyridoxine were supplied in a vitamin supplement.

The best sources of vitamin B-6 in milligrams per less than four ounce portions are: brewer's yeast, 4.0; brown rice, 3.6; whole wheat, 2.9; royal jelly, 2.4; soybeans, 2.0; rye, 1.8; lentils, 1.7; sunflower seeds and hazelnuts, 1.1; alfalfa, 1.00; salmon, 0.98; wheat germ, 0.92; tuna, 0.90; bran, 0.85; walnut, 0.73; peas and liver, 0.67; avocados, 0.60; beans, 0.57; cashews, peanuts, turkey, oats, chicken and beef, 0.40.

Karl Folkers, M.D., who has conducted many studies on pyridoxine, states that carpal tunnel syndrome and associated disorders such as bursitis of the shoulder, diabetes of pregnancy, myxedema, obesity, rheumatoid arthritis, and tennis elbow are so common that almost everybody would benefit from a daily intake of 25 mg of vitamin B-6.[1] This is more than 12 times the RDA and can be obtained in foods by following recipes at the end of this section.

Up-in-years individuals who have run a pyridoxine deficit for years often suffer from carpal tunnel syndrome and seem to benefit from the above supplementation.

Higher Potencies May Be Needed

In his nutritional explorations during the late 1960s and early 1970s, John Ellis, M.D., practicing in a tiny Texas town, observed that carpal tunnel syndrome could often be corrected by 10 to 20 times the RDA level of vitamin B-6.[2]

Dismissed at first as anecdotal, his findings began to attract attention of the medical profession when he and Dr. Karl Folkers conducted more than a dozen careful studies—some double-blind—which showed a direct relationship between a vitamin B-6 deficiency or dependency (a higher than average requirement) and carpal tunnel syndrome.

Ellis and Folkers' biochemical testing of 22 carpal tunnel syndrome patients revealed that all of them were vitamin B-6 deficient and, when given 50 to 300 mg of pyridoxine daily, responded to treatment within 12 weeks.[3]

Not long ago, University of Texas biochemists verified by experiment that a vitamin B-6 deficiency indeed underlies carpal tunnel syndrome.[4]

In an Ellis-Folkers double-blind, controlled study, 100 mg of oral vitamin B-6 daily controlled carpal tunnel syndrome. Look-alike placebo pills didn't![5] Natural foods rich in vitamin B-6 or pills of this vitamin are more appealing to carpal tunnel syndrome sufferers than the surgeon's scalpel.

Stuffed Zucchini

Lentils and onions offer an ideal savory base for tasty, tantilizing overgrown zucchini.

2 ounces brown lentils
1 large zucchini
1 medium onion, chopped
2 T. cold pressed oil
  (or olive oil)

1 medium carrot, grated
1 ounce wheat germ

Prepare lentils ahead by soaking in ample water for 24 hours. Place zucchini (whole) in oven on tray and bake until just tender. Meanwhile, rinse lentils and steam until just tender. Saute onion until golden and transparent. Cut cooked zucchini lengthwise and remove soft intention separating and discarding large seeds. Add grated carrot and lentils to onion. Mix well. Add center from zucchini to mixture, enough to make a well moistened stuffing. Compress stuffing into hollowed zucchini halves and sprinkle with a topping of wheat germ. Turn oven to 300 degrees and cook for 10 minutes. Serves 4.

Hawaiian Chicken Salad

1 c. pineapple (unsweetened), diced
2 c. cooked chicken, diced
¾ c. celery, chopped
½ c. walnuts or cashews, chopped
¼ c. green peppers, diced

½ c. cooked brown rice
½ c. homemade mayonnaise
1 t. season salt
½ t. dill

Mix together and refrigerate for 3 hours before serving. Serve on a bed of lettuce or sprouts. Makes 4 servings.

CHAPTER 60

Hearing Loss (Deafness)

Now, hear this!

Loss of hearing is preventable in most instances—if you know the two major reasons for it—reasons why the number of deaf has more than doubled in the past 40 years:

(1) Bombardment with twice as much ear-punishing noise and (2) nutrient-deficient diets that slowly sabotage the hearing apparatus— improper food selection, excessive junk foods, and unrealistic weight-loss regimes.

Rock music at full volume at home, in the car, and at live concerts probably contributes more to progressive deafness than any other single factor, because it reaches the potentially destructive 120 decibel (db) level.

It's A Matter Of Record

What does this mean? It means that the delicate ear mechanisms can't readily recover from the shock—stress—of super-loud music repeated for hours daily over a long period, as a study in the New England Journal of Medicine revealed.

Frederick L. Dey, M.D., Ph.D, found that at even a level of 10 decibels lower (110), ears of 16 percent of listeners would have difficulty recovering and suffer damage, very likely, permanent damage.[1] Hearing for two percent of the population can deteriorate at sustained noise levels of 100 db.

Imagine the wear and tear on ears of top-of-the-chart rock bands!

The son of an acquaintance of mine plays almost every night in a rock band, and you can't carry on a conversation with him without his asking, "What'd ya say?"..."Huh?"...or "Run that by me again."

The Encyclopedia of Common Diseases (Rodale Press) mentions that when Dr. James Jerger, of the Houston Speech and Hearing Center, tested a five-person rock combo, he found that three of the young men —all in their early twenties—had sustained a small but irreversible hearing loss.[2] After a concert, one of the three showed a temporary 50 db loss.

The sad part of rock is that innocent bystanders who live in the same house with a rock fan sacrifice some of their hearing, too.

Dr. Samuel Rosen, former clinical professor of Otology at Mount Sinai School of Medicine, some years ago told a symposium of the American Association for the Advancement of Science that long-time exposure to even an 85 db level of noise can cause gradual hearing loss.[3]

How We React To Noise Pollution

Further, he explained what happens physically with loud noises. Minute blood vessels in the ear contract—elsewhere in the head and body, too —reducing the flow of oxygen and nutrients to critical areas. When such noises are repeated, it takes even longer for these vessels to relax, causing permanent injury.[4]

Ability to hear high sounds diminishes first. In the cochlea, the snail-shaped part of the ear basic to hearing, little hairs rising from its walls pick up vibrations and change them into electrical impulses which the brain translates into sound or noise.[5]

Phillip Lee, otolaryngologist at the University Hospital in Iowa City, Iowa, fears that many rock fans will destroy the delicate and irreplaceable hairs in their inner ear and soon be unable to enjoy the music they love.[6]

Repeated loud noises and high-pitched sounds also destroy the hairs, and once they are gone, so goes your ability to hear the high-pitched sounds.

Few of us need a refresher course to recall sounds that hurt our ears: the blast of a motorcycle engine, the scream of an emergency vehicle's siren; the nerve-shattering chatter of a jack hammer, the roar of a jet plane taking off; an explosive sonic boom and earth-vibrating thunder.

Add to these the lesser noise pollutants at home and work and you have a harmful accumulation in ears that weren't built for incessant insults: the obnoxious noise of a power lawn mower and leaf blower, the shrill complaint of a food blender, the all-pervasive hum of a vacuum cleaner, the deafening din of industrial machinery, the clatter of typewriters, the whir or whine of computer wheels, the ringing or buzzing of telephones, even the jungle of human voices, the clatter of restaurant dishes, and a hundred other aural offenses that you may ignore, but your ears can't.

You can run or transfer away from some. Ear plugs can drown out part of the din, but they can also block sounds you have to hear. You can buy more quiet household appliances and appeal to the company where you work to install sound-damping equipment on noisy machinery. But, then, you run out of resources.

High-Fat Diet: Enemy Of Hearing?

However, noise pollution isn't the only cause of hearing loss, as stated earlier. Nutritional problems can bring on gradual deafness, too. Deposits of cholesterol and related substances can narrow arteries and capillaries in the ear and brain and cause slow starvation of ear tissue and deterioration of hearing.

A fascinating study of the Mabaan tribe of Africa by Dr. Samuel Rosen revealed that the Mabaans, who subsist mainly on fruits, vegetables and nuts—little saturated fat—rarely experience deafness at any age and no high blood pressure, no artery clogging or dietary deficiencies.[7]

Rosen then studied cardiovascular problems, hearing loss and diet in Finland, a country notorious for its high-fat diet. In a study, he found that hospital patients who followed a low-fat diet had hearing superior to those on the typical Finnish diet who were ten years younger.[8]

James T. Spencer, M.D., writing in the West Virginia Medical Journal, went a step beyond that of Dr. Rosen, restricting his patients' intake of refined sugars and starches, as well as fats, and saw a "phenomenal gain in hearing."[9]

Are You Starving Your Ears?

Can ears be malnourished? Yes, just like any other part of the head or body. Studies show that the hard-of-hearing often have low blood iodine.[10] Pregnant women who are low on iodine can transmit the trait of deafness to the infant.

Inasmuch as iodine is the major food of the thyroid gland (See the section on Low Thyroid Function), a low intake of this chemical element can cause more than 64 symptoms, including poor hearing.

A study in China revealed that in regions where the soil is low in iodine —goiter belts—many children were hard-of-hearing. It took three years of iodine supplementation to bring them back to normal hearing.[11]

Only tiny amounts of iodine are needed. Here are some supplements and foods rich in iodine, listed in milligrams per less than four ounce units: kelp, 180; cod liver oil, 0.84; haddock, 0.31; cod, 0.14; chard and beans, 0.10; perch,, 0.074; sunflower seeds, 0.070 and herring, 0.052.

Most alternative doctors recommend that their iodine-deficient patients take a 225 mcg kelp tablet daily, rather than try to derive iodine from food, because some foods are grown in iodine-deficient soil.

Many Nutrients Influence Hearing

Over and above iodine, several vitamins are needed to preserve normal hearing: vitamin A, B-complex—C and D. In the early 1930s, Sir Edward Mellanby showed with laboratory animals that a deficiency of vitamin A can cause difficulty in hearing and even deafness.[12]

Oswald A. Roels, of Columbia University, disclosed the reason why: with insufficient vitamin A, cell membranes break down. When this breakdown occurs in the ear, it contributes to deafness. Roels concluded that diminished hearing is caused not so much by aging as by a deficiency of vitamin A.[13]

Similarly, too little intake of B-complex vitamins contributes to neuritis, inflammation of the nerves, interfering with sound transmission, making for partial deafness. Several of my alternative doctor friends have helped correct this condition by asking their patients to eat beef liver three or four times a week and take a tablespoon of brewer's yeast daily in freshly squeezed fruit juice. Other physicians I know recommend a vitamin B-complex tablet daily, usually with 50 mg in its major fractions.

Strictly by accident, G. Gordon, M.D., of the Hard-of-Hearing Clinic at the Medical College of Alabama, discovered a formula which dramatically improved hearing. Treating anemia, digestive problems, and nervous exhaustion, Dr. Gordon advised his patients to take brewer's yeast, glutamic acid (a nutrient usually derived from wheat gluten) an important food of the brain, liver extract and vitamin C.[14]

This regime helped the conditions for which it was intended, but also upgraded hearing in 76 percent of the patients, particularly in recovering their ability to hear high tones.[15]

Deficiency Of Vitamin D And Limited Hearing

As in the above study, researchers sometimes come up with unexpected answers to problems. Bone and teeth abnormalities are commonly traced to vitamin D lack, but how can this nutrient possibly have anything to do with hearing loss?

That was what otolaryngologists at London Hospital wondered until they ran into two cases directly related to vitamin D deficiency.[16]

A 35-year old Asian man who had followed a vegetarian diet for some years was found to have a dangerously low blood level of vitamin D and osteomalacia, softening of bones surrounding the middle and inner ear. (See the Section on Osteomalacia.) If these bones are hardened — also apparently too soft — they can't transmit sound properly.[17]

Vegetarianism furnishes very little vitamin D, which comes mainly from fish and fish oils, eggs, liver, and dairy products. About the only food with a fair amount of vitamin D that a strict vegetarian would eat is sunflower seeds. Within two months of vitamin D supplementation, this patient's hearing improved.[18]

A second case on the heels of the first, a 49-year old vagrant who was partially deaf, was found to have low blood levels of vitamin D and osteomalacia of ear bones, as well as muscle weakness. Vitamin D supplementation upgraded his hearing, too.[19]

Certainly there are other causes of hearing loss than long exposure to loud sounds and nutritional deficiencies: inherited ear defects, damage done by bacterial and virus infections, accidents to the ear and accumulation of excessive ear wax, for example. However, most deafness results from noise abuse and nutritional short-changing.

So let's deal with individual nutrients and the foods containing the highest amounts of them. Iodine was covered earlier, so let's begin with vitamin A, hardly an original part of the alphabet for a start. Here are supplements and foods richest in this vitamin or its precursor (in vegetables and fruit) in International Units per portions of less than four ounces:

Cod liver oil, 200,000; sheep liver, 45,000; beef liver, 44,000; dandelion greens, 14,000; carrots, 11,000; yams, 9,000; kale, 8,900; parsley and turnip greens, 8,500; spinach, 8,100; collard greens and chard, 6,500; watercress, 5,000; red peppers, 4,400; squash, 4,000; egg yolk and cantaloupe, 3,400; endive, 3,300; persimmons and apricots, 2,700; broccoli, 2,500; pimentos, 2,300; swordfish, 2,100; whitefish, 2,000; romaine, 1,900; mangoes, 1,800; papayas, 1,700; nectarines and pumpkin, 1,600; peaches and cheeses, 1,300; eggs, 1,200, and cherries, lettuce and cream, 1,000.

So far as B-complex is concerned, it is much easier to take a tablet or capsule with 50 mg in major fractions of this vitamin than supplements or foods. But for those who prefer to go the latter route, let me name seven prime sources of B-complex: brewer's yeast, torula yeast, sunflower seeds, wheat germ, liver, royal jelly and soybeans.

These are the supplements and foods richest in vitamin C in milligrams per less than four ounce units: rose hips, 3,000; acerola cherries, 1,100; guavas, 240; black currants, 200; parsley, 170; green peppers, 110; watercress, 80; chives, 70; strawberries, 57; persimmons, 52; spinach, 51; oranges, 50; cabbage, 47; grapefruit, 38; papaya, 37; elderberries and kumquats, 36; dandelion greens and lemons, 35; cantaloupe, 33; green onions, 32; limes, 31; mangoes, 27; loganberries, 24; tangerines and tomatoes, 23; squash, 22 and raspberries and romaine lettuce, 18.

Best supplement and food bets for vitamin D in International Units per portions of less than four ounces are: cod liver oil, 20,000; sardines, 500; salmon, 400; tuna, 250; egg yolk, 160; sunflower seeds, 92; liver, 50; eggs, 48; butter, 40; cheeses, 30; cream, 15; corn oil, 9.0; human milk, 6.0; cottage cheese and cow's milk, 4.0, bee pollen, 1.6 and bass, 1.0.

CHAPTER 61

Heart Problems

Have a heart for your heart — and your arteries, too!

A little tender, loving care is the best insurance against a heart attack, stroke, or damage to the heart itself. Elsewhere, we have dealt with 20 natural ways to lower cholesterol or to keep it low and with drugless ways of reducing high blood pressure and keeping arteries free-flowing.

One of the key problems is preventing the blood from abnormal clotting and reducing the flow dangerously. Various conditions can cause this: surgery, a break or lesion in an artery, nutritional deficiency, or smoking — or a combination.

A study reveals that patients who were not given supplements of vitamin E and calcium before surgery had twice as many blood clots as those who received these nutrients and six times as many blood clots in the lungs and nine times as many deaths from such blockages.[1]

Folk Remedies To The Rescue

Numerous experiments show that garlic and onions eaten regularly tend to keep blood platelets slippery so that they can't mass together abnormally to form clots. Platelets are disc-shaped parts of blood cells important to clotting. Odorless garlic appears to work as well as the fresh garlic.

Eating cold-water fish—anchovies, cod, herring, salmon and sardines —or consuming Omega 3 oil from these fish also helps to assure slippery platelets.

A deficiency of vitamin C contributes to roughness of the interior (intima) of arteries and to susceptibility to breaks and the rush of clotting agents to cement them over. Sometimes the clotting process continues too long and blockages form.

Dr. Anthony Verlangieri, while at Rutgers University, demonstrated deterioration of arteries by feeding rabbits too little vitamin C and, then, returning them to smoothness by feeding the animals sufficient amounts of this nutrient.[2]

Super-Heavyweights, Beware!

Another enemy to a healthy heart and arteries is obesity — even appreciable overweight, in some instances. Obesity and less extreme overweight can raise cholesterol and triglyceride levels and contribute to high blood pressure. Imagine the stress on the heart of pumping blood through two miles of extra arteries for each pound of fat.

A deadly duo, obesity and high blood pressure, encourage congestive heart failure, coronary heart disease and sudden death. With appreciable weight loss comes reduced blood pressure. Several studies have shown that a concentration of fat in the belly makes a person much more prone to heart attack.

Fewer calories and more exercise—especially bending at the mid-section — is an excellent formula for losing weight and lessening the chance of heart attack.

A tape measure can tell if you're endangered by a big belly. Doctors say that if the circumference of the waist is larger than that of the hips, it's time to work off the suet.[3]

Long-time obesity can exert such stress on the heart that the left ventrical wall thickens, the heart changes dimensions and its stroke volume and blood output are altered. The longer the excess fat stays on, the worse the heart damage becomes.[4]

First-Aid From Carnitine

Now a new supplement that's actually old can help the heart in two ways: by contributing to weight loss and strengthening the Big Pump. I'm talking about L-carnitine, found abundantly in meat ("carne" in Spanish, from which it gets its name.)

Foods richest in L-carnitine are lamb, beef, fish, chicken, brewer's yeast, alfalfa and wheat. How does L-carnitine help burn off excess weight? In a unique manner.

L-carnitine transports fat into the mitochondria, many mini furnaces inside cells, so that it burns and gives us energy and warmth. An enzyme carries the fat to the cell membrane but can't get it through without L-carnitine. A shortage of carnitine can cause fat (triglycerides) to circulate in the blood and be stored, rather than burned.

So the reason for some obesity and overweight is a deficiency of carnitine. A surprising fact about this nutrient is that it can be made by the body from lysine and methionine acted upon by vitamin C, B-6, and niacin.

Then why is it sometimes deficient? Nutrient raw materials aren't always plentiful, due to poor diet or poor absorption or faulty enzymes, among other reasons. This is why carnitine supplements may be necessary — one to three grams daily, my alternative doctors tell me.

In some instances, enough carnitine is in circulation, but, through an abnormality, is not delivered to the cells of muscles, causing weakness in all muscles, including the heart. Supplementary carnitine usually restores muscle strength and, at the same time, burns away fat which has invaded the liver, heart, kidney and muscle tissues.

Without sufficient L-carnitine, the heart can become enlarged and act the same as if it were suffering from congestive heart failure. Maximum heart rate decreases, blood pressure plummets, and the ability of the heart diminishes, sometimes to the point of arrest and death.[5]

A spiritual base in faith, a daily exercise program, a positive outlook and a diet of much raw fruits and vegetables, whole grains and lightly cooked meats and fish help keep my heart strong and efficient and my health excellent.

I have emphasized here natural foods and supplements. In pulling up a zipper on this section, I repeat that garlic, onions, and coldwater fish or fish oils can help to prevent abnormal blood-clotting; vitamin C can contribute to assuring integrity of arteries, and carnitine can guard the heart and arteries of the obese and normal-weights.

Supplements and foods richest in vitamin C in milligrams per units of less than four ounces are: rose hips, 3,000; acerola cherries, 1,100; guavas, 240; black currants, 200; parsley, 170; green peppers, 110; watercress,

80; chives, 70; strawberries, 57; persimmons, 51; spinach, 51; oranges, 50; cabbage, 47; grapefruit, 38; papaya, 37; elderberries and kumquats, 36; dandelion greens and lemons, 35; cantaloupe, 33; green onions 32; limes, 31; mangoes, 27; loganberries, 24; tangerines and tomatoes, 23; squash, 22; raspberries and romaine lettuce, 18 and pineapple, 17.

CHAPTER 62

Hemorrhoids

One of the most misunderstood physical disorders is hemorrhoids. The general impression is that they are varicose veins of the anus, an opinion held for many years.

W.H.F. Thomson, a British physician, blasted this notion when he performed both radiological and other exams of the anal area of 100 babies who had died soon after birth, discovering three small cushions of mucous-like material with blood vessels.[1] Most of today's physiologists believe that these pads help make it possible to keep waste matter contained.

Origin Of Hemorrhoids

Sometimes straining to dislodge hard fecal masses causes super-engorgement of these cushions with blood and swelling of the tissues. Each time a firm fecal mass powers through the anal canal its action is like that of a "ramrod forced down the barrel of a rifle," as stated in the book, Medical Applications of Clinical Nutrition (Keats Publishing, Inc.)[2]

Constant repetition of this action ruptures the attachment of these pads from the muscular valve which opens to permit passage of wastes (the sphincter) and pushes them toward or even out of the anal aperture.[3]

Itching, swelling, pain, and bleeding are the result.

The Sane Treatment

The basic treatment is the same as the best preventive measure: a diet rich in fiber from fresh vegetables, fruits, and bran. (See the section on

Constipation). Sufficient fiber assures the gentle passing through of soft, bulky and moist stools—particularly when the person drinks eight to nine glasses of water daily. Hemorrhoids are a rarity among the Zulus, pastoral people of Africa who eat only unrefined food.[4]

An in-depth University of Edinburgh study of various bran preparations reveals that unprocessed bran (coarse bran) with its sponge-like, water-holding capacity, is the preferred treatment for colonic ailments, which include hemorrhoids.[5]

Relieving Hemorrhoids

Bernard A.L. Wissmer, M.D., of the Medical Policlinic of the University of Geneva (Switzerland), has reported thousands of patients cured with a bioflavonoid compound including rutin, a byproduct of milling buckwheat, and citrus peel bioflavonoid (hesperidin).[6]

Knowing the reputation of bioflavonoids for reducing capillary fragility, Dr. Wissmer set out to relieve discomfort and pain of hemorroid sufferers and to spare them from surgery, if possible.[7] (See the section on Miscarriages in relation to capillary fragility)

He did both. Wissmer initially conducted an experiment with 250 patients who had various types of hemorrhoids—internal and external. His regime was four to six 100 mg capsules of bioflavonoid compounds daily for a week, then two to three daily for three or four more weeks.[8]

Relief from hemorrhaging and pain came in two to five days. Anascopic and rectoscopic exams showed a dramatic change to normal.

Ninety-seven of 148 patients with chronic internal hemorrhoids experienced complete healing with the bioflavonoids.[9] Significant improvement was shown in 32 of the cases, although there remained occasional slight bleeding. Sixteen patients manifested some betterment: less pain and less frequent bleeding. A mere three patients showed no improvement and, in time, had to resort to surgery.

Taming The Toughest Kind

With the same regime, Dr. Wissmer scored phenomenally with the most resistant form of hemorrhoids: external. Twenty-eight out of 32 patients were completely cured.[10]

In another experiment, individuals deprived of vitamin B-6 developed bleeding hemorrhoids, and were cured of them when their diet was supplemented with 10 mg of this vitamin after each meal.[11]

Many preventive medicine practitioners have found pregnant women to be severely deficient in vitamin B-6 and also prone to develop hemorrhoids.

It is difficult but possible to plan meals with a content of at least 10 mg of vitamin B-6 with each one. The following foods and supplements are the richest in this vitamin in milligrams per less than a four ounce serving:

Brewer's yeast, 4.0; brown rice, 3.6; whole wheat, 2.9; royal jelly, 2.4; soybeans, 2.0; rye, 1.8; lentils, 1.7; sunflower seeds and hazelnuts, 1.1; alfalfa, 1.00; salmon, 0.98; wheat germ, 0.92; tuna, 0.90; bran, 0.85; walnuts, 0.73; peas and liver, 0.67; avocados, 0.60; beans, 0.57 and cashews, peanuts, turkey, oats, chicken and beef, 0.40.

Other Tips

Prevention of hemorrhoids and relief from their symptoms can be done in the following ways:

1. By regular exercise to keep bowels moving. (This is in addition to ingesting plenty of fiber.)

2. By a natural supplement. Dr. Linus Pauling says that large amounts of vitamin C will assure taking care of the fundamental problem: keeping stools soft, liquid and easily moved, rather than having to resort to commercial topical salves.[12]

3. By long, healing, warm baths. Alternative doctors often recommend 10 to 20 minutes in the bath three or four times daily. A gentle spreading of the cheeks will allow the water to soothe inflamed tissue and, of course, to cleanse it.

4. By applying vitamin E topically after a cleansing, soothing bath. This is more relieving than using commercial applications, states Dr. Pauling.[13]

Words Of Warning

Rectal bleeding is nothing to treat by yourself—if it is painful or not.

Be sure and see your doctor for a rectal examination. In rare cases, what seems to be a hemorrhoid turns out to be a tumor.

Folklore: you won't find this in any medical book, but applying the inside of a banana peel topically to the hemorrhoid brings instant relief.

CHAPTER 63

Herpes Simplex (Including Genital Herpes)

Only a miracle can cure Herpes Simplex II. Once a person has it, he or she has it for life. But the news isn't totally bad. At least, genital herpes can be kept under control, if managed in the proper way.

This virus is similar to Herpes Simplex I, which causes cold sores and is not sexually transmitted. Genital herpes is passed on mainly by sexual relations. However, it can be transmitted by towels and general physical contact. Genital herpes presents clusters of small blisters on and around the male or female genitals, burning and itching, and a high fever.[1]

These symptoms characteristically disappear in about two weeks, and some patients have a false feeling of security—false, because the virus goes into hiding within the nerve fibers, safe from the immune system army, ready again for attack when the person is struck with emotional stress, deep fatigue, fever or an infection.[2]

Conduct of the herpes virus is strange. It can attack often and with intensity, with blisters appearing at the original site, or only a few more times or even stay dormant for a lifetime.[3]

How To Keep It Under Control

Richard Kunin, M.D., of San Francisco, tells me that he controls patients' Herpes II by natural means:[4]

1. Improving the diet and having the patient take a therapeutic-type daily vitamin to offer the immune system proper support.

2. Cotton swab dabbing of flare-up blisters for five to ten minutes with the sodium ascorbate form of vitamin C with water—other forms could prove irritating—sometimes followed up by dabbing natural vitamin E on the infected areas. His source is a vitamin E capsule cut in two.

3. Recommending that patients who need damaged tissue repaired take vitamin A in slowly increasing doses up to 30,000 I.U. and 100 mg of zinc three times daily for an entire week.

4. Taking a lysine supplement, following the dose mentioned on the bottle.

Lysine, an amino acid, is effective in controlling the herpes virus, but not in lysine-rich foods, because these foods also contain arginine, an amino acid on which the herpes virus thrives.[5]

Much More Than Foods Involved

Stressors of various kinds also tend to depress the immune system and invite attacks of herpes simplex I and II. Numerous studies show that an imminent and feared college exam, fever, physical exhaustion, menstruation or even sunburn can turn on an attack of cold sores, fever blisters or small mouth ulcers.[6]

A continuing study of 10 individuals revealed that repeated attacks of herpes simplex were brought on by conflict, frustration, high anxiety or guilt.[7]

An outbreak of genital herpes blisters and related symptoms often occurred when individuals were threatened by stressful events in the offing, when in negative moods, or lacking social support. Their immune system showed definite depression, too.[8]

An excellent book, Who Gets Sick (Peak Press) by Blair Justice, cites many examples of stressors which depress the immune system and permit outbreaks of latent herpes simplex I and II.

It is important to remember that nutritional support and positivism can often keep the immune system strong enough to prevent or at least minimize the number of attacks of these harmful viruses.[9]

Chicken A La Scheer

2 c. cooked chicken, diced	1 T. vegetable paste
2 egg yolks, hard boiled	½ t. vegetable salt
½ green pepper, diced	½ t. paprika
½ sweet red pepper, diced	3 egg yolks, beaten
1 c. cream	1 t. wheat germ

In a double boiler, make a sauce of the cream, vegetable paste and beaten egg yolks. Add seasonings and other ingredients. Serve very hot.

Tebula
(An unusual salad that will surprise you!)

4 tomatoes, chopped	½ c. lemon juice
2 cucumbers, peeled and chopped	¼ c. olive oil
1 c. Bulgar wheat or cream of wheat	Sea salt to taste

Put wheat in a bowl and cover with boiling water. Set aside for 2 to 3 hours. Drain well. Toss wheat with chopped vegetables, sea salt, lemon juice and oil. Green onions and parsley may be substituted for vegetables as a variation.

The Green Breakfast

1 apple, cored and diced	Spring water or apple juice
(or 1 slice fresh pineapple, cubed)	1½ T. wheat germ
¼ c. soaked raisins	1 T. lecithin granules
¾ c. 5-inch lengths wheat grass,	2 T. unhulled sesame seeds
clipped into 1-inch lengths	1 t. kelp

Put apple, raisins, kelp, wheat grass and enough spring water or juice to blend in blender. Blend until smooth. Combine remaining ingredients in a cereal bowl and pour wheat grass mixture over all. Makes 1 serving.

CHAPTER 64

Hiatus Hernia

To the sufferer from hiatus hernia, it is no comfort that almost half of the U.S. population also experiences this misery: regurgitation of foods and/or liquid, a burning sensation and a pain under the breastbone.

This unpleasant disorder is caused by the upper part of the stomach doing what it's not supposed to do, bulging upward through the diaphragm opening into the esophagus, a long tube for delivering food from mouth to stomach.

Common in the United States and uncommmon in Third World Countries, hiatus hernia seems to have two causes: the low-fiber diet with its consequent constipation and the high pressure exerted to move out waste matter.[1]

Some observers state that straining at the stool exerts more upward pressure on the stomach than weight-lifting. One authority also attributes hiatus hernia to what he considers an abnormal position, sitting on a raised toilet seat, rather than squatting, as is common in Third World countries.[2] Another authority thinks it originates from flabbiness from lack of exercise.[3]

Any Relief In Sight?

This special kind of indigestion grows worse when the patient lies down. A pile of pillows under the head may not alleviate the condition. Some sufferers have gained a measure of relief by sleeping on a recliner chair or a hospital bed which can raise them to almost a sitting position.

Alternative doctors tell me that there is a danger in trying to cope with the burning sensation by taking antacids, which may block hydrochloric acid from digesting food. Eliminating alcohol, coffee and smoking offers relief to some sufferers. Although a low fiber diet helps bring on constipation and hiatus hernia, graduating to a high fiber diet and improving elimination doesn't necessarily bring instantaneous positive results.

Whole grains, vegetables and fruits can help in time. Here are some of the highest fiber foods with ratings according to the percentage of fiber in them: raspberries, 47; pears, 25; melon, 22; strawberries, 19; cabbage, 18; asparagus, 17; cucumber, 14; cauliflower, 13; radishes, 12; apples, 10; carrots, 8.8; green peas, 8.7; spinach, 8.1; onions, 5.0; beans and lentils, 4.1; potato, 3,1; whole wheat, 2.9; brown rice, 0.7 and whole wheat flour, 0.4.

The problem with taking commercial fibers is that, for the most part, they are partitioned products, rather than being derived from whole fruit, vegetables, grains and seeds, as is one fiber formula. Dr. Jonathan Wright describes partitioning of foods in a novel way: "It's like pushing a piece of dry wall through a tomato."

Dr. Robert Downs, who heads the Southwest Center of the Healing Arts in Albuquerque, New Mexico, recommends a special concoction to bring relief from hiatus hernia when sipped often during the day: one part of aloe vera juice and four parts of papaya juice blended fifty-fifty with sugar-free gingerale or club soda.[4]

Cabbage juice may also help the hernia, he says.[5] (See the Section on Ulcers, Stomach.)

Although these recommendations may not clear up hiatus hernia, they can help to bring relief from its most distressing symptoms.

Papaya Fruit Bowl

1 large papaya (½ per person)	6 ounces cashews (almonds or brazil),
3 fresh apricots, diced	ground
6 fresh strawberries, halved	4 raspberries, ground
1 kiwi fruit	

Remove seeds from each papaya half. Place pieces of apricots in papaya shell, followed by strawberries and raspberries. Peel kiwi fruit and slice on top. Sprinkle ground nuts on top of fruit.

Strawberry Fibermilk

2 T. fiber

2 c. blended strawberries

⅓ c. raw honey or 2 very ripe bananas

2 T. nutritional yeast

2 c. certified raw milk

Blend and serve.

CHAPTER 65

Hiccups

Considered to be a nuisance, rather than a legitimate ailment, hiccups can be serious if they persist for more than a few days, using up too much precious oxygen.

Then it's time to visit the Emergency Room of your nearest hospital or your family doctor!

Hiccups is a "too" disorder—caused by eating too fast—gulping food —eating or drinking too much or eating or drinking too cold or too hot foods or beverages.

So Many Remedies, But Do They Work?

In my many years of fascination with folk remedies, I have collected so many hiccups folk therapies that I haven't had hiccups often enough to try them all.

I hate even to tell you the first one, because the food you use is anything but a health food: a teaspoon of dry, granulated sugar. It has worked for me and many in my TV audience.

Recently, I learned that a respected medical doctor, Edgar E. Engleman, M.D., a faculty member of the University of California School of Medicine in San Francisco and two associates tried the sugar cure on 20 patients and scored with a complete and immediate end to the hiccups in 19 patients.[1] This was no small achievement, because many of the patients had hiccupped their way through a number of days—one for six whole weeks.

A venturesome physician who was induced by a friend to eat a slice of lemon soaked in angostura bitters, lost his hiccups and recommended the cure in the letters section of a medical journal.

The Water Cure

The Great Water Cure has several variations. You drink a tall glass of ice cold water. Or you slowly sip a cup of warm water. Now, with either the cold or hot water, you drink with plugs in your ears.

Another version is holding your ears shut with fingers while someone else slowly pours the water into you. Still another variation is sipping honey mixed with a little lukewarm water. No fingers in the ears this time.

One of the oldest home hiccup therapies is breathing into a paper bag held tightly around your mouth. This one has worked for me. Some of my friends have put an end to their hiccups merely by holding their breath as long as they could without perishing.

Very few have perished!

CHAPTER 66

High Blood Pressure, Hypertension

Hypertension is often called the 'Quiet Killer' for the good reason that it gives no sign of the undercover damage it may be doing: (1) weakening blood vessel walls; (2) causing aneurysms, abnormal expanding or hazardous ballooning of the artery wall which, if exploded, can bring on stroke, heart attack and internal bleeding; (3) contributing to congestive heart failure and kidney damage.

The Framingham study found that men with blood pressure higher than 16O/95 were two to three times more prone to suffer stroke or develop heart disease. The first number above is systolic pressure, the amount of force applied to the walls of the arteries when the heart is pumping. The second number is the amount of force applied when the heart is resting between pumpings.

It makes good sense to have your blood pressure checked by your doctor at least twice a year. (Please see the list of alternative doctors in the back of the book.)

Causes Of Hypertension

One or more of the following major factors can boost blood pressure: genetic programming, cigarette smoking, poor diet, stress, under-exercising, overweight or obesity and drinking soft water.

Little can be done about our genes without divine intervention. However, something can be done about the rest of these factors.

Smokers pay for their cigarettes at least twice: in the store and in their hearts, arteries, lungs, and elsewhere in their body. Hypertension is common to cigarette smokers. Individuals who smoke a package daily risk twice the danger of heart attacks as non-smokers.[1] Narrowed arteries caused by smoking force the heart to work harder and raise the blood pressure. Nicotine speeds up the heartbeat, increasing the heart's need for oxygen, while carbon monoxide in the smoke lessens the blood's ability to deliver oxygen. Smoking is slow suicide.[2]

Diet Does It — Or Undoes It!

A generous intake of salt (sodium chloride) remains the major villain in the hypertension scenario, but is this justified? Authorities are almost evenly divided on the subject. Many feel that other issues are far more important.

There is general agreement that the tendency of some to respond to excessive sodium with high blood pressure is inherited.

A generous intake of sodium actually increases the volume of blood, because sodium attracts water to itself, and, therefore, contributes to higher blood pressure. A low-sodium diet does the reverse: it lessens blood volume and, so, lowers blood pressure.[3]

The Case For Potassium

Newest studies point out that sodium intake contributes less to high blood pressure than the ratio of sodium to potassium.[4]

Not long ago, a study by the University of California, San Diego, School of Medicine revealed that a diet high in potassium-rich foods could lower the risk of stroke by as much as 40 percent, regardless of other risk elements such as age, blood pressure, cholesterol level, smoking and weight.

Dr. Elizabeth Barrett-Connor and Kay Tee Khaw, who co-authored a paper based on an ongoing study of 5,000 residents of Rancho Bernardo, a nearby suburb, advised that people take an extra helping of a potassium-rich food, rather than a potassium supplement—for example, an extra banana or some fresh broccoli.[5]

Best Sources

In addition to the two above-mentioned foods, she named other vegetables and fruits with a high potassium content: avocado, Brussels sprouts, cauliflower, potatoes (with skins) cantaloupe, dates, prunes and raisins.

Other potassium-rich foods in terms of milligrams per less than a four ounce serving are: beans, 1,200; parsley, 1,000; peas, 1,000; pistachios, 980; wheat germ, 950; sunflower seeds, 920; chickpeas, 800; almonds, 770; sesame seeds and brazil nuts, 720; peanuts, 670 and pecans, 600.

A fascinating aspect of the Barrett-Connor and Khaw study was that test subjects whose dietary levels of potassium were high had a lower risk of stroke, despite their blood pressure level.[6]

Other tests of rats and human beings show that added potassium can help to lower high blood pressure. Another study reveals that individuals who take in ample amounts of potassium have low blood pressures.[7]

Calcium Helps, Too!

Numerous studies indicate that calcium deficiency has a closer tie-in with high blood pressure than high-sodium or low potassium intakes.[8]

In a health and nutrition study (HANES I), 17 nutrients were examined in relation to 10,372 adults who had no history of high blood pressure and who did not deliberately change their eating habits. Calcium was the only nutrient significantly, consistently and independently associated with blood pressure among persons not previously diagnosed as hypertensives.[9]

Still another study disclosed that when 26 patients with essential hypertension—and no history of hypercalcemia or calcium stones—were given two grams of calcium carbonate daily for three months, 16 of them showed a diastolic decline of at least 10 mm Hg) and reduced blood pressure from an average 160/94 to 128/81.[10]

Calcium And More

Ratio of calcium to phosphorus—ideal is generally 2 to 1 3/4 to one—has a relationship to blood pressure. When calcium ratio to phosphorus is low, hypertension results, reveals a study in Nutrition Reviews.[11]

When a calcium supplement is mated with vitamin D to make sure it is properly absorbed, blood pressure is lowered more than by calcium alone.[12]

In one study of women between 55 and 80, those who took in 800 mg of calcium and 400 I.U. of vitamin D showed a significantly lower systolic blood pressure than those on look-alike placebos.[13]

Marvelous Magnesium

Another study indicates that when the body's magnesium supply runs down and intake of this mineral is low, reversible high blood pressure results. Researchers also discovered that half of magnesium-depleted patients show high blood pressure and that their blood pressure returns to normal with magnesium supplements.[14]

An animal study also bears this out. On a moderate or extremely magnesium-deficient diet for three months, rats showed a significantly raised blood pressure and a decrease of circulation through fine capillaries. Rats on their usual diet (controls) showed no such change.[15]

In a survey of 1,000 essential hypertensives, approximately 4.5 percent had subnormal levels of magnesium. Whatever their potassium levels, these test subjects needed more anti-hypertensive drugs to control blood pressure than hypertensives with normal magnesium levels.[16]

Stress Management

Many studies show that stress elevates blood pressure, sometimes keeping it elevated. So identify your stresses and learn how to cope with them. (See the Section called Stress.) Regular exercise helps to lower blood pressure in many ways: (1) by relieving stress, one cause for elevated blood pressure; (2) by keeping arteries flexible; (3) by circulating blood more widely and evenly, rather than permitting it to put undue pressure in only certain body systems.

An in-depth study of Dr. Jiri A. Kral, a professor at the Charles University in Prague, Czechoslovakia, reported that fifteen to twenty minutes after physical exercise, systolic blood pressure drops and, to a lesser degree, so does the diastolic blood pressure. The decline is more significant in persons with high blood pressure than in those with normal blood pressure.[17]

Dr. Kral concludes that exercise is valuable to preventing and lowering hypertension. Many researchers believe that physical inactivity makes blood vessels less able to adapt to future physical activity. Putting it in another way, the less a person exercises, the less capable he or she is of doing it and the more difficult it is for blood vessels to adapt.

Overweight And Obesity: A Double Burden

A physician friend likens being overweight by 100 pounds to carrying around a 100 pound sack of meal on your back. That's just one of two burdens. The other is the two miles of arteries through which the heart has to pump for each extra pound of fat.

Do you wonder that the heart is stressed and that blood pressure sometimes soars?

Numerous studies reveal a direct relationship between increased body weight and blood pressure. As one loses excess weight, the blood pressure reduces proportionately. Such weight and blood pressure reduction is independent of how much sodium one eats.

Maintaining ideal body weight helps to prevent hypertension, although this is not a gilt-edged guarantee. On the other hand, overweight test subjects are four times more likely to develop hypertension than matched lean persons, discloses one study.

Lean individuals with high blood pressure have been found more likely to gain weight than individuals with normal blood pressure. The reason? Not known at this time. Losing weight isn't the universal answer, although an excellent start, say some researchers. This must be combined with other factors mentioned above.

Sugar And Hypertension

Studies have shown that the incidence of hypertension is low in rural parts of less developed countries, in Africa and India, where refined sugar intake is low. There is also a direct relationship between increased high blood pressure and increased daily sugar intake in advanced countries.

Don't tell Richard A. Ahrens, Ph.D, of the University of Maryland's

College of Human Ecology, that refined sugar has little to do with hypertension. His studies put white sugar on the blacklist. Merely by giving supplemental sugar to lab animals and human beings, he has been able to raise blood pressure at will.[18]

Results of his studies lead Dr. Ahrens to believe that sugar contributes to sodium retention, which, in turn, raises blood pressure.[19]

Beware Of Heavy Meals!

Almost everybody has heard of a person who has suffered a heart attack after the pleasurable gluttony of a Thanksgiving or Christmas feast. Yes, Henry the Eighth-size meals have been shown to boost blood pressure.

Crash dieting—starvation, followed by uncontrolled binge eating—can do the same thing. Animal experiments, more than those with human beings, bear this out, revealing that a repetition of starvation followed by overeating leads to hypertension.

So much emphasis is placed on foods that few writers touch upon something equally important: the water we drink. Numerous studies show that soft water contributes to hypertension and heart attacks. Yet many homes have all their water processed to become soft. In this instance, it is better to switch to bottled spring water.

From this evidence, we readily see that there's a lot more to keeping blood pressure moderate or lowering high blood pressure than just cutting down on sodium intake.

CHAPTER 67

Hoarseness (Laryngitis, Voice Problems)

Yelling at the top of your lungs for hours to cheer the home team on can cost you a raw throat, scratchy vocal cords and difficulty in talking.

Sometimes you can't talk at all, especially if a cold strikes at the same time. This condition is called laryngitis, another word for frustration, because, all of a sudden, you have to communicate in sign language. Ugh!

In more rare instances, hoarseness comes on for no accountable reason and persists, because it originates from a more serious physical condition —a benign or malignant growth in the voice box, or larynx. Then it makes sense to be examined by an alternative doctor.

(Please see the list of such physicians in the back of the book. If there's none near you, write the National Health Federation, which offers a service of listing natural healing doctors throughout the United States: National Health Federation, 212 W. Foothill Blvd., Monrovia, California 91016. Phone: (818) 357-2181.)

Folk Medicine Gargles

However, for routine hoarseness and throat irritation, the practical folk medicine gargles are saltwater—I make mine from sea salt from the health food store — or a honey and lemon combination and one popular in Europe: strained onion syrup with honey and lemon in a glass of warm water.

Here's how I prepare the latter. I slice three large onions into four or five cups of water and simmer them until they become syrupy. After straining, I ladle five to six tablespoons of the onion syrup into a warm glass of water, along with a tablespoon of honey and a dash of lemon.

Of all the home remedy gargles, this works best for me. Even sipped slowly and swallowed, this concoction gives me the quickest and best relief for hoarseness.

Some other gargles (or teas) from out of folklore are: eucalyptus, fenugreek, horehound, and marshmallow. Health food stores carry zinc lozenges which are helpful. A word of caution here. If your sore throat persists and seems to be caused by streptococcal organisms, see a doctor, because this infection could bring on serious ailments such as kidney damage or rheumatic fever.

A Voice Expert's Approach

Dr. Sally Etchelo, a lecturer in music at California State University, Dominguez Hills, in Carson, California and voice coach and vocalist, gets two dimensions of comfort from hot chicken soup when she's hoarse: from ingesting it and from letting its steam moisten her throat.[1] (At the end of this section, you will find the recipe for my favorite chicken soup, loaded with onions and garlic. Bacteria and viruses can't stand it, but I love it.)

Like all of us who make public appearances, Sally has learned many ways to protect her voice from harm.

"I get enough sleep, exercise, eat good food and don't smoke." she says. "If I feel the symptoms of a cold or other respiratory illness coming on, I increase my intake of fluids and increase my dosage of vitamin C."

Sometimes we all have to overwork our voice. Then it's a good idea to substitute paperwork for talking, she suggests. "Think of your voice as if it's a sprained ankle. If you had a sprained ankle, you wouldn't run a race."

Throat Protection

Etchelo offers more major league advice:

If you have a sore throat, avoid crowded, noisy rooms where you are forced to speak loudly and are subjected to lots of smoke.

Don't strain your voice by trying to compete with traffic noise while riding in a car with open windows.

If in a dry environment over a long period—like the cabin of a jet plane —drink plenty of fluids to keep your throat moist.

If you have laryngitis, refrain from using your voice. Write notes instead.

If the weather is dry and your throat is in danger of losing moisture, slowly heat a pot of water and inhale the vapor each time you pass by. A humidifier running in the bedroom at night helps even more, she concludes.

So there you have it, straight from the voice instructor's mouth!

Maureen's Chicken Soup

1 large pullet, cut-up
3 carrots, diced
2 large onions, diced
3 garlic cloves, diced
2 T. liquid garlic

4 celery stalks, diced
1 bunch parsley, chopped
1 large potato (optional)
1 T. sea salt
2 c. spring water

Clean chicken in pot of cold water. Cook all ingredients together, except for potato. Add potato last 30 minutes of cooking. Cook for 1½ to 2 hours. If you desire clear soup, strain it.

CHAPTER 68

Hyperactivity

While alternative doctors diminish or even control hyperactivity naturally by dealing with basic causes, orthodox medical doctors follow a single form of therapy—various stimulating drugs—which deal with symptoms.

Every hyperactive child seems to manifest certain of the following symptoms:

1. Restless, jittery sitting.

2. Difficulty in concentrating or reading. Short attention span.

3. Low-grade school performance characterized by inability to organize work or stay with projects. Impatience.

4. Touching everything and everybody around him or her.

5. Predictably unpredictable conduct in school. Hair-trigger temper. Aggressiveness that sometimes disrupts the class and causes friction with classmates and teachers.

6. Easy tears and depressed states.

7. Being too hyped up to sleep well. Falling asleep with difficulty and waking up often.

Prevention: The Best Cure

Undernourishment in the first three years of life—including time in the womb — can cause severe mental impairment: brain damage, childhood hyperactivity or learning disabilities.

Announcing that sound nutritional practices by the mother-to-be can prevent childhood disorders, the World Health Organization states that more than one-half of the one hundred and sixteen million babies born each year go through their first three years undernourished for protein and with a hypoglycemic mother.[1] (See the Section on Hypoglycemia.)

Danger From Drugs

Carl C. Pfeiffer, Ph.D, M.D., Director of Princeton's Brain Bio Center, writes that parents and physicians, aware of the quick metabolic response of children to stimulant drugs—which, strangely, act as sedatives—take the easy way out. Amphetamines and Ritalin control a hyperactive child's unruly behavior and permit him to concentrate in school.[2]

However, such drugs treat the symptoms only and have the potential of spawning a whole list of adverse side effects: chronic sleeplessness, irritability, loss of appetite and weight, nausea, tactile hallucinations, tics (spasmodic and uncontrollable contraction of muscles).[3]

Pfeiffer's review of medical literature suggests that long-time use of such drugs may result in brain damage, heart and artery disorders, possibly Hodgkin's disease, and—the crowning touch—drug dependency.[4]

Dr. Feingold's Natural Solution

A pioneer in probing to the root of the problem, the late Dr. Ben Feingold, a prominent allergist at San Francisco's Kaiser-Permanente Group Medical Center, investigated hyperactivity for 40 years.

Within a ten year span, the number of hyperactive children in California skyrocketed from two to 25 percent while the use of artificial colorings, flavorings and preservatives in foods soared even higher percentage-wise. Feingold related the two factors, took his young hyperactive patients off junk foods and saw many of them recover dramatically.[5]

Feingold once said that he could switch his kid patients on or off merely by regulating their diet.[6] The major culprits were soft drinks, baked goods, bottled, canned and packaged foods, heavy in refined carbohydrates, and chemicalized with additives.

"Get away from convenience foods," preached Feingold, theorizing that convenience foods were at the heart of inconveniences such as hyperactivity.

His phenomenal track record for controlling hyperactivity attracted worldwide attention and a following. Soon many other doctors were getting similar results with their young patients.

Proved By Test

A double-blind study by C. Keith Conners, Ph.D, while showing that the Feingold system didn't work on all children, found that it had definite value.

Organizations such as the American Council for Science and Health and the Nutrition Foundation responded to Feingold's charges against food additives, reporting on favorable tests to assure the public that all additives are safe and not responsible for hyperactivity.[7]

The late Carlton Fredericks noted that their report somehow had omitted the fact that the amount of additives tested was less than a tenth of what a child ingests daily.[8]

How To Remedy Hyperactivity

In one research project, seventy-six hyperactive children were put on a restricted diet. Sixty-two manifested improvement, and twenty-one realized normal behavior.[9]

Then twenty-eight of the improved children were tested to learn to which dietary items they reacted. Artificial colorings and preservatives triggered their hyperactivity most. An artificial food coloring such as tartrazine brought about 79 percent positive reactions to challenges.

Richard A. Kunin, M.D., grants the importance of food additives to hyperactivity, but claims that this is just a part of the story. "Excessive carbohydrates may be even more so," he writes in his book, "Mega-Nutrition." (New American Library) Kunin feels strongly that it is also a case of too much refined sugar and flour. And he could be right.[10]

In several cases of hyperactivity, Kunin slashed the intake of refined carbohydrates—candy, cookies, sugared cereals and soft drinks—from 300 grams a day to 125 to 130. The patients made an about-face, scored in school, improved in physical coordination and moved from being ignored by classmates to being sought-after as friends.[11]

Other Causes For Hyperactivity

A diet high in refined carbohydrates triggers low blood sugar—a condition called hypoglycemia. In a large-scale study—200 hyperactive children—more than 60 percent were found by glucose tolerance tests to have low blood sugar, which hit the switch that started or aggravated typical hyperactive behavior.[12]

Many of these same children had brain allergies to common foods—usually to those they favor and eat whenever possible—which set off behavior which they can't control. (For more information, see the Section on Food Allergies.)

Why Does Vitamin B-6 Seem To Work?

Certain nutrients seem to control hyperactivity. A fortunate accident led to the discovery that vitamin B-6 might be useful in coping with hyperactivity.[13] In measuring blood levels of serotonin — a key neurotransmitter—in thirty mentally retarded, severely overactive and emotionally disturbed institutionalized patients, Mary Coleman and Alan S. Greenberg, two medical doctors, found that 83 percent showed below-normal levels of serotonin.

Dr. Coleman tried numerous drugs to improve the condition of the patients, finding that only those which raised serotonin levels worked.

Later investigation revealed that as many as 88 percent of hyperactive children showed depressed levels of serotonin. Knowing that vitamin B-6 activates enzymes which convert tryptophan, an amino acid, into serotonin, she and colleagues administered high dosages of vitamin B-6 and found that they really do raise blood serotonin levels, whatever the intitial blood levels in test subjects: low, normal or high.

This led Coleman to test six hyperactive children comparatively over 21 weeks. Three were placed on one of the following for seven three week periods: placebo, low-dose vitamin B-6; high dose vitamin B-6; placebo; low-dose Ritalin, high dose Ritalin and then a placebo. The three others were put on a similar regimen, varying only in that they were given Ritalin before vitamin B-6.

The doses of vitamin B-6 were 10 to 15 mg of B-6 per kilogram of body weight: about 425 mg a day for a 75-pound child. The high dose was 15 to 30 mg per kilogram of body weight: about 750 mg a day for a 75-pound child. (THESE ARE HIGH POTENCIES AND SHOULD BE

TAKEN ONLY UNDER SUPERVISION OF A NUTRITION-
ORIENTED MEDICAL DOCTOR).

Based on a behavior rating scale, the high dosage of vitamin B-6 proved
to be the most effective treatment. The lower potency of this vitamin
proved ineffective—no better than the placebo. Ritalin came in second.
Vitamin B-6 raised the blood serotonin levels. Ritalin didn't. The positive
influence of the B-6 lasted for almost three weeks after the vitamin was
no longer given.

Evening Primrose Oil May Help

Many children have difficulty translating essential fatty acids (EFAs)
in vegetable oils into prostaglandins (PGs), present in every human cell
and vital to the function of every human organ.

Some authorities hold that hyperactivity may be caused by too low an
intake of EFAs.[14] (Animal experiments show that thirst is an indication
of EFA deficiency. It is one symptom of diabetes, as well.) Hyperactive
boys outnumber hyperactive girls three to one, supposedly because boys
have far more difficulty in converting EFAs to PGs. Therefore, boys
appear to require three times as much EFA as girls.[15]

Joint studies of hyperactive children by clinicians in the United States,
Canada, South Africa and the United Kingdom reveal that almost two-
thirds of the test participants show improvement after taking two to three
500 mg capsules of evening primrose oil each morning and evening and,
after six to eight weeks, one in the morning and one in the evening.[16]

An oddity of the experiments was the fact that some children responded
better to evening primrose oil if it was rubbed into their skin. Those who
conducted the study felt this was true because certain individuals have
poor intestinal tract absorption.[17]

Another Strategem Against Hyperactivity

Warfare on two fronts against hyperactivity worked wonders for
Matthew Venuti, a graduate student in health services at Columbia Pacific
University: upgraded diet, featuring natural, whole foods, and daily
aerobic exercise.[18]

Venuti selected seven super-tough cases: hyperactive boys in Cincinnati's St. Aloysius Orphanage—boys with consistently anti-social behavior: punching others, defiant of authority, abnormally over-active, sleeping poorly and often ill.

He created a new diet low on sugar and eliminating foods with chemicals and artificial colors and flavors and a 15 minute program of nonstop, daily running, selling the plan on the basis that it would improve the boys' health. Vernuti persuaded national and local companies to supply whole grain cereals, bakery products and natural spring water for the experiment.

Nothing positive happened the first week. The children showed their usual unruly, undesirable traits, creating disturbances at the dinner table.

"By the second week, the children were capable of serving themselves (previously impossible), and reduced disruptive behavior to a minimum," says Venuti. "By week number three, disturbances and complaints were practically non-existent."

Initially, the boys complained because they couldn't run nonstop for even five minutes. Soon, by encouraging each other to keep up the pace, they became serious joggers, and their health improved markedly, along with their conduct.

Once the experiment was over, and the boys stopped exercising and returned to their former diet, they soon reverted to their aggressive and hostile behavior.

Considering the evidence of various studies and experiments, hyperactivity can be controlled by various individual means and combinations of them.

Dwight's Brown Rice Casserole

3 c. chicken broth	½ c. onions, chopped
1 t. salt	1 T. liquid garlic or garlic clove
½ t. basil	2 T. brewers yeast
½ t. thyme	1 c. sliced zucchini
1 c. brown rice, uncooked	1 c. green pepper, chopped
2 T. olive oil	1 large tomato, cubed
1½ c. egg plant, diced	2 c. swiss cheese, shredded

In medium sauce pan, heat chicken broth to boiling. Add salt, basil, thyme, brewers yeast and rice. Reduce heat to low. Cook covered for 1 hour. In medium skillet, heat oil. Add eggplant, onions and garlic. Saute for 5 minutes. Grease casserole dish. Preheat oven to 350 degrees. Mix all vegetables, onion and garlic with rice. Spoon half of rice-vegetable mixture into casserole. Sprinkle on all, but 2 tablespoons of cheese. Top with remaining rice-vegetable mixture. Sprinkle on remaining cheese. Bake covered for 25 minutes. Makes 6 servings.

Zonelle's Apple-Banana Salad

6 lbs. sweet apples,
  some red and some yellow
3 to 4 bananas
1 c. toasted peanuts

Home-made mayonnaise or
  salad dressing
12 boston lettuce cups

Core apples, but do not peel. Cut into bite-size pieces and place in salad bowl. Slice bananas and add to apples. Sprinkle with nuts and toss with mayonnaise or dressing. Serve in lettuce cups. Makes 12 servings. NOTE: The contributor's orchard is organically maintained.

Home-Made Mayonnaise

2 fresh egg yolks
2 T. fresh lemon juice

¾ c. cold-pressed vegetable oil
½ t. fine mixed herbs

Place eggs, herbs and lemon juice in blender. Add oil slowly as you blend. Chill in refrigerator until ready to serve.

CHAPTER 69

Immune System Problems

After a Sunday morning service at my home church, the Cathedral of Faith in San Jose, when I had finished chatting with Pastor Kenny Foreman, a middle-aged, heavy-set woman of the congregation, stopped me to talk about her health.

"Maureen, I have one cold after another. Maybe it's the same one that never ends. I'm so tired it's hard for me to drag through a day, and the wound on my right arm from surgery is taking forever to heal. I asked my doctor whether or not he thinks my immune system is declining."

"What did he say?" I asked.

"That immune function does decline with added years and that I should learn to live with it."

"Sure, the thymus gland, a major part of the immune system, does shrink with age, but we don't just have to sit idly by and watch our immune function shrink along with it," I replied.

Aging Or Nutrient Deficiency?

Then I recommended a nutrition-oriented medical doctor in the area and urged her to make an appointment with him and get supplementation to bolster her thymus gland and immune function and to have him give her a five-hour glucose tolerance test for possible low blood sugar. When she promised to do this, I made another point:

"A decline in the immune function is not always due only to the aging process. It often happens because one is vitamin and mineral-deficient and/or under severe and continuous stress. The immune army can't fight off infection or contribute to efficient wound-healing if it is ill-fed."

This made sense to her. And she asked where in the body the thymus

319

gland is located and what nutrients are particularly important to keeping it healthy and vigorous.

I indicated the thymus's location by some Tarzan thumping on the upper front region of my chest and then told her the results of several studies. In one of them, patients who were highly susceptible to infection were tested and found deficient in zinc. When they took a zinc supplement, their resistance to infection increased measurably. [1]

The Thymus Declines But Doesn't Have To Fall

Yes, the thymus gland declines sharply by the time we are fourteen years old and continues to waste away slowly. One study indicates that this process is hurried along by nutritional deficiency. [2]

Just thirty days of taking an oral zinc sulphate supplement improved the immune system response of every one of 15 seventy year old patients. [3]

Not only has zinc supplementation helped the thymus gland, but also the immune function at the level of individual cells and body fluids — blood as well as lymph. When patients took in 22.7 mg of zinc daily for three weeks, their impaired cell immune function dramatically returned to normal. [4]

For a better understanding of how nutrients influence our glorious, God-given, in-built defense system against invading germs and viruses, as well as cancer cells, let's look at the immune system and exactly what it does.

A Biochemical Work Of Art

An awesome creation — particularly to the scientists probing its mysteries — the immune system has been characterized as follows in Time Magazine by Nobel Laureate Baruj Benacerraf, president of the Dana Farber Cancer Institute in Boston: "It is an enormous edifice, like a cathedral."

Indeed, in design, it is an intricate biochemical cathedral with the most spectacular features of Westminster Abbey, St. Paul's Cathedral and Notre Dame. In function, it is like the world's best-trained, most intelligent, most efficient army for defense.

The soldiers are variations of two kinds of cells: T-cells—those which go through basic training while stationed in the thymus gland—and B-cells—white blood cells recruited from the bone marrow.

T-cell officer scouts patrolling body fluids and cells suddenly sense an enemy invader—a harmful virus—which has managed to penetrate the body's various ports of entry: ears, eyes, mouth and nose.

Who Goes There?

The protein molecules on the surface of the viruses are unique as they are in every kind of cell—as unique as fingerprints. So the T-cells (T-lymphocytes) sense that they are different, that they are outsiders. They produce and attach special identifying tags on the invaders. These spell out the word "enemy," and, on the basis of this information, B-cells custom design weapons (antibodies) to annihilate this specific kind of enemy. And special immune system cells even dispose of their remains.

If the same virus attacks again, the process is shortened, because the pattern already exists for the enemy dogtags. Therefore, the type of illness brought about by that virus might not even be sensed by you or me.

Hardly a minute can go by without our being exposed to some foreign substance in the food we eat, the water we drink and the air we breathe. Some may be harmless, others may be harmful. However, your immune system officers must be able to tell which are which and alert the defense forces to what kind of enemy it is and issue orders to attack.

Immunity Gone Wrong

Sometimes these T-cell officers are inefficient or even defective, through inherited traits, through nutritional deficiencies, or through the body being under endless stress. Then they order attacks on harmless substances — foods such as eggs and milk, for instance—as well as animal danders, molds and pollens. And immune system soldiers blindly obey, attacking them as if they are true enemies.

Such attacks show up as disorders such as allergies, asthma, eczema and headaches. If frequent and persistent, such warfare against a non-enemy can wear down the immune system so that it is weakened when a real enemy invades. (See the Section on Allergies for identifying and eliminating substances that weaken your immune system.)

A second helpful measure to take is assuring intake of sufficient zinc and other nutrients to assure a strong immune system.

Several paragraphs ago, we mentioned defective T-cells. In a controlled experiment, patients with an acute zinc deficiency were found to have developed abnormal T-cells — officers unfit for duty. Then for 12 days, these patients were injected with 12 mg of zinc daily. Controls were given a placebo injection. Those who received zinc showed a return to normality with improved T-cell function by 139 to 221 percent above that of controls.[5]

From Z To A

Vitamin A, too, is an immune system booster. For many decades, vitamin A has been effective in battling infection, but its relation to immune function was not clearly established. Recently a study showed that vitamin A-deficient children without overt symptoms proved to be infection-prone.[6]

Now a study at the University of Wisconsin reveals that the immune system's T-cells can't work efficiently unless supplied with sufficient vitamin A.[7] In animals deficient in vitamin A, T-cell activity was depressed by 70 percent. When the researchers made good the deficiency, T-cell activity returned to normal.

Dr. Eli Seifter, of Albert Einstein Medical College, demonstrated that vitamin A guards the thymus gland from shrinking under stress and restores it to normal after the stress is over.[8]

Another of the fat-soluble vitamins, vitamin E, and its mineral mate selenium, increase immune system effectiveness, as do the lipotropics.[9] So what is a lipotropic? A substance that regulates or reduces the accumulation of fat — in the liver, for instance. And what are some of them? Betaine, a nutrient found in beets; choline, a B vitamin in soy lecithin, egg yolk, lentils, rice, split peas and wheat germ; inositol, a B vitamin in barley, brown rice, lentils, soy lecithin and wheat germ and methionine, an essential amino acid richly present in eggs.

A lipotropic encourages the production of antibodies and stimulates the growth and aggressiveness of phagocytes, Pac-Man cells which gobble up and destroy bacteria, viruses, and abnormal or foreign tissue.[10]

AIDS Beats The System

The immune system is tough on invaders, but one invader is so tough on the immune system that it disables the body's defenses: the AIDS virus, which destroys T-cells and disarms the body's defenders. Usually when a virus tries to establish a beachhead in the body, T-cells produce gamma interferon, a powerful chemical which slows the speed at which viruses can reproduce in the cells and stimulates the efficiency of macrophages to kill. Vitamin C stimulates the production of gamma interferon.[11]

With the leadership and the power of the T-cells knocked out, the body is at the mercy of the AIDS virus and micro-organisms which multiply faster than body cells can be replaced and is an easy mark for infectious ailments such as tuberculosis and pneumonia and degenerative diseases such as cancer.

Autoimmune diseases, in which immune system cells improperly identify a part of the body as an enemy and attack it are best handled by a nutrition-oriented endocrinologist, whose approach is usually to normalize function of T-cells.

Your Mind Can Help You Stay Well

Even a normal immune system can be thrown off balance by emotional stress. The most powerful example of this is the death of a person within six months of his or her spouse's death.

Combine the stress of bereavement with the nutritional one of zinc deficiency and you see a strong suppression of the immune function.

Men in unhappy marriages, separated or divorced were found to have weakened immune systems and to be more susceptible to two common forms of herpes virus infections than those happily married, say researchers Janice Kiecolt-Glaser and Ronald Glaser, of Ohio State University.[12]

This study followed another by the same team with unhappily married women, who also were discovered to have weakened immune systems.[13]

"Confession is good for the soul," states an old proverb. It can also be good for the immune system and the body, indicates another study by the Glasers in collaboration with psychologist Jamie Pennebaker, of Southern Methodist University in Dallas.[14] Twenty-three students were asked to write about intensely personal problems—unhappy relationships, family difficulties or homesickness. Twenty-three others were asked to write about trivial subjects.

Those who unburdened themselves on personal subjects showed stronger immune response in blood samples taken shortly after the experiment and six weeks later.

In still another experiment, the Glasers discovered that medical students on the verge of an examination revealed decreases in a form of T-cells.[15] When half of the group practiced relaxation exercises, their T-cells increased. Inasmuch as stress reduces immune function—a fact established by much research—the Glasers believe that deliberate relaxation of stress may have an influence on discouraging disease or changing its course.

An arresting study on a far more serious subject indicates that a positive attitude may be able to prolong the life of cancer patients.[16] Dr. Lydia Temoshok, of the University of California in San Francisco, found that the 50 percent survivors of malignant melanoma were upbeat, compared with the half that died, individuals who manifested almost twice the levels of depression-dejection, fatigue-inertia, tension-anxiety, confusion and distress.

In Love, Medicine and Miracles (Harper & Row), Dr. Bernie Siegel observes that patients who respond to cancer with anger had a far greater life-expectancy than those who passively followed doctor's orders or who became helpless and hopeless.

A 20-year rat experiment conducted by Martin Seligman, Ph.D and associates at the University of Pennsylvania, demonstrates that helplessness made one group of animals more than twice as vulnerable to tumor than the others.[17]

The latter group learned how to control electric shocks to which they were exposed by pressing a bar and, therefore, had mastery over them. The second group had no way to control the shocks and experienced helplessness, which made them more cancer prone. Several researchers have found that helplessness made already established cancer in lab animals grow faster.

Without question, the mind and emotions exert a strong influence on the immune system and predict, to a great degree, the wellness or sickness in a person's future. This puts us in a position of power, for we can virtually select the state by our mental and emotional life.

Following are the key nutrients mentioned above for strengthening the immune system: zinc and vitamins A, E an C. And here are the foods and supplements richest in zinc in terms of milligrams per unit of less than four ounces: herring, 110; wheat germ, 14; sesame seeds, 10; torula yeast, 9.9; blackstrap molasses, 8.3; maple syrup, 7.5; liver, 7.0; soybeans, 6.7; sunflower seeds, 6.6; egg yolk, 5.5; lamb, 5.4; chicken, 4.8; regular molasses, 4.6; brewer's yeast, 3.9; oats, 3.7; bone meal, 3.6; rye, 3.4; whole wheat, 3.2; corn, 3.1; coconut and beef, 3.0; beets, turkey and walnuts, 2.8; barley, 2.7; beans and avocados, 2.4; peas, 2.3; blue cheese, 2,2; eggs, 2.1; buckwheat, 2.0; mangoes, 1.9 and millet, brown rice and almonds, 1.5.

Following are the foods and supplements with the largest amounts of vitamin A or its precursor in terms of International Units per less than four ounce units: cod liver oil, 200,000; sheep liver, 45,000; beef liver, 44,000; calf's liver, 22,000; dandelion greens, 14,000; carrots, 11,000; yams, 9,000; kale, 8,900; parsley and turnip greens, 8,500; spinach. 8,100; collard greens and chard, 6,500; watercress, 5,000; red peppers, 4,400; squash, 4,000; egg yolk and cantaloupe, 3,400; endive, 3,300; persimmons and apricots, 2,700; broccoli, 2,500; pimentos, 2,300; swordfish, 2,100; whitefish, 2,000; romaine, 1,900; mangoes, 1,800; papayas, 1,700 and nectarines and pumpkin, 1,600.

These are the supplements and foods richest in vitamin E in terms of International Units per less than four ounce units: wheat germ, 160; safflower nuts, 35; sunflower seeds, 31; whole wheat, 30; sesame oil, 26; walnuts, 22; corn oil and hazel nuts, 21; soy and peanut oil, 16; almonds, 15; olive oil, 14; cabbage, 7.8; brazil nuts and peanuts, 6.5; cod liver oil, 5.4; cashews, 5.1; soy lecithin, 4.8; spinach, 2.9; asparagus, 2.5; broccoli,, 2.0; butter, 1.9; parsley, 11.8 and oats, barley, and corn, 1.7.

Best supplement and food sources of vitamin C in milligrams per less than four ounce units are: rose hips, 3000; acerola cherries, 1100; guavas, 240; black currants, 200; parsley, 170; green peppers, 110; watercress,

80; chives, 70; strawberries, 57; persimmons, 52; spinach, 51; oranges, 50; cabbage, 47; grapefruit, 38; papaya, 37; elderberries and kumquats, 36; dandelion greens and lemons, 35; cantaloupe, 33; green onions, 32; limes, 31; mangoes, 27; loganberries, 24; tangerines and tomatoes, 23; squash, 22 and raspberries, romaine lettuce and pineapple, 17.

CHAPTER 70

Impotency

No single influence can make a man feel like a fraction of himself more than learning that he's impotent—incapable of carrying out the sexual act.

Now the good news is that, in most instances, impotency need not be a life sentence. In men over 40 at least 60 percent of cases have a physical cause. There are some 200 different causes, most of them correctable by a urologist fully conversant with male sexual dysfunction.

Even among diabetics who are impotent, half of them can be helped by medical treatment, states Loren Lipson, M.D., chief of the Division of Geriatric Medicine at the University of Southern California, based on his own research.[1]

Don't Call A Spade "An Implement For Digging"

Dr. Beverly Palmer, a psychology professor at California State University, Dominguez Hills, who teaches a course in human sexuality and serves as a clinical psychologist to a medical doctor specializing in male sexual dysfunction, says it's a mistake for a man to think of his condition as "impotency," because this makes him seem powerless and devastated.[2]

"The man's whole concept of himself gets tied up with his sexual performing. It is better to call this disorder 'erectile dysfunction,' " she says. "That sticks to the specific part of the body having the problem, rather than to the man's conception of himself."

Takes Two To Tango

The man blames himself, and his mate wonders what she did wrong. "It doesn't necessarily take two to create the problem, but it does take two to treat it," says Palmer.

Inability to perform can result from tension which reduces blood flow to vessels of the male organ. An engorgement of blood in the penis is essential to its becoming rigid. Anxiety, anger, fatigue, stress, depression and distraction can cause the problem.

Many Other Causes

Some of the causes of erectile dysfunction are side effects of other physical conditions: overwork and fatigue, alcoholism, obesity and — among others—various medications: anti-hypertensive medications, anti-ulcer drugs, lithium, anti-depressants and many tranquilizers.

Fundamental to recovering is the knowledge that temporary dysfunction can happen even to young men and that neither mate should give it over-concern, which could mar future encounters, states Palmer.

"Erectile dysfuntion can be cured. However, no one should delay. Delay only increases the problem in the relationship and the problem with self-esteem," Palmer says. "We're not talking about long term therapy, only straightforward communication and medical and surgical management, no matter what the cause."

Back Into Circulation

Perhaps the major physical cause is impairment of blood circulation to the penis, due to cholesterol, calcium and other substances which narrow the arteries. Is this hopeless? Not any more.

Practitioners of alternative medicine tell me that many of their patients have been returned to full sexuality after a series of chelation treatments, which dissolve blockages in the tiny capillaries of the penis. The American College of Advancement in Medicine (ACAM) has members in all parts of the nation who practice chelation. A letter or phone call to this society can help you locate an ACAM member near you.

Just write or phone, The American College of Advancement in Medicine: ACAM, Suite 204, 23121 Verdugo, Laguna Hills, California 92653. Phone: (714) 583-7666.

Are there any foods that chelate? In Sexual Nutrition (Coward-McCann),

Dr. Morton Walker and Joan Walker mention that certain tropical fruits —bananas, kiwi, mangoes and papaya—have a high content of chelating minerals and an enzyme called bromelain, which creates a chelation-like effect. The Walkers write that bromelain "acts like a pipe cleaner" for blood vessels.[3] (Warning: A heavy intake of bromelain may delay healing of a stomach ulcer.)

Is It True What They Say About Ginseng?

If you believe locker room talk, ginseng is supposed to be an aphrodisiac that fires up the libido and boosts erectile efficiency.

Not so. Ginseng can help one develop more well-being and rev up energy and contribute to endurance, as Russian experiments show. And energy and endurance are important to sexual competency, but ginseng is no aphrodisiac.

Think Zinc!

Like ginseng, the trace mineral zinc has a reputation for firing up sexuality and renewing a man's capability.

True or false? True to a degree. Impotent young males with a zinc deficiency, when given a daily zinc supplement, usually become capable for sex within four or five months, writes Carl C. Pfeiffer, M.D., Ph.D in Mental and Elemental Nutrients (Keats Publishing, Inc).

Pfeiffer has found that the most common nutritional cause of impotency in young men is deficiency in both zinc and vitamin B-6. With adequate intake, potency should return in one to two months, he writes.[4]

Biochemist DeWayne Ashmead, Ph.D's review of the literature on zinc reveals that there may be a direct link between the output level of testosterone (a major male hormone) and the amount of zinc in the body.[5]

Sperm could not be produced in adequate amounts without enough zinc intake, adds Ashmead. A high level of erectile dysfunction and inadequate sperm generation could relate to the fact that United States soils are zinc-deficient. Michael Lesser, M.D., testifying before the Senate Select Committee on Nutrition and Human Needs, exploded the blockbuster that the soil of thirty-two states is zinc-deficient and that commercial fertilizers provide no zinc.[6]

Ashmead refers to a four-year study of 11 midwest states in which several thousand grain samples revealed that zinc levels in corn dropped 10 percent during the study.[7]

As fundamental as two and two equalling four is the fact that if soil is short of zinc, so is the plant grown in it, and so is the animal that eats the plant, and so are you if you eat that animal or that plant.

Many alternative medical doctors feel that zinc deficiency is at the bottom of much erectile deficiency. University tests show that chelated zinc is better absorbed in the intestine than zinc sulphate—127 percent better.

Other Causes

Pfeiffer states that sexual impotency in older males could also result from deficiency of the trace mineral molybdenum.[9] Best food and food supplement sources of molybdenum are seaweeds, soybeans, lima beans, peas, lentils, wheat germ, rye, honey, liver and dill.

Earlier Dr. Louis Lipson mentioned that half of the sexual dysfunction of diabetics—that which is not relatable to their disease—is treatable.[10]

"Many diabetics with sexual problems can be helped but fall in the trap of thinking the situation is hopeless," he says. In a study of 320 diabetic men, Lipson traced half of the impotency to three causes other than diabetes: psychological factors (20 percent); medications (20 percent) and other diseases (10 percent).

"Sometimes, psychological impotence occurs, because the patient is told that sexual dysfunction is common with diabetes. He's expecting it to happen, so it becomes a self-fulfilling prophecy," says Lipson, indicating that psychological factors can be treated with psychotherapy or sex therapy.

Lipson states that alcoholism is a major cause of impotency. "Even social drinking can cause impotency," Lipson comments. "For many people, the solution is to stop drinking."

Medications can bring on sexual dysfunction, which may be corrected by changing prescriptions, he says. Even when impotence is a direct cause of diabetes, there is some hope, although the problems are of an organic type, involving damage of arteries and nerves.

"The important point for diabetes patients is not to resign themselves to sexual difficulties. Too many suffer needlessly."

The same goes for anyone with erectile dysfunction. Often the family doctor may not even be totally aware of the many ways by which urologists can help solve this problem, so he could be needlessly discouraging. The best place to start, then, is with a urologist who specializes in male sexual dysfunctions, with an authority familiar with all options.

Please read the Section on Infertility. Many of the points apply also to erectile dysfunction.

CHAPTER 71

Infertility
(Female and Male)

"Put the blame on Mame!"

Lay a guilt trip on the woman when a wanted pregnancy fails to occur. This has been the custom throughout the centuries.

Thank goodness, many studies have punctured the big, fat balloon of a myth that the woman is always the one at fault. Now it turns out that the male is responsible about half the time.

So let's deal with what can be done by both sexes to convert infertility to fertility. All sorts of factors can keep males from doing their share: environmental conditions, lifestyles and under-nutrition.

Low sperm count—which lessens the odds of conception—can result from workplace exposure to chloroprene, lead, microwaves, PCBs, DBCP, and, among other major environmental negatives, superheat.

Be Cool, Man!

Long-time workers in the blistering heat of a foundry or under a melting tropical sun show unusually low sperm counts, because there's an intense heat buildup in their scrotum, the area where sperm is secreted. The scrotum is a pouch intended not only to hold the testicles in place, but also to insulate them from excessive heat. For sperm to be produced, the interior scrotum temperature must be a bit lower than normal body temperature.

One of the greatest enemies of fertility and conception today is the onipresent and popular hot tub, as well as hot baths and showers, saunas and steam baths. Excessive bedclothes and the electric blanket during sleeping hours also elevate inner-scrotal temperatures.

Other enemies are tight-fitting, overheating jockey shorts, athletic supporters, and close-fitting, dark trousers. Natural, air-conditioned kilts and generally cool temperatures in Scotland are said to contribute to high fertility in Scotsmen. Around-the-house wearing of loose-fitting shorts sometimes helps increase male fertility.

Modern science has come up with a device to enhance evaporative cooling of the testicles—a special device called the scrotal pouch, which a Lancet article indicates works. The quality of semen in five out of six men improved after they wore the scrotal pouch for 12 weeks. Three of their wives proved the point by becoming pregnant.

Self-Defeating Lifestyles And More...

Some of the most notorious killers of sperm count are alcohol, cigarettes, excessive caffeine and various prescription drugs for ulcers and ulcerative colitis.

Upwards of a billion dollars a year is spent trying to achieve pregnancy. One of the areas of counsel most neglected by medical doctors is the upgrading of patients' nutrition.

Over and above low sperm count are various problems with sperm itself —clumping (agglutinization in medical jargon) and low ability to move (motility). If more than 20 percent of the sperm clumps, a man is considered infertile. Thirty-five men with an average of 33 percent sperm agglutinization were fed 1,000 mg of vitamin C for three weeks, and their sperm clumping dropped a sharp 67 percent to 11 percent.[1]

In a study by Earl B. Dawson, Ph.D, at the University of Texas Medical Branch, Galveston, 12 of 20 men with sperm-clumping who could not make their wives pregnant were given 500 mg of vitamin C every 12 hours. Eight took a placebo.[2]

After 60 days, the sperm of all 12 vitamin-takers showed a dramatic drop in clumping and other improvements—including greater animation and motility—and every one of their wives became pregnant. None of the placebo-takers showed sperm improvement, and not one of their wives became pregnant.

Big Assists From Vitamin E And Zinc

Additional studies also show the effectiveness of vitamin C in sperm enhancement. Other nutrients, too, have been shown to improve impregnation qualities of sperm: vitamin E and zinc.

In several studies, men who could not produce normal sperm were given 150 to 300 International Units of vitamin E daily for from eight to 40 weeks and many developed normal sperm, impregnating their wives.[3]

Many human and animal studies show that the mineral zinc can often restore the sperm cells to normal. There is a greater concentration of zinc in sperm cells than in any other kind of cell in the body.

Women, Attention Please!

It is more than obvious that men can make key adjustments to contribute to a successful pregnancy. So can women—particularly in making certain that they are eating enough foods containing vitamin B-6. (See list at chapter's end.)

Two gynecologists, Joel T. Hargrove, M.D., Columbia, Tennessee, and Guy E. Abraham, M.D., Torrance, California, studied 14 women—ages 23 to 31—who suffered premenstrual tension and could not explain their inability to become pregnant.[4]

Almost all of the women had been unable to become pregnant for anywhere from 18 months to seven years. On a long-range regime of taking from 100 to 800 milligrams of vitamin B-6 daily, 11 of the 14 women became pregnant inside of six months. One more pregnancy happened in the seventh month and still another at the 11th month.

Two more major factors may prevent pregnancy: too little or too much body fat, conditions which upset normal ovulation, as well as overstrenuous exercise.

Women who take the Pill often cannot become pregnant until a year after discontinuing this oral contraceptive. Ninety-eight percent resumed menstruation and became pregnant within 24 months.[5]

So far, I have mentioned vitamins and a mineral essential to fertility. Now there are two folk medicine items said to be helpful to fertility of both males and females: the herb Dom Oui and red raspberry tea.

Nutrient-Containing Foods

Supplements and foods richest in vitamin C in milligrams per less than four ounce units are: rose hips, 3,000; acerola cherries, 1,100; guavas, 240; black currants, 200; parsley, 170; green peppers, 110; watercress, 80; chives, 70; strawberries, 57; persimmons, 52; spinach, 51: oranges, 50; cabbage, 47; grapefruit, 38; papaya, 37; elderberries and kumquats, 36; dandelion greens and lemons, 35; cantaloupe, 33; green onions, 32; limes, 31; mangoes, 27; loganberries, 24; tangerines and tomatoes, 23; squash, 22 and raspberries and romaine lettuce.

Best supplement and food sources of vitamin E in terms of International Units per less than four-ounce units are: wheat germ, 160; safflower nuts, 35; sunflower seeds, 31; whole wheat, 30; sesame oil, 26; walnuts, 22; corn oil, 21; soy oil and peanut oil, 16; almonds, 15; olive oil, 14; cabbage, 7.8; almond oil, 7.5; brazil nuts and peanuts, 6.5; cod liver oil, 5.4; cashews, 5.1; soy lecithin, 4.8; spinach, 2.9; asparagus, 2.5; broccoli, 2.0; butter, 1.9; parsley, 1.8; oats, barley and corn, 1.7 and avocados and pecans, 1.5.

Highest zinc-content foods and supplements in milligrams per less than four ounce units are: herring, 110; wheat germ. 14; sesame seeds, 10; torula yeast, 9.9; blackstrap molasses, 8.3; maple syrup, 7.5; liver, 7.0; soybeans, 6.7; sunflower seeds, 6.6; egg yolk, 5,5; lamb, 5.4; chicken, 4.8; brewer's yeast, 3.9; oats, 3.7; bone meal, 3.6; rye, 3,2; whole wheat, 3.2; corn, 3.1; coconut and beef, 3.0; beets, turkey and walnuts, 2.8; barley, 2.7; beans and avocados, 2.4; peas, 2.3; blue cheese, 2.2; eggs, 2.1 and buckwheat, 2.0.

Richest food and supplement sources of vitamin B-6 in milligrams per less than four ounce units are: brewer's yeast, 4.0; brown rice, 3.6; whole wheat, 2.9; royal jelly, 2.4; soybeans, 2.0; rye, 1.8; lentils, 1.7; sunflower seeds and hazelnuts, 1.1; alfalfa, 1.00; salmon, 0.98; wheat germ, 0.92; tuna, 0.92; tuna, 0.90; bran, 0.85; walnuts, 0.73; peas and liver, 0.67; avocados, 0.60; beans, 0.57; cashews, peanuts, turkey, oats, chicken and beef, 0.40; halibut, 0.34 and lamb and bananas, 0.32.

Carla's Papaya Fruit Bowl

One of the most nutritious of all fruits is papaya. It is richer in Vitamin C than are oranges.

1 large papaya (½ per person)	1 kiwi fruit
3 fresh apricots, diced	6 ounces brazil nuts, ground
6 fresh strawberries, halved	

Remove seeds from each papaya. Place pieces of apricots in papaya shell, followed by strawberries. Peel kiwi fruit and slice on top. Sprinkle ground nuts on top of the fruit.

CHAPTER 72

Intestines (Toxic)

Although you can't see inside your intestines to know when they need cleansing, you can feel it by means of one or more of ten common symptoms: bloating, bad breath — your best friend will tell you — diarrhea, fatigue, gastrointestinal pain, gas (flatulence), headaches, kidney disorders, nervousness, or breaking out of the skin.

If some of these conditions persist, what do you do about them? First, get to know more about your intestinal plumbing and what's happening down under.

The stomach lining secretes hydrochloric acid, a mini lake of fire, that starts digestion of food, continued by powerful pancreatic enzymes in the duodenum, the horshoe-shaped first part of the small intestine.

The Inside Story

Muscle contractions (peristalsis) move the food mass downward, in contact with multi-billions of brush border cells on the intestinal wall. Tiny, hairlike appendages reach out and draw in desired nutrients and pass them into the bloodstream, while rejecting toxic particles.

Poisons such as partially digested and putrefying food, alcohol, and various drugs and medicines can damage the hyper-sensitive, intestinal mucous lining and reduce its ability to sense the difference between nutrients and toxins. So harmful toxins are often absorbed into the bloodstream with nutrients.

Problems start in other ways, too. Some individuals don't secrete enough hydrochloric acid—especially the middle-aged and beyond—so food is not sufficiently digested.

However, the major problem is usually a diet too low in fiber, and, consequently, too slow in moving waste matter from the body, permitting putrefying to take place. Then toxins invade the blood and create symptoms mentioned above.

Rapid Transit Time

The time from intake of food to outgo of wastes is called transit time. Most authorities say that this should be no more than 24 to 36 hours. Yet for some individuals, it might be 72 hours to a week—so long that transit time almost becomes "parking time".

Just as over-parking on the street brings a penalty, so does over-parking in the last five feet of the intestine, the colon—anything from toxicity to colon cancer. (See Section on Cancer, Colon.)

Then enemy bacteria called Clostridium have more time to work—to work their harm. In the hardened waste matter impacted against the colon walls, they attack remaining nutrients and substances such as bile acids, cholesterol and fatty acids and change them into poisons and cancer-causing chemicals.

The best defense against this condition is a strong offense: fiber-rich foods. Like thousands of tiny sponges, bits of dietary fiber increase the amount of water the stool can hold, provide bulk and speed up the transit time. Some fibers also detoxify the intestinal tract: agar, cellulose, pectin, psyllium husk, guar gum and oat bran fiber.

Guar Gum: Fantastic Fiber

Aside from its value in bulking the diet and detoxifying the colon, guar gum is a secret weapon against overweight and obesity.[1] In experiments, it reduced hunger better than bran, raised the body's ability to burn off carbohydrates and fats, lowered blood sugar after meals (decreasing the need for insulin in diabetics), lowered blood cholesterol after long use and significantly reduced weight of obese persons who stayed on their usual diet.[2]

Even this is not the end of the guar gum story. This fantastic fiber, along with pectin, can help detoxify the body by throwing off some of the poisonous heavy metals to which we are subject today: lead and cadmium, among them.[3]

However, a total intestinal cleansing program also involves the Italian folk medicine treatment: taking olive oil. In the booklet "Intestinal Toxicity And Inner Cleansing," (Keats Publishing, Inc.), biochemist Jeffrey Bland, Ph.D states that an olive oil flush seems to bring about two detoxification benefits: causing the pancreas gland to secrete more digestive enzymes and bicarbonate and the gall bladder to contract and release more bile.

Dr. Bland mentions an internal cleansing program evaluated at the Linus Pauling Institute of Science and Medicine. Twelve human subjects, some with chronic constipation, were tested prior to and after taking the Yerba Prima Internal Cleansing Program: a blend of healing herbs, more fluid intake, the olive oil flush, malt extract and soluble fiber.

During the three month program, the volunteers found definite improvement: quicker bowel transit time, more effective peristaltic action, less constipation, and, as a consequence, fewer of the toxic bacteria Clostridium. In addition, urine samples showed less of a chemical (indican), indicating decreased intestinal toxicity. The crowning benefit was evidence that nutrients were better absorbed after the cleansing.

Some long-time folk remedies to relieve constipation are nature's sauer kraut (one cup daily) or sauer kraut juice (one glass daily). Prunes and prune juice, too, are prime movers. However, these folk remedies are more in the nature of laxatives than colon cleansers. It is far better to eat natural roughage every day: large amounts of fresh vegetables, some fruit and fibers mentioned above, not only for their laxative effect but also for their ability to detoxify the intestinal tract and make the small intestine more able to receive health-building nutrients.

CHAPTER 73

Itch,
Rectal
(Pruritus Ani)

Flat on a chair, bent over a drawing board day after day, Estelle, a commercial artist, suffered tormenting rectal itch. Too embarrassed about her condition to tell her male boss, she made frequent trips to the ladies' room to scratch, often to the point of bleeding.

Her doctor had given her a succession of salves. However, none of them had worked—even cortisone. Frustrated, upset and being driven crazy, she followed my recommendation and saw an alternative doctor who insisted on dealing with causes, rather than symptoms.

By in-depth questioning, he discovered the basic problem, a perfumed toilet tissue which Estelle had used, then put her on a regime of three warm baths daily to soothe and heal the inflammation, using a bland soap (aloe vera-based from the health food store) rinsing well and then drying fully. Living near the office, she could bathe at noon.

He put her on a diet including foods high in vitamin A and iron and a 50 mg vitamin B-complex tablet. Within two days, she felt relieved and, within 10 days, she was completely healed and happy.

How Does Rectal Itch Start?

Many things touch the anal area: clothing, waste matter, toilet paper, oral antibiotics and laxatives passing through, enema appliances, sanitary napkins and suppositories.

Further, the area by its very nature is an ideal breeding ground for bacteria and fungus: often moist with perspiration, warm and dark. Two other factors make the anus vulnerable to attack by pruritus ani: the abundance of nerves there and the high sensitivity of the skin.

A great deal of dietary refined sugar leads to a heavy concentration of sugar in the skin—a perfect environment for fungus to colonize. This is particularly true in the diabetic, who often has a rectal fungus infection.

Common Contributors

Alternative doctors report that the intake of certain foods encourages pruritus ani: excessive fruit juices and even fruit; cola drinks, and chocolate, including cocoa.

Smoking can bring on this ailment, too, for logical reasons. Smoking narrows the arteries, diminishing blood circulation to the entire body, but, especially to the genital and anal area. This can cause intense itching. Many a sufferer of pruritus ani has slowly recovered from this condition after stopping smoking.

The Practical Encyclopedia of Natural Healing (Rodale Press, Inc.) by Mark Bricklin and associates, states that individuals may get relief by careful washing, rinsing and drying of afflicted parts and then applying wheat germ oil or vitamin E oil.[1]

As stated earlier, foods rich in vitamin A and iron and a vitamin B-complex tablet with 50 mg of the major B fractions have been found by alternative doctors to help alleviate pruritus ani.

Best food sources of vitamin A in international units per less than four ounce units are: cod liver oil, 200,000; sheep liver, 45,000; beef liver, 44,000; calve's liver, 22,000; dandelion greens, 14,000; carrots, 11,000; yams, 9,000; kale, 8,900; parsley and turnip greens, 8,500; spinach, 8,100; collard greens and chard, 6,500; watercress, 5,000; red peppers, 4,400; winter squash, 4,000; egg yolk and cantaloupe, 3,400; endive, 3,300; persimmons and apricots, 2.700; broccoli, 2,500; pimentos, 2,300; swordfish, 2,100; whitefish, 2,000; romaine, 1,900; papayas, 1,700; nectarines and pumpkin, 1,600; peaches and cheeses, 1,300; eggs, 1,200; cherries, lettuce and cream, 1,000.

These are the best of food sources of iron in milligrams per less than four ounce units: kelp, 370; torula yeast, 18; brewer's yeast, 17; kidney, 13; soy lecithin and caviar, 12; pumpkin seeds, 11; sesame seeds, 10; wheat germ, 9.4; blackstrap molasses, 9.1; liver, 8.8; pistachios, egg yolks and sprouts, 7.2; sunflower seeds, 7.1; chickpeas, 6.9; millet, 6.8; lentils, 6.7; molasses and walnuts, 6; parsley, 5; almonds, 4.7 and oats, 4.1.

A word of caution. Unlike the situation with many vitamins, more is not always better with minerals such as iron. In fact, it is easy to take an excess of minerals.

So far as iron is concerned, the RDA is 10 mg for men and 18 for women. Actually, we absorb about six percent of the iron eaten in foods. A diet with considerable vitamin C in it—say 500 mg per day—raises the absorption rate considerably, as various experiments show.

Richest supplement and food sources of vitamin C in milligrams per a unit of less than four ounces are: rose hips, 3,000; acerola cherries, 1,100; guavas, 240; black currants, 200; parsley, 170; green peppers, 110; watercress, 80; chives, 70; strawberries, 57; persimmons, 52; spinach, 51; oranges, 50; cabbage, 47; grapefruit, 38; papaya, 37; elderberries and kumquats, 36; dandelion greens and lemons, 35; cantaloupe, 33, green onions, 32; limes, 31; mangoes, 27; loganberries, 24; tangerines and tomatoes, 23; squash, 22 and raspberries and romaine lettuce, 22.

A consensus of leading alternative doctors suggests taking a vitamin B-complex with a potency of 50 mg to satisfy requirements for this family of vitamins, backed by whole grain cereals and breads, sunflower seeds, lentils, peas, liver and eggs.

Chicken Livers with Yogurt—Mustard Sauce

2 T. rye flour	1 to 2 T. butter
2 T. wheat germ	2 t. prepared mustard
¼ t. dried tarragon	1 c. yogurt
¼ t. pepper	Freshly chopped parsley
1 lb. chicken livers	

On a flat plate or piece of wax paper, combine wheat germ, flour, tarragon and pepper. Add livers and roll and toss until livers are coated evenly. Melt butter in large skillet over medium heat. Add livers and cook until browned on both sides and pink in the center, about 10 minutes. Remove livers from pan and keep warm. Remove pan from heat. Add mustard and yogurt to pan juices and stir until mixture is well blended and hot. Add livers and toss until well coated with sauce. Serve immediately. Top with parsley. Delicious served over cooked brown rice. Makes 4 servings.

Pumpkin Seed Salad

1 c. fresh asparagus,
  steamed until just tender
1 c. fresh brussel sprouts,
  trimmed and steamed
1 raw beet, grated

2 stalks celery, chopped
½ c. alfalfa sprouts
3 lettuce leaves, torn in pieces
½ c. raw pumpkin seed kernels,
  ground

Scrub all vegetables. Steam asparagus and brussel sprouts. Chop all vegetable into bite-size chunks. Tear lettuce into small pieces and toss all ingredients together in salad bowl. Sprinkle ground pumpkin seeds over top. Seeds will absorb a great deal of moisture making a kind of paste. This makes a delicious salad cream.

CHAPTER 74

Jet Lag

A flight attendant in the days when we were called stewardesses, I have known the disorder called jet lag too many times.

Picture this scene. It's nine A.M. when the airplane lands in the U.S.A. Friends will be there to meet me, and I've got to look alive, and yet my drowsy head and sleep-walking body tell me it's four in the morning London time.

What did I do? Toughed it through with coffee, because I didn't know then what I know now. Eventually, I learned to take a warm epsom salts bath the first chance I had. That worked!

Then, by experimentation, I found that a hearty meal of fresh eggs, a ground beef patty, whole wheat toast, and half a grapefruit helped. This was long before experiments by M.I.T.'s Dr. Richard Wurtman revealed that a high protein meal charges up alertness and ability to think efficiently.[1]

Individuals who had been stewardesses far longer than I realized that jet lag is a stress and advised me to take B-complex vitamins, as they did. This helped, too — especially with 1,000 mg timed release vitamin C. Fortunately, now health food stores carry several brands of excellent anti-stress vitamins.

More Than Adjusting To Time Changes

Jet lag is a far more complex disorder than just trying to get in gear with time changes. The body takes some severe stressing from flying at altitudes far higher than the protective atmosphere, and being more vulnerable to radiation from outer space: cosmic, gamma, ultraviolet, and x-rays.

Further, pressurized cabins offer an environment with slightly less oxygen, a high positive to negative ion ratio and unusually low humidity. Even frequent flyers often neglect drinking enough water in flight—and also after.

These factors all tilt the balance of our trillions of body and brain cells, contributing to the forming of free radicals. "Radicals" is the right name for them. These molecules are short one electron and literally run amuck, trying to pick up another electron and getting back in harmony. So they strong-arm an electron from a nearby cell. The next cell steals an electron from the cell adjoining it and on and on it goes—a chain reaction—until the body's defenses can stop it.

I help these defenses by taking free radical quenchers, certain enzymes, vitamins and minerals carried by health food stores: catalase, glutathione peroxidase, methionine reductase, and superoxide dismutase, in the first group; and anti-oxidant vitamins A, C, E, and the anti-oxidant mineral selenium.

These nutrients supply the missing electron to free radicals without themselves becoming free radicals and stop the chain reaction.

Anti-jet lag tips learned from flight attendants, pilots, and biochemists have helped me immeasurably. I no longer dread transcontinental flights for fear of being undermined by jet leg, because I now know how to handle this complex form of stress.

CHAPTER 75

Low Blood Pressure (Hypotension)

Once a rarity in the doctor's office, low blood pressure (hypotension) is becoming a more common disorder these days with so many women and girls on semi-starvation diets to make themselves slender. (This happens to some men, too.)

Marginal to poor nutrition causes the walls of blood vessels to become relaxed, leading to less oxygen and nutrients being supplied to tissue throughout the body.

Consequently, individuals experience the following symptoms: a blood pressure reading below 100/70, fatigue or even exhaustion, little or no endurance, depression, hyper-sensitivity to heat or cold, a rapid pulse after exertion, sometimes even dangerous heart arrhythmias, and no interest in sex.

Low blood pressure can be brought on by many factors: heavy alcohol intake, anorexia, medicines for depression, bulimia, chronic diarrhea, diuretics abuse, prolonged fever (causing dehydration); heart disease, hypothyroiodism (low thyroid function); hypoadrenalism (too little adrenal function) and exercise extremes.

The Key Vitamin

As many research projects indicate, diets low in calories, protein, B vitamins and vitamin C bring on low blood pressure.[1]

The most critical vitamin shortage which invites low blood pressure is that of pantothenic acid. A deficiency of pantothenic acid blocks production of adrenal hormones. Under this condition, salt and water are extravagantly thrown off and blood volume is reduced along with blood pressure.

Nutritional stress plus emotional stress which it helps to bring makes the need for pantothenic acid more acute and leads to even lower blood pressure. Sometimes a 50 mg pill of pantothenic acid daily can normalize blood pressure.

By proper choosing, it is possible to take in 50 mg of pantothenic acid daily in food and food supplements. Here's the Who's Who of pantothenic acid foods in terms of milligrams per less than a four ounce serving: royal jelly, 35; brewer's yeast, 11; torula yeast, 10; brown rice, 8.9; sunflower seeds, 5.5; soybeans, 5.2; corn, 5.0; lentils, 4.8; egg yolk, 4.2; peas, 3.6; alfalfa, 3.3; wheat, 3.2, peanuts, 2.8; rye, 2.6; eggs, 2.3; bee pollen and wheat germ, 2.2.

Water, Salt And Vitamins

Inasmuch as malnutrition often contributes to low blood pressure, this condition usually responds to increased calories, protein, the entire vitamin B family, and vitamin C.

A northern California doctor has had great success treating hypotension with increased intake of water — eight or more glasses daily — a half teaspoon of salt in a glass of water to swell the volume of the blood; two to three capsules of an amino acid supplement; six to eight grams of vitamin C; a vitamin B-complex capsule with 100 mg of the major factors and an addition of 500 mg each of vitamins B-5 and B-6 each day.

Because low blood pressure can originate from any of the many causes mentioned above, it is best to enlist the help of a nutrition-oriented doctor to get at the root of the problem and to guide a recovery regime.

Bean Soup with Vegetables

1 c. dried kidney beans	¼ lb. spinach
2 garlic cloved, pressed	⅓ c. long grain brown rice
2 T. liquid garlic	2 tomatoes, cut in wedges
1 onion, chopped	½ c. parsley, chopped
2 potatoes	½ T. celery salt
2 carrots	¼ t. marjoram
2 zucchini	1 t. oregano
2 leeks	2 T. brewers yeast

Place beans in pot with two quarts spring water. Bring to a boil. Remove from heat and let stand for 1 hour. Add onion, brewers yeast, garlic, tomatoes, spinach and simmer for 1½ hours. Chop potatoes in large chunks. Do not peel. Slice carrots ½ inch and zucchini 1 inch thick. Scrub, do not peel. Slice leeks and cut beans into 1 inch pieces. Add to soup along with seasonings. Simmer for 1 hour longer. Thinly slice cabbage and add to soup along with rice (or spaghetti). Simmer another 20 minutes. Add more water if too thick.

Sunflower Seed Milk

Soak 3 ounces sunflower seeds overnight in 5 ounces of spring water and blend in blender for 2 to 3 minutes. Flavor with honey and carob powder to taste.

CHAPTER 76

Low Blood Sugar (Hypoglycemia)

Ever since 1924 when the disorder called low blood sugar (hypoglycemia or hyperinsulinism) was first announced, orthodox medicine has insisted that this ailment is all in the mind, that it didn't exist, that people who claimed to have its symptoms were hypochondriacs with "nothing organically wrong."

Now, many decades later, some orthodox medical practitioners concede that it exists, "But that very few people have it."

However, to the millions who experience many of the vast range of hypoglycemia's physical symptoms, their "imaginary" illness is all too real.

O.K., what is hypoglycemia, what are its major symptoms, and what can be done about it?

First Things First

Hypoglycemia is a disorder in which the level of blood sugar (glucose) is too low, because the body processes sugars and starches (carbohydrates) in a faulty way. A person eats a meal top heavy in carbohydrates or a junk food snack rich in refined sugar and his or her blood sugar soars, then, a few hours later, plummets.

This condition is called reactive hypoglycemia, and here's how it works. A hungry hypoglycemic downs a candy bar and his or her pancreas suffers shock and over-responds, spurting so much insulin into the bloodstream that sugar is drawn out too quickly, contributing to a glucose deficiency and new hunger.

Such frequent refined carbohydrates assaults (cake, candy, coffee cakes, cookies, sweet rolls, ice cream or granulated sugar snowed over breakfast cereals or stirred into coffee or tea) make the pancreas even more trigger-happy and over-reactive. First, the blood sugar vaults high and the person feels great. The resulting insulin charge causes the blood sugar to drop fast. Then the person falls from the mountain peak to the pits.

More To Hypoglycemia

It would be an over-simplification to say that all low blood sugar results from carbohydrate shock to the pancreas. Hypoglycemia can originate from many causes: a deficiency of certain vitamin B complex fractions— mainly B-1, B-2 and niacin, necessities for efficient carbohydrate metabolism; too little intake of protein added to a deficiency of the B-vitamins pantothenic acid and B-2 (make it difficult to impossible for the liver to remove excess insulin); continuous stress, overworked adrenal glands, a tumor of the pancreas (a stimulant to insulin secretion); food allergies and low thyroid function.

When stress doesn't let up, the adrenal glands, overworking to secrete adrenalin to prepare for "fight or flight," set off a gland-to-gland relay that leads to turning liver-stored glycogen into blood sugar, triggering the pancreas to pour out more insulin. (See Section on Stress.)

Stressors such as alcohol, chewing tobacco, caffeine-rich colas, and smoking also rev up the adrenals to over-production with hypoglycemia the consequence.

Low thyroid function also interferes with the working of the adrenal glands. Too little thyroid hormone in the bloodstream reduces the secretion of cortisol, a hormone which stimulates the liver to produce glycogen. A shortage of glycogen, then, can cause hypoglycemia. (See Section on Low Thyroid Function.)

Hypothyroidism can contribute to low blood sugar in still another way. Remember, hypoglycemia is the faulty processing of carbohydrates. In low thyroid function, the liver operates sluggishly, storing glucose too slowly. This makes blood sugar look deceptively high in a fasting glucose tolerance test. This excess glucose, then, may be spilled into the urine, making it look as if the person is a pre-diabetic, when he or she is actually a hypothyroid.

The Test And Symptoms

And, speaking of the glucose tolerance test, a reading between 35 to 50 milligrams of glucose per 100 milliliters of blood is considered low blood sugar.

If you have certain common symptoms of hypoglycemia, you might wish to apply to your doctor for a glucose tolerance test to confirm your condition—preferably to an alternative medical doctor, because he or she recognizes low blood sugar as a real disorder.

A prominent Jacksonville, Florida physician, Stephen Gyland, M.D., made a major study of 600 well-documented hypoglycemics and listed 39 symptoms of this ailment, starting with those found most frequently in the group[1]:

Nervousness, irritability, exhaustion, faintness and dizziness, depression, vertigo, drowsiness, headaches, digestive disturbances, forgetfulness, sleeplessness, constant worrying, mental confusion, heart palpitation, muscle pains, numbness, undecisiveness, unsocial, asocial and antisocial behavior; crying spells, lack of sex drive (females); allergies, lack of coordination, leg cramps, blurred vision, twitching and jerking of muscles; itching and crawling sensation of skin; gasping for breath; smothering spells, staggering, sighing and yawning, impotence (males); unconsciousness, night terrors and nightmares; rheumatoid arthritis, phobias and fears; neurodermatitis, suicidal intent, nervous breakdown, and convulsions.

Eating To Beat Hypoglycemia

If you think you're hypoglycemic and want to confirm it, you can buy a glucometer, a very low cost, portable instrument for measuring blood sugar at any time that you experience symptoms. If you require more information on this device or other home tests, you might wish to check the best book on this subject: Do-It-Yourself Medical Testing (Over 160 Tests You Can Do at Home) by Cathey Pinckney and Edward R. Pinckney, M.D. (Facts on File).

Dozens of discussions with alternative medical doctors have given me a list of major foods and food groups for beating low blood sugar. Here they are: All vegetables (low carbohydrate)

Beef, lamb, poultry
Butter (provided you are not hypercholesterolemic)
Cheese, milk, yogurt, kefir
Eggs (provided you are not hypercholesterolemic)
Fish
Low carbohydrate fruits
Nuts (preferably unsalted)
Soybeans and their products
Whole grain cereal and bread

(Nothing omitted from this list is permitted, including sugar in all forms, candies, pastries, macaroni, spaghetti, white rice, sweetened soft drinks, alcohol, coffee and processed cereals, canned fruits or vegetables, because they contain some form of sugar.

At the start, at least, it's best to stay with produce in the five to 10-percent carbohydrate groups. So skip items of produce not mentioned, because they are in the 15 percent to 20 percent carbohydrate content group — or above. Fruits and vegetables with the lowest carbohydrate content follow. First is the five percent or less category: beans, carrots, cauliflower, lettuce, onions, okra, pepper, pumpkin, radishes, string beans, and watercress. (No fruits in this bracket.)

In the seven percent category are grapefruit, lemons, strawberries and watermelon and avocados and olives.

Featured in the 10 percent group are: cantaloupe, oranges, peaches, raspberries, Hubbard squash and turnips.

Nine times out of ten, alternative doctors successfully cope with hypoglycemia by putting patients on a medium to high protein diet and complex carbohydrate food items in the above list. The secret to success is eating five or six evenly spaced small meals, rather than the usual three, so that sugar level will be sustained.

Foods Containing Key Vitamins

These are supplements and the foods richest in vitamin B-1 in terms of milligrams per less than four ounce units: brewer's yeast, 16; torula yeast, 15; sunflower seeds, 2.2; wheat germ, 2.0, royal jelly, 1.5; pinon nuts, 1.3: peanuts, 1.2; soybeans, 1.10; sesame seeds, 0.98; brazil nuts,

0.96; bee pollen, 0.93; pecans, 0.86; alfalfa and peas, 0.80; millet, 0.73; beans, 0.68; buckwheat and oats, 0.60; wheat, 0.57; hazelnuts, 0.46; rye, 0.43; lentils and corn, 0.37; brown rice, 0.34; walnuts, 0.33; egg yolk, 0.32; chickpeas, 0,31; blackstrap molasses, 0.28; liver 0.25; almonds, 0.24; barley and salmon, 0.21; eggs, 0.17 and lamb and mackerel, 0.15.

The following supplements and foods have the most liberal amounts of vitamin B-2 in milligrams per less than four ounce servings: torula yeast, 16; brewer's yeast, 4.2; liver, 4.1; royal jelly, 1.9; alfalfa, 1.8; bee pollen, 1.7; almonds, 0.92; wheat germ, 0.68; mustard greens, 0.64; egg yolk, 0.52; cheeses, 0.46; human milk, 0.40; millet, 0.38; chicken, 0.36; soybeans and veal, 0.31; eggs and sunflower seeds, 0.28; lamb, 0.27; peas, blackstrap, molasses, parsley and cottage cheese, 0.25; sesame seeds, 0.24; eggwhite, lentils, rye and beans, 0.22; spinach, turkey, broccoli and beef, 0.20 and corn, 0.19.

Best supplement and food sources of niacin in milligrams per less than four ounce units are: torula yeast, 100; brewer's yeast, 38; bee pollen, 19; peanuts, 17; liver, 16; salmon. 13; chicken and tuna, 12; swordfish and turkey, 11; halibut, 9.2; royal jelly, 8.2; veal, 7.8; sunflower seeds, 5.6; sardines and sesame seeds, 5.4; beef and alfalfa, 5.0; potatoes, 4.8; brown rice and wheat bran, 4.7; pinon nuts, 4.5; buckwheat and whole wheat, 4.3; wheat germ, 4.2; barley, 3.7; almonds, 3.5; peas, 2.6; beans, 2.4; millet, 2.3; soybeans and corn, 2.2; blackstrap molasses, 2.1; lentils and chickpeas, 2.0 and cashews, 1.8.

Richest supplements and foods in pantothenic acid in milligrams per less than four ounce units are: royal jelly, 35; brewer's yeast, 11; torula yeast, 10; brown rice, 8.9; sunflower seeds, 5.5; soybeans, 5.2; corn, 5.0; lentils, 4.8; egg yolk, 4.2; peas, 3.6; alfalfa, 3.3; whole wheat, 3.2; peanuts, 2.8; rye, 2.6; eggs, 2.3; bee pollen and wheat germ, 2.2; bleu cheese, 1.8; cashews, 1.3; chickpeas, 1.2; avocado, 1.1; chicken, sardines, turkey and walnuts, 0.90 and perch, and salmon, 0.80.

Sunshine Salad

4 c. mixed greens
1 c. celery, thinly sliced
1 c. zucchini, cut lengthwise in half, then thinly sliced
1 c. cucumber, cut lengthwise in half, then thinly sliced
½ c. parsley, coarsely chopped
2 T. pumpkin seeds
2 T. oat bran

2 T. grated Parmesan cheese
1 T. sunflower seeds
1 T. sliced almonds
4 radishes, sliced
1 c. cottage cheese (raw certified)
1 c. raw beets, grated
1 c. carrots, grated
1 c. alfalfa sprouts
Garnishes: lemon slices and parsley

Toss together the first twelve ingredients. Place on four separate plates. Top with ¼ cup cottage cheese and surround with ¼ cup beets, carrots and sprouts. Garnish with lemon slices and parsley sprigs. Serve with favorite dressing. Serves 4.

CHAPTER 77

Memory Loss (See Alzheimer's Disease)

References to the guy who forgot to go to his memory class or to the gal who will never forget "what's his name?" — may still draw a laugh.

However, memory loss is no laughing matter to the person losing it and to those living with him or her. And the saddest part of it is that so many people—young adults, middle-agers and seniors—sigh with resignation and cop out with the remark, "I guess I'm getting old."

Some individuals with a diminishing memory and many birthdays behind them jump to the usually unwarranted conclusion that they are in the beginning of Alzheimer's disease. Yet the chances are that they are just malnourished in vitamins and minerals which help sustain mental functions.

Declining memory could result from a deficiency in vitamin B-1, vitamin B-12, choline, lecithin and the mineral magnesium—as well as from low thyroid function (hypothyroidism) or low blood sugar (hypoglycemia) or even long-term stress. Possibly it results from a combination of these factors.

Consider Vitamin B-1

Faulty memory—as well as low energy, lack of appetite, and emotional excesses—are all symptoms of vitamin B-1 deficiency.[1] Individuals who eat many foods containing refined sugar and flour or other processed foods, who drink alcohol regularly, or are addicted to coffee literally drain the vitamin B-1 from their system.

An experiment with rats demonstrated with force that vitamin B-1 lack can sabotage the memory. Rats trained to get through a maze were divided into two groups, one given a nutritionally complete diet and the other a

355

diet totally lacking vitamin B-1.[2]

Twenty days later, the rats were tested. The group on the good diet made it through in an average of 22 seconds. The vitamin B-1-deprived rats took 55 seconds — almost three times as long. Put on a diet rich in the previously missing vitamin, the rats made a startling recovery in memory and ability to speed through the maze.

Human experiments have revealed similar results. Many individuals who seem senile are just lacking in vitamin B-1. Doctor friends of mine have seen vitamin B-1 bring incredible recoveries of memory, usually by means of a daily B-complex supplement with 50 mg of major fractions, including B-1. (A list of vitamin B-1 rich foods will come later.)

Vitamin B-12 and Choline: memory-enhancers

A deficiency of vitamin B-12 brought on devastating memory loss and ability to think, plus a swarm of emotional problems such as depression, confusion, delusions and hallucinations, in an experiment by Dr. J. MacDonald Holmes reported in the British Medical Journal.[3]

Another high-powered food supplement for boosting flagging memory is choline, a nutrient in lecithin, derived from soybeans, liver and egg yolks. Choline becomes changed at the ends of certain brain cell nerves into acetylcholine, a chemical messenger which is lacking in the brain of Alzheimer's disease victims.

Half of the Alzheimer's patients in a six-month London study were given large doses of lecithin. The lecithin-takers made a deinite improvement in memory, related functions, and ability to care for themselves, while the other half stayed the same.[4]

Other studies of young and old with faulty memory have shown that lecithin can work wonders.

The memory center of the brain, the hippocampus, has a special affinity for the mineral magnesium. Individuals who have trouble learning and a sieve-like memory may be lacking magnesium, as various experiments demonstrate.[5]

Hypothyroidism and Hypoglycemia: memory-underminers

Low thyroid function can deprive the brain of oxygen in several ways: by slowing down the blood circulation and delivery of oxygen and nutrients and by reducing the rate at which blood sugar "burns" to nourish brain cells—also by depressing the production of red blood cells, the mini freight cars that deliver oxygen, and by encouraging hardening of the arteries. (See the Section on Low Thyroid Function).[6]

Iodine-rich kelp usually helps correct this condition in first generation hypothyroids. A prescribed thyroid supplement is necessary for second generation hypothyroids and beyond.

Like hypothyroidism, hypoglycemia can make forgetting far easier than remembering. Stephen Gyland, M.D., a prominent Jacksonville, Florida physician, made a study of 600 well-documented sufferers from hypoglycemia and found faulty memory to be a symptom in 67 percent of the cases.[7]

How to correct low blood sugar level? Lay off refined sugar and flour products, include more protein in the diet, and eat five or six small meals a day instead of the standard three. (See Section on Low Blood Sugar.)

Stress: a memory thief

One of the best reasons for avoiding or adjusting to stress in a positive way is a little known factor: sustained stress can destroy brain cells in the hippocampus and kill off memory.

This was demonstrated by a research project at the Salk Institute for Biological Studies in San Diego. Here's what happens. Under severe and unyielding stress, adrenal hormones (corticoids) seal off the entry of blood sugar (glucose) into many brain cells, reserving it for physical action such as muscle movements in what appears to be an emergency. Glucose is the single source of energy and life for the brain cells. With their sugar supply cut off, they starve and die.[8]

Unforgettable Memory Foods

Richest food and supplement sources of vitamin B-1 in milligrams per less than four ounce servings are: brewer's yeast, 16; torula yeast, 15; sunflower seeds, 2.2; wheat germ, 2; royal jelly, 1.5; pinon nuts, 1.3; peanuts, 1.2; soybeans, 1.10; sesame seeds, 0.98; brazil nuts, 0.96; bee pollen, 0.93; pecans, 0.86; alfalfa and peas, 0.80; millet, 0.73; beans, 0.68; buckwheat and oats, 0.60; whole wheat, 0.57; hazelnuts, 0.46; rye, 0.43; lentils and corn, 0.37; brown rice, 0.34; walnuts, 0.33; egg yolk, 0.32; chickpeas, 0.31; liver, 0.25; almonds, 0.24; barley and salmon, 0.21 and eggs, 0.17.

Best food sources of vitamin B-12 in milligrams per less than a four ounce portion are: liver, 0.086; sardines, 0.034; mackerel and herring, 0.0100; red snapper, 0.0088; flounder, 0.0064; salmon, 0.0047; lamb, 0.0031; swiss cheese, 0.0021; eggs, 0.0020; haddock, 0.0017; muenster cheese, 0.0016; swordfish and beef, 0.0015 and bleu cheese, 0.0014.

Richest sources of choline in milligrams per less than four units are: soy lecithin, 2900; egg yolk, 1700; chickpeas, 780; lentils, 710; split peas, 700; brown rice, 650; liver, 550; caviar, 540; eggs, 500; wheat germ, 400; soybeans, and green beans, 340; green peas, 270; cabbage and torula yeast, 250; spinach, peanuts and brewer's yeast, 240; sunflower seeds, 220; blackstrap molasses, 150 and alfalfa, bran and barley, 140.

Noteworthy foods for high lecithin content are scarce: soy beans, organ meats and eggs.

Best sources of magnesium in milligrams per less than four ounce units are: kelp, 740; blackstrap molasses, 410; sunflower seeds, 350; wheat germ, 320; almonds, 270; soybeans, 240; brazil nuts, 220; pistachios and soy lecithin, 160; hazelnuts, 150; pecans and oats, 140; walnuts, 130; brown rice, 120; chard, 65; spinach, 57; barley, 55; coconut, 44; salmon, 40; corn, 38; avocados, 37; bananas, 31; cheeses, 30 and tuna, 29.

Superior sources of iodine in milligrams per less than four ounce units: kelp, 180; iodized salt, 10; cod liver oil, 0.84; haddock, 0.31; codfish, 0.14; chard, 0.10; beans, 0.100; sea salt, 0.095; perch, 0.074; sunflower seeds, 0.070; herring, 0.052; turnip greens, 0.047; halbut, 0.046; peanuts and cantaloupe, 0.020; liver, 0.019; soybeans, 0.017; pineapple, 0.016; potatoes, 0.015; cheeses, 0.011 and lettuce, 0.010.

CHAPTER 78

Menopause (Change of Life)

One of the most difficult phases of a woman's life is the menopause (change of life), characterized by various unpleasant to painful symptoms: backaches, breathing difficulties, depression, dizziness, excessive menstrual flow, fatigue, headaches, hot flashes and inordinate sweating, nervousness and palpitations and dry vaginal tissues.

While female hormones are often used to relieve such symptoms—with the risk of contributing to cancer—certain safe nutrients have been shown to be helpful.

An experimental study revealed the greater effectiveness of the citrus-derived bioflavonoids hesperiden and hesperiden methyl chalcone in relieving certain symptoms of menopause—mainly flushing—than sub-therapeutic dosages of estrogen and two other similar treatments.[1]

"E" For Excellent

Much more experimentation, including a single blind study, showed that vitamin E supplementation may also be helpful in reducing symptoms of menopause.[2]

Administering of 100 I.U. of vitamin E three times daily by H.A. Gozen, M.D., lessened symptoms in 16 out of 35 menopausal women in three months. Gozen stated that results might have been even more impressive if a higher amount of vitamin E had been used.[3]

N.R. Kavinoky, M.D. scored impressive results supplementing the diet of 92 menopausal patients with 10 to 25 I.U. of vitamin E daily.[4] This diminished the copious menstrual flow in 16 of 34 test subjects; relieved all 37 subjects troubled with hot flashes and alleviated backache of 16 women.

The Versatile Vitamin

Kavinoky upped the amount of vitamin E to 50 to 100 I.U. daily in another group of 79 menopausal women.[5] Seventy-five percent of the patients with hot flashes and profuse sweating showed improvement. More than half of them reported less fatigue, nervousness, disturbed sleep and sleeplessness. In almost all of these women, dizziness, heart palpitation and shortness of breath disappeared in from two weeks to two or three months.

C.J. Christy, M.D. supplemented the diet of 25 women with unremitting hot flashes with 10 to 30 I.U. of vitamin E daily for from one to six weeks.[6] Due to their history of cancer, these women were given alternative therapy, rather than risk estrogen treatment. Every one manifested marked improvement or total relief from hot flashes, with the bonus value of brightening of characteristic moods.

In an experimental single-blind study, 66 patients with vasomotor problems (inadequate regulation of expansion and contraction of blood vessels) received an average of 30 I.U. of vitamin E daily for an average of one month.[7] R.S. Finkler, M.D., found that 31 had positive results —good to excellent—and sixteen had fair response. (Symptoms returned when supplementation was discontinued.)

Unknown to them, seventeen patients were then given placebo substitutes and again experienced previous symptoms, only to lose them shortly after vitamin E was resumed.

The Fredericks Regime

In Carlton Fredericks' Nutritional Guide For The Prevention & Cure of Common Ailments and Diseases (A Fireside Book, Simon and Schuster), Dr. Fredericks writes that emotional storms in menopause— and this would include nervousness and depression—are often quieted with vitamin B-complex (plus brewer's yeast, liver, other organ meats, wheat germ and whole grains), bioflavonoids, lecithin, calcium and vitamin E.

The Fredericks menopausal regime called for two to three grams of bioflavonoids daily, preferably the kind derived from citrus fruit.

Although he didn't specify the amount of lecithin, he stated that the phosphatidyl choline form was three times as rich as the ordinary kind. He suggested 1,000 to 1,500 mg of calcium daily. (A quart of milk contains 1,000 mg.) The amount of vitamin E (mixed tocopherols) recommended was 400 I.U.

Dr. Fredericks writes that vitamin E is also helpful for the last menopausal complaint on the list: dry or atrophied vaginal tissues, whose symptoms are lack of lubrication, itching and pain in sexual intercourse.

Medical reports indicate that vitamin E, as an alternative to estrogen creams, is helpful in relieving this condition and also reduces hot flashes, states Fredericks.

Alternative doctors cite studies reported here as evidence that menopausal problems can often be handled without using female hormones, which can over-stimulate responsive tissues such as breast and uterus, contributing to cancer.

Several of the key nutrients helpful in dealing with menopause and the foods richest in them have been mentioned. However, vitamin E and calcium remain to be covered.

Following are the supplements and foods with highest ratings of vitamin E in International Units per less than four ounce portions: wheat germ, 160; safflower nuts, 35; sunflower seeds, 31; whole wheat, 30; sesame oil, 26; walnuts, 22; corn oil and hazelnuts, 21; soy oil and peanut oil, 16; almonds, 15; olive oil, 14; cabbage, 7.8; brazil nuts and peanuts, 6.5; cod liver oil, 5.4; cashews, 5.1; soy lecthin, 4.8; spinach, 2.9; asparagus, 2.5; broccoli, 2.0; butter, 1.9; parsley, 1.8; and oats, barley and corn, 1.7.

Best supplement and food sources of calcium are: bone meal, 40,000; dolomite, 21,000; sesame seeds, 1,200; kelp, 1.100; cheeses, 700; brewer's yeast, 420; sardines and carob, 350; molasses, 290; caviar, 280; soybeans and almonds, 230; torula yeast, 220; parsley, 200; brazil nuts, 190; watercress, salmon, and chickpeas, 150; egg yolk, beans, pistachios, lentils and kale, 130; sunflower seeds and milk, 120; buckwheat, 110; maple syrup, cream and chard, 100; walnuts, 99; spinach, 93; endive, 81: and pecans, 73.

Sunflower-Carrot Casserole

1½ lbs. turkey, ground
½ c. onion, chopped
½ c. celery, chopped
2 garlic cloves, minced
4 c. carrots, thickly sliced

3 c. tomatoes
½ t. sea salt
1 c. sunflower seeds or
    chopped almonds
2 T. wheat germ

Preheat oven to 300 degrees. Brown meat with onion, celery and garlic. Combine with remaining ingredients in large baking dish. Sprinkle chopped nuts or seeds on top. Bake at 300 degrees for ½ hour. Serves 8. Serve with fresh lightly steamed asparagus covered in butter.

Avocado with Fruit

Avocado pears
Soy cottage cheese
French dressing
Sesame crackers

Seedless grapes or berries
Grapefruit wedges
Plums

Select ripe small avocado pears. Peel and cut in half. Put 2 tablespoons Soy Cottage Cheese in each pear and place any of the above fruits over the top. Add a little French Dressing and serve surrounded by crackers and more fruit as a garnish.

CHAPTER 79

Migraine
(And Lesser Headaches)

"A very severe illness that does not get the sympathy it deserves!"

This is how a migraine headache is described by an authority on the subject, K.M.A. Welch, M.D., of Baylor College of Medicine, who, with co-workers at the Baylor-Methodist Center for Cerebrovascular Research in Houston, Texas, has made an intensive study of the phenomenon.[1]

Dr. Welch says that the migraine should no longer be regarded a benign disease, inasmuch as there is often a degree of depressed blood flow to the brain as severe as in a stroke.[2]

And he refers to findings of Sir Charles Symonds, an authority of another generation — that frequent migraines could lead to cumulative neurological deficits.[3]

Warning Signs And Symptoms

One of my friends tells me, "You've never had a headache until you've had a migraine."

"No, thanks."

All sorts of alarms go off when a migraine is imminent. Hands get cold to icy. Lights flash inside the head (sometimes like zig-zags of lightning). Nerves seem raw. Depression and an overwhelming fatigue weigh you down.

Then, after this drum-roll, comes the main event: throbbing pain that settles down to a persistent dull ache and, sometimes, a queasy feeling, a pain in the abdomen, vomiting or diarrhea.

Female migraine sufferers outnumber males.

363

Triggers of Every Sort

What causes migraines? The dilation of blood vessels in the head. But what pulls the trigger? One or more of the following: a nutrient called tyramine, food additives, low blood sugar, sticky blood platelets, oral contraceptives or supplemental estrogen, or emotional stress.

Foods and beverages which contain tyramine, an agent powerful in dilating blood vessels, are well-documented for triggering migraines: aged cheese, bananas (I hate to list this fruit, one of my favorites); beef and chicken livers, chocolate, eggplant, pickled herring, soy sauce, sour cream, cured meats such as ham, hot dogs, salami and beer, certain champagnes and red wine.

Some food additives—monosodium glutamate (MSG), and nitrate and nitrite used to preserve bacon, ham, hot dogs, salami and various other types of sausage—are also activators of migraines, particularly when in tyramine-containing foods. Many Chinese restaurants still use MSG as a flavor-enhancer.

Other Prime Suspects

Low blood sugar (hypoglycemia), too, can bring on migraines. An article in the New England Journal of Medicine tells of 35 migraine patients who, during migraine attacks, were shown by encephalograms to have low blood sugar.[4] The lower the blood sugar, the worse their migraines.

When a high protein, sugar-free regime was substituted for the patients' previous heavy-in-refined- carbohydrate diet, they all were delivered of their migraines.

In another study of hypoglycemics, this one reported in the medical journal Headache, 118 migraine patients were put on a high-protein, low-carbohydrate diet. Their daily food was distributed over six feedings, rather than the customary three to keep their sugar level properly elevated. When the test ended 90 days later, most of patients— 85 in all —were improved by at least 75 percent.[5]

Sticky blood cells that bunch together (platelet aggregation) also contribute to migraines. In one study, 77 percent of migraine patients had excessively high rates of platelet aggregation.[6] Fish oils—mainly Omega-3— have been found to make the platelets less sticky. So has garlic—fresh and liquid or odorless capsules.

Both the pill and supplemental estrogen are suspect when a woman taking them has migraines. Lee Kudrow, M.D., of the California Medical Clinic for Headache (Encino, California) discovered that women taking estrogen in the Pill or otherwise have twice the migraines than non-takers.[7] When 239 patients cut out their supplemental estrogen, they reported a marked reduction in migraines.

Emotional Causes, Too!

Some decades ago, a popular song told us that love and marriage "go together like a horse and carriage."

Now two medical doctors say that marriage—the stressful kind—goes together with something that fails to rhyme: migraine headaches.

Harvey J. Featherstone, an internist, and Bernard D. Beitman, a psychiatrist at the University of Washington School of Medicine in Seattle, have found that persons who suffer daily migraines which painkillers cannot diminish, let alone relieve, are either involved in a stressful marriage or in some other discordant personal relationship.

How can they beat their migraines? With something less drastic and more successful than ridding themselves of their mates: marriage counseling or psychotherapy.

Other Ways of Handling Migraines

Many successful ways of coping with migraines have been mentioned above: avoiding tyramine-containing foods and food additives such as MSG, managing low blood sugar, preventing abnormal platelet aggregation, avoiding the Pill or supplemental estrogen, and resolving personal conflicts in marriage and, of course, otherwise, too.

Now there are several other routes to travel: exercising, taking alternate hot and cold showers, and using a folk medicine called feverfew.

Numerous qualified sources mention the merit of feverfew in coping with migraines. As a matter of fact, the Harvard Medical School Health Letter offered a comprehensive writeup on the subject, indicating that it is, indeed, legitimate. [8]

Made from the leaves of the feverfew plant, a member of the chrysanthemum family, feverfew can be found in health food stores. Another folk medicine therapy for migraines and lesser headaches is hyssop, which comes from a fragrant, blue-flowered, mint-family plant. For one of my rare headaches, I chew on a sprig of hyssop or rub it on my forehead like Mary did in the Bible: Fable says it was she who named it the "blessed plant." At all times, I keep a hyssop plant growing in a flower pot in the backyard.

About exercise, University of Wisconsin Biodynamics Lab researchers found walking, jogging or running for 30 minutes three times weekly over 15 weeks worked wonders for the Migraine Miserable. [9] They suffered only half as many migraines.

A UCLA School of Medicine neurologist claims that the hot-cold shower routine has called an abrupt halt to many a murderous migraine and ordinary headaches, as well. [10]

Ordinary Headaches Are A Pain, Too!

While an airline stewardess, I met an excellent folk therapy for common headaches: rubbing my hands and arms in a basin of hot water to draw the blood away from my head. Soon my headaches seemed to follow the released water down the drain.

Food and environmental alergies (See the Section on Allergies with its list of most common food alergens) are notorious for setting off common headaches, too. Other triggers for common headaches are emotional stress, low blood sugar, bright lights, drinking too cold liquids, withdrawing from coffee or other caffeine sources, sulfites in enhancers, and monosodium glutamate disguised in many of our foods as "hydrolized protein or "natural flavoring."

Another successful folk medicine therapy stewardesses use for headaches is placing an ice bag on the forehead or the back of the neck.

Resolving tension of stressful relations brings relief from ordinary headaches as well as those extraordinary migraines. It pays to seek peace in our time and remember what the Bible says about loving "thy neighbor," even if he or she happens to be your spouse.

Love not only banishes fear, but also migraines. Isn't that worth a shot?

CHAPTER 80

Milk Intolerance (Lactose Intolerance)

Physicians constantly hear patients complain, "I like milk, but milk doesn't like me!"

Many patients still think they are allergic to milk. Some may be, but most of them have a physical deficiency that makes them intolerant of milk — rather, to its content of lactose, milk sugar.

Most adults lose the ability to produce lactase, an enyzme required for breaking down milk sugar. So the lactose escapes the stomach undigested, meets intestinal bacteria which feed on it and cause fermentation, and these milk-drinkers actually feel like a war zone with cramps, diarrhea and gas.

Blacks, Hispanics, Jews and Orientals are particularly prone to lactase deficiency. What to do about it? Here are some solutions—drastic to not so drastic:

1. Avoid milk, cream and cheese.

2. Use small amounts of milk products. Some of us produce a little lactase.

3. Use milk which comes with lactase added.

4. Buy lactase enzymes—available in health food stores—to accompany milk-drinking and cheese-eating.

5. Eat a high grade of lactobacillus acidophilus-cultured yogurt. Top quality yogurts do not contain fillers, to which some people are allergic. Experiments by Dr. Joseph Kolars, at the University of Minnesota, revealed that seven out of 10 persons who could not tolerate milk, were able to eat yogurt without discomfort. The yogurt appears to digest its own lactose.[1]

6. A small quantity of milk or cheese can often be tolerated when taken along with yogurt.

7. Raw certified milk—unpasteurized—seems better tolerated than pasteurized. It is available in California. (The Wulzen factor, an anti-stiffness element, is abundant in raw certified milk, but not in the pasteurized form. (See the Section on Arthritis.)

8. Don't depend entirely on dairy products for your calcium for strong bones and teeth and steady nerves. Lactose intolerance and allergy to milk may bring on digestive problems which could cause intestinal inflammation or bleeding and, as a result, inefficent digestion, and, lead to a calcium deficiency.

Following are some excellent alternative food sources of calcium, starting with the highest number of milligrams per less than four ounce servings: sesame seeds, 1,200; kelp, 1,100; brewer's yeast, 420; sardines and carob—not a very tasty combination—350; molasses, 290; caviar, 280; soybeans and almonds, 230; parlsey, 200; Brazil nuts, 190; watercress, canned salmon and chickpeas, 150; egg yolk, beans, pistachios lentils and kale, 130; sunflower seeds, 120; buckwheat, 110; chard, 100 and walnuts, 99.

Milk Substitute Drinks

Almond Milk
Soak 3 ounces almonds overnight in 5 ounces of apple juice. The next morning add 3 to 5 ounces of spring water and blend in blender for 2 to 3 minutes. Flavor with honey and a banana, or carob powder to taste. Delicious over cereal or just to drink.

Sunflower Seed Milk
Use the same recipe as above, but with sunflower seeds.

Soy Milk Powder
Add 2 tablespoons soy milk powder to one pint water. Sweeten with honey. Add a pinch of sea salt or kelp. Add carob powder or fruit (black currants) for a change. Use in any recipe that would normally call for milk.

Keeps just a few days.

Rice Milk

4 c. water

1 c. brown rice (cooked)

1 t. vanilla (optional)

Place all ingredients in blender and process until smooth.

CHAPTER 81

Miscarriage

Expulsion of the fetus from the womb before it is far enough developed to live is one of the definitions of miscarriage.

One bit of advice some medical doctors offer women who are habitual miscarriers is to spend a great deal of time in bed. This is good advice for women who can afford a housekeeper. But what about the vast majority who can't?

Perhaps the solution is in several nutrients, one of which is considered a non-essential nutrient, a substance not known to be necessary for human function: bioflavonoids.

Bioflavonoids are substances derived mainly from citrus fruits — the white underskin of the peeled orange or grapefuit, and the segment parts — from apricots, blackberries, black currants, cherries, grapes, and lemons.

Convincing Studies

Two prominent researchers — Dr. Carl Javert, of Cornell University, and Dr. Robert Greenblatt, of the Medical College of Georgia, independently discovered the same thing: that bioflavonoids and vitamin C can prevent miscarriage.

Javert tested 1,334 women with a history of habitual abortion and found 45 percent deficient in vitamin C. Over and above a diet which supplied 350 mg of vitamin C daily, he gave 100 pregnant women from this larger group a bioflavonoid-vitamin C pill (with 150 mg of vitamin C). Ninety-one percent experienced successful pregnancies![1]

Dr. Greenblatt placed 13 habitual aborters on a similar regime. Eleven who had had two miscarriages previously gave birth to live infants.[2]

Why Bioflavonoids Seem To Work

Bioflavonoids appear to be important, because of their contribution to capillary integrity. (The body has vast networks of capillaries.) Through capillary walls pass life-giving oxygen and nutrients, as well as waste materials to be transported by the blood and thrown off.

Cement binding cells of capillaries together—all other body cells, too — has an important ingredient of vitamin C and, presumably, bioflavonoids also. If this cement does not bind properly, oxygen and nutrients can't be delivered to the hungry cells as efficiently as needed. The state of the capillaries in the womb is the key consideration in miscarriages, say authorities.

Does Spontaneous Abortion Indicate a Defective Fetus?

Some physicians feel that spontaneous abortions are nature's way of rejecting a defective fetus? True?

A loud and clear "No!"

The one study we find in medical literature, in the American Journal of Obstetrics and Gynecology (44: 973, 1942), offers statistics on threatened miscarriages in 12,000 cases. Only 1.5 percent of the fetuses had major birth defects—excellent odds for having a normal baby.

A Boost From Wheat Germ Oil

Writing in the Ohio State Medical Journal, Wynne M. Silbernagel, M.D. and James B. Patterson, M.D. express strong feelings that any woman threatening to abort deserves some kind of help.

In a survey of almost 3,000 pregnant women—most of whom chose not to be treated—and those who chose to take wheat germ oil daily—the untreated had miscarriages in 15 percent of the cases. In sharp contrast, women on the wheat germ oil aborted in only 3.7 percent of the cases.[3]

Untreated mothers had premature infants in 7.1 percent of the cases in contrast with 3.7 percent for the women treated with wheat germ oil.[4]

A word of caution comes from Gary Gordon, M.D. of Sacramento, California, about wheat germ oil.

"Buy it only in small bottles, recap it quickly after use, and refrigerate it. Wheat germ oil soon becomes rancid. Rancidity defeats the whole purpose."

Vitamin E's Track Record

The late Evan Shute, M.D., who with his brother Wilfrid, is famous for brilliant pioneering work with vitamin E, kept records on 4,141 consecutive cases of women who received a daily supplement ranging from two drams of wheat germ oil to 50 to 450 mg of vitamin E — alpha tocopherol — from pregnancy to delivery.[5]

Just 5.2 percent of the women experienced miscarriages, as compared with almost twice that amount according to reports in medical literature.

A Negative Influence

Just as the supplements reported exert a positive influence, smoking exerts a strong negative influence. Dr. Jay Zabriskie made a study of 2,000 consecutive births in an Army hospital and learned that miscarriages were almost 50 percent more common in smoking mothers-to-be than in non-smokers.[6]

Further, smoking women had two and one-half times more premature babies than non-smokers and their babies averaged a half pound lighter in weight.

How does smoking cause harm? The carbon monoxide which it supplies displaces necessary oxygen. It delivers toxic chemicals to the cells, decreases blood circulation and depletes the available vitamin C, which, as stated earlier is so important to avoiding miscarriages and having full term babies.

Research cited offers valuable guidelines for preventing miscarriage— the loss of a fetus which might have become a full-term baby, if proper nutritional options were exercised.

Alternative doctors know about most, if not all, of the research reported here.

Apple-Banana Salad
with Boston Lettuce Cups

3 lbs. sweet apples,
  some red and some yellow
3 bananas
1 c. macadamia nuts
2 T. instant mayonnaise

2 fresh egg yolks
2 T. fresh lemon juice
¾ c. cold pressed sunflower oil
2 t. C-kist lemon flavored granules

Core apples, but do not peel. Cut into bite size pieces and place in a salad bowl. Slice bananas and add to apples. Sprinkle with nuts and toss with mayonnaise or with whipped nut cream. Serve in lettuce cups. Sprinkle with lemon flavored C-kist granules (found at health food stores). Makes 6 servings.

Chinese Chicken Salad

4 baked chicken breasts, shredded
1 package chinese vermicelli noodles
Chinese spice
Cinnamon salt
1 t. soy seed oil

½ c. sesame seeds
1 bunch chinese parsley
Cilantro (tough to find,
  but worth the trouble)

Saute shredded chicken in soy oil and sesame seeds. Mix sauted chicken with all other ingredients, seasoning with spice and cinnamon salt.

Super "C" Fruit Salad

10 ounces raw pecan pieces
½ lb. cherries
½ pint strawberries
3 nectarines

3 tangerines
6 plums
2 t. wheat germ

Grind nuts to suitable fineness. Wash fruit thoroughly and cut into bite-size pieces. Sprinkle ground nuts and wheat germ over fruit pieces and serve.

Apple-Banana Salad

6 lbs. sweet apples,
  some red and some yellow
3 to 4 bananas

1 c. toasted peanuts
Home-made mayonnaise or salad dressing
12 boston lettuce cups

Core apples, but do not peel. Cut into bite-size pieces and place in salad bowl. Slice bananas and add to apples. Sprinkle with nuts and toss with mayonnaise or dressing. Serve in lettuce cups. Makes 12 servings. NOTE: The contributor's orchard is organically maintained.

CHAPTER 82

Mononucleosis (Overwhelming Viral Fatigue)

Not many years ago, when told they had mononucleosis, patients faced the dismal prospect of having to withdraw from society and vegetating for months or years, because they were disabled by fatigue and unable to attend school or work.

Today there's bright hope from alternative doctors who use the Cathcart method of subduing this strength-sapping disease. (See list of alternative doctors in the back of the book. If none is close enough to you, ask your local health food store for a referral.)

Stubborn mononucleosis will not yield even to an excellent diet of natural food. However, I decided to include the Cathcart strategy, because, if there's a non-medicinal solution to a devastating health problem, it should be presented. That solution is massive doses of Vitamin C.

Robert Cathcart, M.D. patterned his therapy on Dr. Linus Pauling's findings of the early 1970s and those of the late Dr. Fred Klenner, who accomplished phenomenal cures with injections of vitamin C.

Massive Doses

Prior to a telecast on which I interviewed Dr. Cathcart, I learned from him that his therapy subdued mononucleosis in numerous cases in a very short time.[1] Vitamin C doses used would frighten the average doctor who knows little about mega-vitamin therapy: anywhere from 60 to 100 grams daily—that's 60,000 to 100,000 milligrams.

How does this work? The doctor has his own theory. It all begins with free radicals, which in human cells are molecules that have an odd electron. They form from radiation and oxidation that goes on constantly in cells, from chemicals in air, food and water and also from exercise.

These oddball free radicals almost run amuck looking for another electron with which to pair and, in the process, damage or destroy healthy cells. Many authorities feel that they contribute to weakening the immune system and to rapid aging.

Viruses such as the Epstein-Barr which appears to cause mononucleosis actually suppress the immune system, says Dr. Cathcart.

Vitamin C is an anti-oxidant and a free radical scavenger. On encountering a free radical, the vitamin C says, "Here, have the electron you need and don't cause any more destruction."

The free radical is tamed into an orderly, law-abiding cell citizen, but the Vitamin C is destroyed in the process and thrown off in body wastes.

Dr. Cathcart says that when a disease such as mononucleosis strikes, there are far more free radicals within the tissues than the body can handle. Super-high doses of Vitamin C, supplied regularly, quench free radicals generated by mononucleosis or other diseases.

Many patients are intimidated by such tremendous doses of vitamin C until Dr. Cathcart tells them about another patient, a 23-year old, 98-pound lady librarian who wanted to get over severe mononucleosis in a hurry. "She ate a whole pound of ascorbate in two days," he told me. "That's more than 200 grams in a 24-hour period, 200,000 milligrams. Four hundred grams, 400,000 milligrams in a 48-hour period."

Yes, she accomplished her purpose.

Massive doses of vitamin C often cause diarrhea. However, the sicker the person is, the more vitamin C he or she can take before diarrhea strikes, says Dr. Cathcart.

"The reason for this is that a patient with mononucleosis or another severe illness draws off ascorbate from the stomach and intestines so quickly and efficiently to destroy free radicals that little of it reaches the rectum," explains Dr. Cathcart.

Colds, flus, and mononucleosis can actually be cured in a short time with gigantic doses of vitamin C, states the doctor. "Now Epstein-Barr syndrome is another story. We can clear up the symptoms, but not the disease itself." (See the Section on Epstein-Barr.)

Any regime of this kind should be followed in cooperation with an alternative medical doctor familiar with the methods of Dr. Cathcart.

All right. How can one possibly down enough tablets of vitamin C to reach the staggering amount of 60,000 to 100,000 milligrams? Not by means of 500 milligram units. That would mean swallowing 120 to 200 tablets and much inflating air and making a career of vitamin taking.

So Dr. C advises using powdered or granulated ascorbate. This is purchasable from any local health food store. One level teaspoon is the equivalent of 4 grams, 4,000 milligrams.

Now, instead of exercising patience and waiting until mononucleosis leaves of its own accord, the patient, with cooperation of his or her doctor, can speed its departure with massive doses of vitamin C.

Here are the supplements and foods richest in vitamin C for individuals who wish to form a solid base for heavy supplementation. They are listed in milligrams per units of less than four ounces: rose hips, 3,000; acerola cherries, 1,100; guavas, 240; black currants, 200; parsley, 170; green peppers, 110; watercress, 80; chives, 70; strawberries, 57; persimmons, 52; spinach, 51: oranges, 50; cabbage, 47; grapefruit, 38; papaya, 37; elderberries and kumquats, 36; dandelion greens and lemons, 35; cantaloupe, 33; green onions, 32; limes, 31; mangoes, 27; loganberries, 24; tangerines and tomatoes, 23; squash, 22, and raspberries amd romaine lettuce, 18.

Peggy's Vitamin Caesar Salad

½ c. parsley, chopped	¼ t. fresh cayenne pepper
½ c. green pepper, chopped	1 garlic clove, finely chopped
¼ c. lemon juice	1 T. anchovy paste
¼ c. spring water	1 T. honey
¼ c. cider vinegar	2 T. Romano Cheese, grated
¼ to ½ t. vegetable salt	¾ c. olive oil

Put all ingredients, except oil, in blender. Blend until smooth. While blending, add oil gradually in medium speed until mixture thickens. Chill well. Serve on romaine lettuce.

CHAPTER 83

Motion Sickness (And Morning Sickness)

An old folk remedy scored a dazzling triumph over the drug considered the best on the market to cope with motion sickness. Ginger root beat Dramamine in a double-blind study conducted by researchers at Brigham Young University.[1]

Students chosen because of their susceptibility to motion sickness were divided into three groups: those given a gingerroot capsule (about a half teaspoon of powdered ginger) Dramamine, or a placebo. Test volunteers did not know which product they had taken.

All participants were blindfolded and then spun around in a tilting chair for as long as they could take it up to six minutes. Half of the gingerroot takers endured the test for six minutes. Not one of the Dramamine or placebo takers was able to stay aboard for six minutes.

Health food stores sell ginger root capsules, most of whose labels advise taking one capsule three times daily. Not being subject to motion sickness, I have never taken gingerroot capsules or Dramamine. However, my motion sickness-prone friends have played guinea pig with gingerroot capsules and have found them effective whether for a harbor cruise or an ocean voyage.

I am told it's most advantageous to take gingerroot an hour before meeting with potentially upsetting motion. Peggy Boyd, owner of Peggy's Health Center, where I shop in Los Altos (northern California), advises against taking gingerroot by the teaspoon. "It burns like fire," she tells me. "It's best to mix it in fruit juice or to take it by the capsule.[2]

Peggy reminds me that gingerroot is an old folk remedy for women experiencing morning sickness. "More women buy it for that than for motion sickness," she says.

Another Preventive (Not So Folksy)

A formerly pregnant friend beat morning sickness by taking a vitamin B-complex tablet (with 100 mg of B-6) each morning and night. Highly susceptible to motion sickness, she found that this supplement also protects her against motion sickness.

Unfortunately it would take bales of food to supply 200 mg of vitamin B-6 daily and few of us are equal to that so we'll have to settle for the vitamin B-6.

Ginger Sauce for Brown Rice

½ c. Tamari Soy Sauce   1 small onion, sliced
¼ c. vinegar   1 small piece of fresh gingerroot, minced

Place all ingredients in blender at high speed for 2 minutes. Serves 6.

Ginger Tea

Stir ¼ Tsp powdered ginger into 1 Cup hot water. Add honey to taste and lemon, if desired. Makes 1 serving.

CHAPTER 84

Osteomalacia (Bone Softening)

The frightening experience occurred in the front seat of my middle-aged neighbor's foreign car!

As Marge leaned far to her right to flip open the door lock for a lady friend to enter, her rib cage pressed against the arm rest, and she felt her ribs give way, bending inward as if they were rubber.

Tears in her eyes and holding her side, she rang my doorbell in panic, pouring out her story almost faster than I could hear.

"Maureen, what's wrong with me? What should I do?"

As I invited her and her friend into the living room, I replied:

"Sounds like osteomalacia, softening of the bone, but I'm no doctor."

"What should I do?" she pleaded.

"Nothing much now. Let me call an alternative physician for you."

Regimen For Osteomalacia

Marge was so nervous about her condition that I wangled an emergency appointment for her between a doctor friend's other appointments. Yes, the diagnosis was osteomalacia. The doctor gave her a mild pain-killer, told her that the ribs would slowly come back into place, but that she should immediately follow his special daily regime: 400 I.U. of Vitamin D; and a calcium-magnesium supplement (three tablets with 1,000 mg of calcium and 500 mg of magnesium); 50 mg of manganese, 1,000 mg of vitamin C and 10,000 I.U. of vitamin A.

The doctor also gave her a list of natural foods containing the minerals and vitamins in the paragraph above. And they worked for her!

About the same time, I ran across an article in Science News which told about 142 elderly patients confined at Massachusetts General Hospital in

Boston with hip fractures.[1] Seventy-five percent turned out to have osteomalacia. All of them were checked for vitamin D levels.

A researcher named Samuel H. Doppelt and associates found that more than 40 percent were deficient in this vitamin.[2] This came as no great surprise, because many elderly individuals live almost exclusively indoors — shielded from sunlight, which, with cholesterol, forms vitamin D in the skin.

Failure to take a fish liver oil supplement (which provides vitamin D); calcium, magnesium, manganese, vitamin C and other raw materials needed for keeping bones strong, contributed to their condition.

Middle-eastern women who wear veils, keeping the sunlight off their skin, frequently suffer from osteomalacia, have painful backs and develop spontaneous fractures, I observed when in that area. A local doctor told me that they often make striking recoveries when given fish liver oils.

Various products and drugs can create a condition similar to a deficiency of vitamin D even when there is enough of this vitamin: frequent use of cathartics which irritate the intestinal wall or increase peristalsis (wavelike contractions and expansions of intestines); use of the cholesterol-lowering drug cholestyramine for a number of years; long-term taking of anti-convulsant drugs and ingesting mineral oil.

Getting Physical

In addition to proper diet, weight-bearing exercise can often help to renew the bones of senior women, reveals a study by Peter Jacobson and co-workers at the University of North Carolina, Chapel Hill.[3]

Aware of the risk of uterine cancer when women take estrogen for post-menopausal bone loss, Jacobson and associates sought an alternative, discovering that tennis, jogging or running helps cope with this condition.[4]

Eighty women, ages 35 to 65, who played tennis three times a week, were compared with 400 non-exercising women of the same age group. Tennis players in the 35 to 55 age bracket had just a trifle more bone mass than the non-exercisers—as the researchers suspected, because excessive bone loss is not common before menopause.

However, tennis players in the 55 to 65 age group had far more bone than the non-exercisers. The researchers, reporting on results, stated that weight-bearing exercise either prevents or slows bone loss.[5]

Needed Nutrients In Foods

Regular weight-bearing exercise can make a dramatic contribution to stopping bone loss, but offering the right food raw materials for bone-rebuilding is also necessary.

Best supplement and food sources of vitamin D in International Units per units of less than four ounces are: cod liver oil, 20,000; sardines, 500; salmon, 400; tuna, 250; egg yolk, 160; sunflower seeds, 92; liver, 50; eggs, 48; butter, 40; cheese, 30; cream, 15; corn oil, 9.0; human milk, 6.0; cottage cheese and cow's milk, 4.0; bee pollen, 1.6 and bass, 1.0.

Richest sources of calcium—supplements and foods—in milligrams per units of less than four ounces are: dolomite, 21,000; sesame seeds, 1,200; kelp, 1,100; cheese, 700; brewer's yeast, 420; sardines and carob, 350; caviar, 280; soybeans and almonds, 230; torula yeast, 220; parsley, 200; brazil nuts, 190; watercress, salmon and chickpeas, 150; egg yolk, beans, pistachios, lentils and kale, 130; sunflower seeds and cow's milk, 120; buckwheat, 110; maple syrup, cream and chard, 100; walnuts, 99; spinach, 93; endive, 81, pecans, 73; wheat germ, 72 and peas, 70.

Here are the top supplement and food sources of magnesium in milligrams per less than four ounce units: kelp, 740; blackstrap molasses, 410; sunflower seeds, 350; wheat germ, 320; almonds, 270; soybeans, 240; brazil nuts, 220; bone meal, 170; pistachios and soy lecithin, 160; hazelnuts, 150; pecans and oats, 140; walnuts, 130; brown rice, 120; chard, 65; spinach, 57; barley, 55; coconut, 44; salmon, 40; corn. 38; avocados, 37; bananas, 31; cheese, 30; tuna, 29 and potatoes and cashews, 27.

Best foods for deriving manganese are the following in terms of milligrams per units of less than four ounces: tea leaves, 28; cloves, 26; ginger, 8.7; buckwheat, 5.1; oats, 4.9; hazelnuts, 4.2; chestnuts, 3.7; whole wheat, 3.6; pecans, 3.5; barley, 3.2; brazil nuts, 2.8; sunflower seeds, 2.5; ginseng, watercress, peas and beans, 2.0; almonds, 1.9; turnip greens and walnuts, 1.8; brown rice, 1.7; peanuts, 1.5; honey, 1.4; coconut, 1.3; pineapple, 1.1; parsley, 0.94; spinach, 0,82, grapefruit and lettuce, 0.80; bananas, 0.64; carrots, 0.60; berries, 0.55, brewer's yeast,

0.53 and yams, 0.52.

Highest vitamin A and the vitamin A precursor content supplements and foods in International Units per less than four ounce units are: cod liver oil, 200,000; sheep liver, 45,000; cow liver, 44,000; calf's liver, 22,000; dandelion greens, 14,000; carrots, 11,000; yams, 9,000; kale, 8,900; parsley and turnip greens, 8,500; spinach, 8,100; collard greens and chard, 6,500; watercress, 5,000; red peppers, 4,400; winter squash, 4,000; egg yolk and cantaloupe, 3,400; endive, 3,300; persimmons and apricots, 2,700; broccoli, 2,500; pimentos, 2.300; swordfish, 2,100; romaine lettuce, 1,900; mangoes, 1,800; papayas, 1,700; nectarines and pumpkin, 1,600; peaches and cheese, 1,300; eggs, 1,200 and cherries, lettuce and cream 1,000. Richest supplement and food sources of vitamin C in milligrams per units of less than four ounces are: rose hips, 3,000; acerola cherries, 1,100; guavas, 240; black currants, 200; parsley, 170; green peppers, 110; watercress, 80; chives, 70; strawberries, 57; persimmons, 52; spinach, 51; oranges, 50; cabbage, 476; grapefruit, 38; papaya, 37; elderberries and kumquats, 36; dandelion greens and lemons, 35; cantaloupe, 33; green onions, 32; limes, 31; mangoes, 27; loganberries, 25; tangerines and tomatoes, 23; squash, 22 and raspberries and romaine lettuce, 18.

Crunchy Tuna Casserole

13 ounce can flaked tuna	1 c. milk
4 c. chopped spinach, fresh	½ t. dill
2 c. broccoli, chopped	½ t. oregano
½ c. green pepper	¼ t. nutmeg
1 c. celery, sliced	½ c. cashews, chopped
1 c. carrots, sliced	4 T. wheat germ
¼ c. spring water	3 T. oat bran
2 T. butter	2 T. sesame seeds
3 T. whole wheat flour	2 T. parmesan cheese, grated

Drain tuna. Combine spinach, broccoli, green pepper, celery and carrots with ¼ cup water in a skillet. Cook covered for approximately 2 minutes. Remove vegetables, but save liquid. Combine vegetables with tuna. Set aside. In a sauce pan, melt butter. Stir in flour until blended. Combine water from vegetables with milk (should make 1½ cups liquid). Add liquid gradually to sauce pan and cook until thickens. Add dill, oregano, nutmeg and nuts. Fold sauce into vegetables and tuna. Pour into a quart-size baking dish. Top with mixture of wheat germ, bran, sesame seeds and parmesan cheese. Bake at 350 degrees for 30 minutes. Serves 4 to 6.

Almond Milk

Soak 3 ounces almonds overnight in 5 ounces apple juice. In the morning, add 3 to 5 ounces spring water and blend in blender for 2 to 3 minutes. Flavor with honey and carob powder to taste.

CHAPTER 85

Osteoporosis
(Weak, Honeycombed Bones)

All sorts of information has been given out about preventing and coping with osteoporosis — some oversimplified, some incomplete, some downright wrong:

(1) It's just a normal part of the aging process. (2) Don't do a thing until your blood has been tested for calcium. (3) Get your doctor to prescribe estrogen (if you're a woman in or beyond menopause). (4) Increase your intake of calcium. (5) Exercise more—particularly the weight-bearing bones.

Let's take a close look at these items: (1) Osteoporosis is not a normal part of aging. It is a normal part of degeneration, which comes about for numerous reasons to be covered later. Many seniors in their sixties, seventies or eighties still have solid bones. (2) Results of blood tests for calcium level mislead you. The body's first priority is to keep the blood serum well supplied with calcium. If your diet is low in calcium, the body robs from your calcium banks—the teeth, bones and spine. Robbery on a steady basis over a long period can cause the banks to collapse. (3) Extra estrogen after menopause is a definite plus which helps bones maintain themselves or rebuild, but it is also a possible minus. There's no gilt-edge guarantee that it won't contribute to cancer. (4) A calcium deficiency is the most likely cause of osteoporosis, but, by far, not the only cause. (5) More exercise may indeed help the person whose bottom rarely detaches itself from the top of the chair seat, provided his or her weakened bone structure can sustain physical activity. More on this subject later.

Symptoms And The Safe Approach

Remember that bones are living objects, constantly losing and gaining

385

calcium and other minerals. The important thing is to keep a balance—not losing more than you gain and weakening your bones.[1] Women tend to lose bone three to four times faster than men.[2]

If a blood test won't reveal whether or not osteoporosis is doing a number on you, how can you find out for sure? X-rays cannot usually reveal such degeneration until at least 30 percent of the bone is gone.[3] Some bone-scanners in large medical centers can detect bone deterioration early. Then there's nuclear magnetic resonance (NMR), a way of learning the truth without danger of radiation.

Self-diagnosis of osteoporosis poses a tough challenge, because when symptoms become obvious, difficult-to-correct degeneration has already taken place. The patient becomes shorter, develops a dowager's hump, an assortment of bone or joint pains that seem like arthritis, and — the most telltale sign — translucent skin on the back of her or his hands.[4] Deterioration of bone structure supporting the teeth also reveals that osteoporosis is occurring. (See Section on Tooth and Gum Problems.)

Various surveys have shown that almost 10 percent of individuals over 50 years of age have osteoporosis.[5] Why so many? Some nutrition-oriented doctors feel that the cholesterol phobia has reduced the intake of one of the best sources of calcium: milk and other dairy products without replacing them with calcium food sources of similar value.

Others feel that eating many man-made foods—virtually foodless foods — have deprived many Americans of calcium and other minerals and vitamins that team with calcium to make strong bones and teeth.

Where Do We Start?

For many individuals, more calcium is an excellent start in preventing or managing osteoporosis. A study by Dr. Charles H. Chesnut, professor of medicine and radiology at the University of Washington, reveals that the best time for taking calcium to insure against osteoporosis after menopause is the teen years when the skeleton reaches the greatest bone mass in size and density.[6]

The amount of calcium taken daily during the teen years determines how sturdy or porous the bones will be forty years later, he says.[7]

Although the Recommended Daily Allowance (RDA) for calcium is

1,200 mg, thirty-one 14-year old girls interviewed by Chesnut were taking it in tablet form or from dairy products — anywhere from 200 to 1,600 mg daily, with the average at almost 1,000 — 200 mg under the RDA. One quarter of the girls ingested less than 800 mg daily and were found to be calcium-deficient.[8]

A glass of milk — there are four glasses in a quart — provides approximately 250 mg of calcium. (See the section on Milk Intolerance.)

Richest food sources of calcium in milligrams per less than four ounce units are: sesame seeds, 1200; kelp, 1100; cheeses, 700; brewer's yeast, 420; sardines and carob, 350; caviar, 280; soybeans and almonds, 230; torula yeast, 220; parsley, 200; brazil nuts, 190; watercress, salmon and chickpeas, 150; egg yolk, beans, pistachios, lentils, and kale, 130; sunflower seeds and cow's milk, 120; buckwheat, 110; maple syrup, cream and chard, 100; walnuts, 99; spinach, 93, endive, 81; pecans, 73; wheat germ, 72; peas, 70; peanuts, 69; eggs, 54 and oats, 53.

Elemental, My Dear Watson!

The Recommended Daily Allowance (RDA) for calcium seems reasonable at 1,200 mg, in terms of food and supplements. However, at the higher limit of 1,500 to 1,600 mg, the girls surveyed by Dr. Chesnut absorbed more calcium and retained more in their bones — a key consideration.[9]

Some individuals are confused about the term "elemental" on the label of various minerals. If the label indicates 500 mg of elemental calcium, that is the exact amount delivered. If your supplement is not marked "elemental," only a large fraction of the milligrams on the label will be assimilated.[10]

So, if you're buying, get exactly what you pay for.

Even in these days, many individuals—young to aged—take in enough calcium, but are still not enriching their bone structure efficiently, because they may be short on vitamin D, which has much to do with calcium being absorbed and used in our trillions of cells.

Blocks To Calcium

One major source of vitamin D is sunlight or skyshine on our skin. However, with strong warnings against sun-bathing, due to a skin cancer threat, many persons avoid or sharply reduce direct exposure to sunlight or skyshine. Sometimes they don't make up this deficit by eating Vitamin D-rich foods.

Probably the best known source of vitamin D is cod liver oil. Before you say, "Ugh," and refuse to take the fishy stuff, remember that cod liver oil now comes in many pleasant and even tasty flavors — citrus, cherry, mint and strawberry. A tablespoon supplies as much as the RDA of 400 I.U.

Best foods for vitamin D content in terms of I.U.s per less than four ounce servings are: sardines, 500; salmon. 400; tuna, 250; egg yolk, 160; sunflower seeds, 92; liver, 50; eggs, 48; butter, 40; cheeses, 30; cream, 15; mother's milk, 6; cottage cheese and cow's milk, 4 and bee pollen, 1.6. Both a deficit and an extreme excess of vitamin D can keep calcium from being absorbed. However, too much phosphorus—a diet heavy in meat, eggs, sardines and liver—can cause needed calcium to be lost. When excess phosphorus is thrown off, it strong-arms calcium out of the body.[11]

A rich intake of protein — 100 or more grams a day — can also cause needed calcium to be flushed out of the body, although a moderate allowance of protein — 40 to 60 grams — does not.[12]

It's easy to eat 100 grams of protein in the following common foods: a breakfast of two eggs, a couple pieces of toast; a lunch of chicken salad, and a dinner of a moderate serving of salmon (five ounces) or a six-ounce beef patty. A protein deficit—less than 40 grams daily—can also deplete calcium stores.

Drains On Bone Calcium

When magnesium is deficient — at a ratio of less than one part magnesium to two parts calcium—calcium is lost. Calcium is also thieved from the body by the following: (1) caffeine in coffee and soft drinks. (One cup a day doesn't seem to hurt, but, beware, above that point.);[13] (2) refined sugar (not lactose, milk sugar) interferes with calcium entering the bones;[14] (3) Alcohol, as a sugar, limits the making of the stomach's hydrochloric acid and also encourages the loss of magnesium.[15] Magnesium leaves quietly enough but not without taking calcium along. (4) A deficiency of hydrochloric acid in the stomach blocks calcium absorption and increases excretion of calcium in the urine.[16] Forty percent of post-menopausal women have no gastric juice secretion and, therefore, absorb less calcium and discharge more of it in the urine. (5) A deficiency of vitamin B-6, a close associate of magnesium, can also cause the departure of needed calcium from the body.[17] (6) Another nutritional nuisance combines with calcium and ushers it out of the body: oxalic acid[18] in beet tops, chard, chocolate, cocoa, rhubarb, parsley and spinach. (7) Smoking causes excessive loss of calcium by bringing on an earlier menopause, which hastens bone loss. (8) Menopause, however early or late, means a loss of estrogen, which permits excessive amounts of calcium to leave the bones. (9) Other enemies of calcium use or retention are antacids,[19] aspirin, mineral oil—taken orally or in cosmetics—a large intake of fluids, cortisone (the natural kind brought on by stress or the prescribed hormone) or ACTH, drugs for epilepsy, excessive sweating due to sustained, gruelling exercise or long hours of work in torrid temperatures, and, of course, nursing an infant.

Use It Or Lose It

A little-considered enemy of our bones needs attention: physical inactivity—being laid up in bed, confined to a wheelchair, or immobilized in a cast.[20]

Confinement and physical inactivity actually pull the calcium from our bones, as shown by tests of astronauts in their space vehicle who urinated away an average of 200 mg of calcium daily.

In experiments, when healthy individuals were held rigid in casts from waist to ankles, they continuously lost vast amounts of calcium, phosphorus, and other nutrients.

How can you stop calcium loss due to immobilization? By more calcium intake or in-bed-exercise? Strangely, neither one! When research subjects just stood for a few hours daily, excessive mineral loss ended, convincing the experimenters that the force of gravity is a key to calcium balance.[21]

Calcium Stop-Loss Mineral: Boron

Being able to keep most of the bone calcium you now have appears to be as vitally important as taking in more of this mineral.

And how can you accomplish this in the daily diet? By taking 3 mg of boron, a trace mineral not even established as essential to human nutrition, as revealed by a U.S. Department of Agriculture study.

Eight days after taking three mg of boron daily, a group of post-menopausal women lost far less of the major minerals which make up bones: about 40 percent less calcium, 33 percent less magnesium and about 30 percent less phosphorus.

In terms of milligrams, they retained 52 mg more calcium daily. That's a gram every 20 days! Why? In the complex process of absorbing calcium, sex hormones—particularly estrogen—are a must. After menopause, the ovaries no longer produce estrogen. Therefore, most dietary and supplementary calcium is lost in the urine.

A Boron Boost

So estrogen replacement is a widely used osteoporosis treatment for post-menopausal women. This is where boron comes in. The researchers discovered that, by taking boron, the women tested had double the blood level of the most active form of estrogen.

An eminent biochemist, Dr. Mark Hegsted, Professor of Nutrition at Harvard University, says that osteoporosis, appears to be more than just a calcium problem. Actually, it is a total nutrition problem also involving magnesium, boron, phosphorus and silicon. (It is even more than that. See the reference to manganese a few paragraphs down.)

Only minute amounts of boron are found in foods. And only minute amounts are needed. Agriculture Department researchers estimate the daily human requirement for boron—based on animal experiments—is one to two mg. Significant traces of boron are found in apples, legumes, nuts, pears and vegetables — particularly leafy ones.[22]

Other excellent sources are: soy meal, prunes, raisins, almonds, peanuts, hazel nuts, dates and honey. Boron supplements come in capsules of three mg each, and it is wise to take no more than one daily, state nutritional medical doctors, because excess boron can be toxic.

An often overlooked mineral in the war to prevent osteoporosis—sadly, so—is manganese. Therefore, I am including a list of the best manganese-containing foods in milligrams per a unit of less than four ounces:

Tea leaves, 28; cloves, 26; ginger, 8.7; buckwheat, 5.1; oats, 4,9; hazelnuts, 4.2; chestnuts, 3.7; whole wheat, 3.6; pecans, 3.5; barley, 3.2; brazil nuts, 2.8; sunflower seeds, 2.5; ginseng, watercress, peas, and beans 2.0; almonds, 1.9; turnip greens and walnuts, 1.8; brown rice, 1.7; peanuts, 1.4; honey, 1.4; coconut, 1.3; pineapple, 1.1; parsley, 0.94; spinach, 0.82; grapefruit and lettuce, 0.80; bananas, 0.64; carrots, 0.60, berries, 0.55, brewer's yeast, 0.53 and yams, 0.52.

Exercise: A Bone Builder

Numerous experiments have established the fact that a non-nutritional factor can preserve bone mass and volume and, in some instances, even rebuild bone.

Regular exercising of weight-bearing bones, in particular, helps to retain and, frequently, to build bone volume and density.[23]

Recently, it was found that even regular vigorous exercise of non-weight-bearing bones can preserve bone mass and integrity.

Today the outlook for coping with osteoporosis, even in the latter years, is growing more positive and hopeful.

The Jayne Sousa Special Salad

1 c. cottage cheese (raw certified)	Pinch black pepper
⅓ c. sour cream (raw certified)	Salad greens
3 T. scallions, finely minced	2 hard boiled eggs, chopped
3 T. radish, finely minced	½ can flaked tuna (in spring water)
3 T. cucumber, peeled and finely minced	

Combine cottage cheese, sour cream, scallions, radish, cucumber, pepper, eggs and tuna. Mix thoroughly. Serve scooped onto salad greens. Garnish with a little paprika.

CHAPTER 86

Overweight
(How To Be A Good Loser)

Sounds too good to be true!

You can lose unwanted weight the no-diet way: the same foods and the same number of calories. All you have to do is eat your heaviest meal at a different time of day.

This is one of the major thrusts of the book, How To Win At Weight Loss by Stephen Langer, M.D. and James F. Scheer (Thorsons).

Five hundred and ninety-five overweight patients in reasonably good health were asked to stay on their usual number of daily calories, but to eat a substantial breakfast, a modest lunch and a light dinner.[1]

What's the big idea? To take in the most calories at the time of day when the most energy is spent. This is the hard part. Patients were asked to breakfast early, to lunch in mid-morning and to have dinner at noon (at least no later than 3 P.M.) so that there would be at least an 8 1/2 hour interval between the day's last meal and bed-time.[2]

Everybody Is A Winner

Each person who followed the ground rules to the letter lost weight. However, those who concentrated all their calories at breakfast time lost the most — an averge of 10 pounds per month. Individuals who ate all three meals lost an average of five to six pounds in the same period.[3]

Over the span of the program, not a solitary soul felt a negative side effect. Persons who dropped 20 to 30 pounds experienced a gain in their blood's hemoglobin level. Among those who shed 30 or more pounds, diabetics revealed a drop of blood sugar to normal. Then, too, low thyroid patients who melted away at least 30 pounds were able to cut back on their thyroid supplementation.[4]

Other similar experiments with people and animals brought almost the same results, so such a program seems worth trying. What have you got to lose but weight?

Detailed instruction which enables you to stay slim and healthy for the rest of your life is in my book "The Diet Bible" McGraw Hill.

CHAPTER 87

Premenstrual Syndrome (PMS)

Only in recent years have male medical doctors begun to accept the fact that premenstrual syndrome (PMS) is a real, rather than an imaginary disorder.

Meanwhile, women — ever since Eve — have suffered an incredible spectrum of physical and emotional symptoms: anxiety, anti-social behavior, bloating, breast-swelling and sensitivity, confusion, cramps, cravings for certain foods (particularly salty or chocolaty ones); crying spells, depression, dizziness, exhaustion, fluid retention — especially in the legs — headaches, irritability, sleeplessness, and, among others, wide mood swings.

Every PMS-prone woman can add her own unique symptoms to the above list, but every one is not fully familiar with natural ways of alternative doctors for preventing or relieving some or all of the symptoms.

Doing What Comes Naturally

Vicki Georges Hufnagel, M.D., an obstetrician-gynecologist, told the 14th Annual California Dairy Council Nutrition Conference, that two of the major causes of PMS are strict dieting, which deprives women of needed nutrients, and eating junk foods, which stresses body and mind.[1]

Dr. Hufnagel warned that frequent and rigid dieting may invite PMS, which is related to hormonal changes influencing brain and body functions. Over-dieters don't have enough fat left for the brain to use in "burning" and utilizing food and may develop an acid imbalance and, possibly, faint.[2]

Hormone fluctuations take place in the brain as well as the body, she explained. Fluid accumulates there, making the blood vessels swell. Such fluctuations bring on psychological and physical changes.[3]

Dr. Hufnagel advises PMS-prone women to review their diet and limit or eliminate empty-calorie foods, which essentially starve body and mind and contribute to premenstrual syndrome: junk foods, refined sugar and sugary foods, salt and carbonated soft drinks.[4]

Some Answers: Protein And Complex Carbohydrates

Urging women with PMS to make sure of eating at least 50 grams of protein daily—that's about two ounces—she recommends turkey white meat or red meat during PMS time.[5]

Additionally, she suggests upping the intake of complex carbohydrates —cereals, fruits, legumes, vegetables and whole grains—cutting down on sharp cheeses and adding milder ones, such as cottage and cream cheese.[6]

An effective nutritional weapon during PMS is unsweetened yogurt blended with a small amount of brewer's yeast, which contains glutamic acid, food for the brain.[7]

Low blood sugar (hypoglycemia) is a major contributor to PMS. (See the Section on Low Blood Sugar, Hypoglycemia.) This is why Dr. Hufnagel recommends that patients eat a mid-morning snack—wheat or bran in milk—to satisfy hunger and increase fiber and calcium. PMS sufferers should keep their blood sugar level up by eating six small meals a day, instead of three large ones, refrain from adding salt to foods and eat more potassium-rich fruits, vegetables, nuts, seeds and legumes: bananas, cantaloupe, parsley, peas, avocados, potatoes, cabbage, almonds, peanuts, pecans, sunflower and sesame seeds, and lentils.[8]

Individuals with PMS should consider alcohol, caffeine, chocolate and some teas as No-No's, says Dr. Hufnagel.[9]

Other Routes To Relief

In addition to an improved diet, alternative doctors recommend nutritional supplements, regular exercise and better stress management.

One specific supplement which holds promise in preventing PMS symptoms is evening primrose oil.[10] In an experiment at St. Thomas

Hospital in London, one of the world's largest PMS clinics, M.G. Brush, M.D. gave primrose oil to 70 women who had failed to get relief from one or two other kinds of treatment.

Two capsules of evening primrose oil three times daily brought full relief from PMS symptoms to 67 percent of the women. Twenty-two percent got partial relief, making a total of 89 percent of treatment-resistant women who achieved partial to full relief.

One hundred women participated in a placebo-controlled, double-blind, crossover study, trying evening primrose oil capsules to treat breast pain.[11] Many of the women experienced worse pain premenstrually, but a majority experienced significant pain relief.

Zinc and vitamin E also seem to lessen cramping. Added magnesium in foods or supplements serves two purposes, alternative doctors tell me. It is a diuretic for removing retained fluids and decreasing the desire for chocolate. A supplement of vitamin B-6 (usually, 50 mg) is sometimes needed to increase magnesium absorption.[12]

Exercise Can Help

Alternative doctors and PMS-plagued women say that daily exercise lessens pre-menstrual and menstrual pain and cramping, chases depression and brings on a state of well-being.

Conservative outside exercise—no tennis or volley ball—can encourage relaxation, particularly fast walking, twenty-five to thirty minutes twice daily.[13]

Such physical activity also tends to lower the stress burden. The very prospect of the premenstrual period brings on stress and tension. So a relaxed, positive attitude coupled with exercise can diminish the symptoms of PMS.

Exercise and stress management along with dietary recommendations mentioned above form a winning combination against PMS.[14]

Food Fare

Foods richest in vitamin B-6 in milligrams per less than four ounce units are: brewer's yeast, 4.0; brown rice, 3.6; whole wheat, 2.9; royal jelly,

2.4; soybeans, 2.0; rye, 1.8; lentils, 1.7; sunflower seeds and hazelnuts, 1.1; alfalfa, 1.0; salmon, 0.98; wheat germ, 0.92; tuna, 0.90; bran, 0.85; walnuts, 0.73; peas and liver, 0.67; avocados, 0.60; beans, 0.57; cashews, peanuts, turkey, oats, chicken and beef, 0.40; halibut, 0.34; lamb and banana, 0.32; blackstrap molasses, 0.31 and corn and egg yolk, 0.30.

Best sources of vitamin E in terms of International Units per less than four ounce units are: wheat germ, 160; safflower nuts, 35; sunflower seeds, 31; whole wheat, 30; sesame oil, 26; walnuts, 22; corn oil and hazel nuts, 21; soy and peanut oil, 16; almonds, 15; olive oil, 14; cabbage, 7.8; brazil nuts and peanuts, 6.5; cod liver oil, 5.4; cashews, 5.1; soy lecithin, 4.8; spinach, 2.9; asparagus, 2.5; broccoli, 2.0; butter, 1.9; parsley, 1.8; oats, barley and corn, 1.7 and avocados and pecans, 1.5.

Supplements and foods richest in magnesium per milligram in less than four ounce units are: kelp, 740; blackstrap molasses, 410; sunflower seeds, 350; wheat germ, 320; almonds, 270; soybeans, 240; brazil nuts, 220; bone meal, 170; pistachios and soy lecithin, 160; hazelnuts, 150; pecans and oats, 140; walnuts, 130; brown rice, 120; chard, 65; spinach, 57; barley, 55; coconut, 44; salmon, 40; corn, 38; avocados, 37; bananas, 31; cheeses, 30; tuna, 29; potatoes and cashews, 27 and turkey, 25.

Richest food and supplement sources of zinc in milligrams per less than four ounce units are: herring, 160; wheat germ, 14; sesame seeds, 10; torula yeast, 9.9; blackstrap molasses, 8.3; maple syrup, 7.5; liver, 7.0; soybeans, 6.7; sunflower seeds, 6.6; egg yolk, 5.5; lamb, 5.4; chicken, 4.8; brewer's yeast, 3.9; oats, 3.7; bone meal, 3.6; rye, 3.4; whole wheat, 3.2; corn, 3.1; coconut and beef, 3.0; beets, turkey, and walnuts, 2.8; barley, 2.7; beans and avocados, 2.4; peas, 2.3; bleu cheese, 2.2; eggs, 2.1; buckwheat, 2.0; mangoes, 1.9; millet, rice and almonds, 1.6 and salmon, 1.4.

Banana Delight

4 bananas, firm but ripe
1 c. unsweetened shredded coconut
1 c. natural plain yogurt

1 c. pecans, chopped
½ c. kiwi fruit, skinned

Blend yogurt and kiwi fruit. Cut each banana into thirds. Dip each banana in yogurt. Roll in yogurt, then roll in coconut, then pecans. Store in refrigerator. Serves 10 to 12.

CHAPTER 88

Prostate Problems (Enlargement, Inflammation, Cancer)

Enlargement of the prostate gland, inflammation (prostatitis) or cancer can cause any of the following typical symptoms:
1. Difficulty in starting to urinate.
2. Increased urge to urinate.
3. Burning or painful voiding of urine.
4. Dribbling and difficulty emptying the bladder.
5. Frequent or continuous lower back pain.

Why are these symptoms common to all three major prostate disorders?

Before answering, it is necessary to describe the prostate, its location and size. This gland, whose purpose is to secrete a milky white fluid to transport sperm cells out of the penis, surrounds the narrow neck of the bladder, the urethra), a flexible tube at the base of the penis through which urine is discharged.

In many men, the prostate enlarges with advancing age, becomes inflamed in a non-cancerous way — this condition is called prostatitis — or develops cancer (usually a slow-growth type). All of these conditions cause swelling which makes the prostate tighten like a noose around the urethra, bringing about the above symptoms.

Risks of Conventional Treatment

Surgery is the usual treatment for enlarged prostate or cancer, and part or all of the prostate is removed. Antibiotics can clear up prostatitis caused by bacteria, but not by viruses.

Neither of these therapies guarantees success. So, prevention is the best bet. Does non-cancerous prostate enlargement make the development of cancer more probable?

398

Yes. Researchers in epidemiology at Johns Hopkins University and the department of Biostatics at Roswell Park Memorial Institute studied 1,200 case histories and found that prostate enlargement patients are four times more likely to develop cancer than others.[1]

Preventive Measures

Patients with prostate disorders usually show a low measurement of zinc in their semen and prostate gland, as discovered in examining 755 prostate patients by Irving M. Bush, M.D. and fellow researchers at Cook County Hospital in Chicago.[2]

A super-high level of zinc is normally found in the prostate gland and in the semen.

Dr. Bush surprised the national American Medical Association convention of 1974 with his findings: patients given zinc tablets of a potency which can be offered in anyone's daily snacks and foods showed remarkable improvement.[3]

Nineteen patients with noncancerous enlarged prostate glands were given a 34 mg zinc pill daily for 60 days and then put on a maintenance program of 11 to 23 mg daily. All of them reported a reduction of pain. Examination revealed that the prostate of 14 had decreased in size. Measurement of semen levels of all patients showed increased zinc.[4]

Two hundred patients with infectious prostatitis took 11 to 34 mg of zinc daily for as much as 16 weeks with 70 percent finding relief from symptoms and higher amounts of zinc in their semen.[5]

Getting Zinc From Foods

Here's how it's possible to add the highest amount of zinc used in the above study (34 mg) to a day's meals and snack—even slightly more. Two ounces of herring alone will provide 55 mg; a lamb chop (5 mg); two ounces of wheat germ (7 mg); two ounces of sesame seeds (5 mg); two ounces of sunflower seeds (3.3 mg); a bowl of oatmeal, (3.5 mg); three ounces of chicken (3.2 mg); two ounces of soybeans (3.4 mg); two slices of whole grain wheat bread (2.1 mg); a medium size beet (1 mg) and an ounce of walnuts (1 mg). Skip the herring and all the rest of the foods listed will go slightly over 34 mg.

Help From Another Quarter

Dr. Jonathan Wright tells his patients that another help for enlarged prostate is essential fatty acids (EFAs), substances which cannot be made by the body and are found in highest concentrations in vegetable oils and seeds—safflower, sesame, and pumpkin.[6] Pumpkin seeds is an old folk remedy for enlarged prostate.

His recommendation that prostate patients use EFAs is based on a study published before World War II by medical doctors James P. Hart and William L. Cooper, who fed EFAs to 19 men with an enlarged prostate.[7] Every one of them experienced a reduction in size.

Dr. Wright had his prostate patients take one 400 mg capsule of EFAs three times daily.[8] This is the equivalent of the EFAs in two handfuls of pumpkin or sunflower seeds. He makes the telling point that the EFAs taken or the seeds eaten must be fresh—not rancid. Otherwise, they may cause harm.

Clues To Prostate Cancer Prevention

Peter Hill, Ph.D, of New York City's American Health Foundation, conducted an unusual study based on the observation that South African blacks whose diet consists of low-fat whole foods — whole grains and vegetables and fruit—have little prostate cancer.[9]

Dr. Hill and co-workers fed a typical western diet—heavy on fat and meats—to black, volunteer South Africans and the typical low-fat, lower-calorie diet of the South Africans to black and white American volunteers.

Then he measured excreted hormones usually associated with the development of prostate cancer. Within three weeks the South Africans on the Western diet were excreting markedly more of the telltale hormones than before, and the Americans on the low-fat diet, were throwing off markedly less.[10]

The preliminary indication is that the lower calorie diet replacing animal calories with vegetables and fruit changed a group at high risk for prostate cancer to a low-risk. [11]

Warning

Sometimes people who know symptoms of a disorder and have them are tempted to be their own doctor. This could be dangerous with many ailments. It is particularly so with prostate problems, because the symptoms are the same for all three disorders and the condition could be cancer. Warning: be examined, by your alternative doctor! (See the list in the back of the book.)

Lamb with Seed and Sprout Salad

2 lamb chops   3 lemons, cut in half
3 garlic cloves

Put ½ of lemon in hot water and drink while preparing this meal (helps digestion). Soak lamb in puree of lemon and garlic for 1/2 hour or longer.

Seed and Sprout Salad

1 c. fresh asparagus,   1 raw beet, grated
  steamed until tender   2 celery stalks, chopped
1 c. fresh brussels sprouts,   ½ c. alfalfa sprouts
  trimmed and steamed   ½ c. raw pumpkin seed kernels, ground

Scrub all vegetables. Steam asparagus and brussels sprouts. Chop all. vegetables into bite-size pieces. Tear lettuce into small pieces and toss all ingredients together in salad bowl. Sprinkle ground pumpkin seeds over top. Seeds will absorb a great deal of moisture, making a kind of paste. Serves 4.

Raw Fruit Cake

1 c. raisins, ground   1 c. whole wheat bread crumbs
1 c. dates, chopped   1 c. fruit juice (pineapple)
2 c. dried apricot   1 c. sunflower seed
¾ c. spring water

Soak dried fruits in water and fruit juice for 2 hours. Add crumbs and seed. Pack into floured mold. Set for one or more days in refrigerator. Unmold, slice and serve with Soy Yogurt.

CHAPTER 89

Psoriasis (Skin Disorder)

A long-lasting and frequently recurring skin disorder identified by round or oval red patches covered with tiny, silvery scales, psoriasis usually shows up on the back, buttocks, elbows, knees, palms, scalp or soles of the feet of children ten years of age to adults up to their forties. However, it is not limited to these areas or age groups.

This ailment usually appears—or worsens—after some form of stress: physical or emotional: a general infection (like the flu), a strep throat, an injury to the skin, a severe emotional jolt like the death of a loved one, being fired from a job, or losing a life's savings.

Is A Food Allergy To Blame?

Improvements and even permanent disappearance of this condition have been scored as much by skipping certain foods as by eating certain others.

Researchers in France discovered that by removing gluten from the diet —a sticky, protein substance in grains such as wheat, barley, oats and rye which gives elasticity to dough — many patients showed remarkable improvements.[1]

Contrary to these findings, some authorities feel that breads and cereals, as well as fruits, vegetables and fish, can decrease the occurrences of this disorder.

Another theory holds that the liberal amount of arachidonic acid in dairy products, eggs, meat and poultry contributes to psoriasis, as shown in the journal Cutis.[2]

Reporting in the Western Journal of Medicine, John M. Douglas, M.D. cleared up his wife's psoriasis when she cooperated and omitted foods to which she was sensitive or allergic: corn, fruits — mainly citrus — nuts, and milk.[3] His patients improved by avoiding acid-containing beverages and foods such as coffee, soft drinks, pineapple and tomatoes. Other skin disorders were also helped by cutting out acids.

Certain Kinds of Fish Help, Too

Experiments of S.S. Bleehen, M.D., professor of dermatology at the Royal Hallamshire Hospital, Sheffield, England, show that Omega-3 oil in five and a half ounces of mackerel, sardines, or salmon eaten daily can significantly lessen the itching, redness and scaling of psoriasis.[4]

Omega-3 oil probably makes the body more efficient in processing arachidonic acid — mentioned earlier as a possible villain — theorizes Dr. Bleehen, who used 10 fish oil capsules of Omega-3 daily for 12 weeks on patients, whose itching, redness and scaling reduced markedly.[5]

Dr. Vincent Ziboh, a dermatology professor and biochemist at the University of California, cites a similar research project conducted by both U.C. and the University of Michigan in which sixty percent of psoriasis patients experienced reduced itching, redness and scaling by taking Omega-3 capsules daily.[6]

Lecithin Seems To Work

Based on the fact that 254 psoriasis patients taking four to eight tablespoons of lecithin each day recovered in five months,[7] some alternative doctors have urged patients to eat lecithin-rich foods: soy beans (a major source of lecithin); wheat germ, nuts, seeds (sunflower and pumpkin) whole grains and cold-processed vegetable oils: soy, safflower, and oils made from the seeds mentioned above.

Otherwise, the family chef includes from four to eight tablespoons of soy lecithin granules in oil dressings for salads or sprinkled on whole grain cereals or cooked oats. Results have been encouraging — well worth the effort.

Anita Smith's Cashew Oat Waffles

2½ c. water
1¾ c. old fashioned oats
⅓ c. raw cashews

½ t. sea salt
2 T. wheat germ

Blend all ingredients until smooth. Bake in preheated medium hot waffle iron 10 to 12 minutes. Do not open before time is up.

Carob Drink

2 c. soy or nut milk
¼ t. vanilla

2-4 T. carob
Pinch sea salt

Place all ingredients in blender until smooth. Serve hot or cold. Makes 4 small servings.

Soy Milk

Add 2 T. soy milk powder to one pint spring water. Sweeten with honey. Add pinch of sea salt or kelp. Add carob powder.

CHAPTER 90

Shingles (Herpes Zoster)

The virus that causes chicken pox in children seems responsible for shingles (herpes zoster), an infection of a major spinal nerve which semi-circles the body and brings with it severe neuralgic pain and a skin rash of small, round blisters (vesicles) on both sides of the waist or chest.

The unique pattern of the rash gives this disease the name herpes zoster. "Zoster" is Greek for "girdle". Adults exposed to children with chicken pox often become infected with shingles. Likewise, children, exposed to adults with shingles frequently come down with chicken pox.

Apparently adults who have had chicken pox carry the dormant virus, which can flare into action when the immune system defenses are weak from fighting off a serious illness such as cancer, from severe stress, critical injury, heavy environmental pollution, and, among other major causes, drugs which suppress the immune system.

Sometimes the blisters disappear in a matter of months, but their departure doesn't always take away the neuralgic pain connected with shingles. At other times, they persist for endless years. About the only medications which orthodox medicine has for shingles is pain-killers. Neurosurgery is a last desperate measure.

Quick Relief

My friend Jonathan Wright, M.D. told me about a make-it-yourself salve that he says brings almost instant relief to the discomfort or pain of the rash.

It is made of zinc ointment, an over-the-counter product, a tablespoon of aloe vera (available at any health food store) and the content of one 1,000 I.U. capsule of natural vitamin E (d-alpha tocopherol, NOT

DL-alpha tocopherol) mixed together and applied to the vesicles.

Beyond Natural Foods

It would be unfeeling toward persons who have shingles to omit certain therapies from this book just because they go somewhat beyond the abilities of natural foods to help: for instance, supplements such as vitamins B-12, C and E.

Researchers A.K. Gupta and H.S. Mital, both medical doctors, revealed in the Indian Practitioner their successful method of managing herpes zoster: a daily injection of 500 micrograms (mcg) of vitamin B-12, a nutrient important to nerve health, to thinking and remembering and to various emotional disorders and to energy.[1]

Injected with 500 mcg of vitamin B-12 daily, 21 shingles patients showed progress by the second or third day and made "dramatic" gains in relief from pain and the drying up of the rash. Further, none of the patients developed neuralgia — its medical name is "post-herpetic neuralgia" — which often occurs after the vesicles disappear.[2]

Usually oral vitamin B-12 is sold in pills with a 500 mcg potency, but no studies are available to show whether this form of the vitamin would bring relief from shingles. In any event, the 500 mcg injection would be far more potent, because it bypasses the stomach and intestinal tract, which exact their toll from nutrients passing through.

Vitamin C Meets Shingles

Vitamin C also has brought about quick turn-arounds from herpes zoster. The late Fred Klenner, M.D., made an experimental study of eight patients, injecting them with two to three grams every 12 hours and having them take a gram of vitamin C by mouth every two hours. Seven of them reported the end of pain two hours after the first injection, the drying up of vesicles inside of one day and their total disappearance in three days.[3]

The eighth patient, a diabetic, needed 14 injections — the others averaged six — but was completely free of symptoms in two weeks. Following the Klenner regime, a researcher in France treated 327 shingles and herpes patients, and every one of them lost all symptoms within three days, as reported in the medical publication, Journal des Practiciens.[4]

The Clean-Up Man: Vitamin E

Remarkable results followed the treatment of stubborn and long-lingering post-herpetic neuralgia with vitamin E. Nine of 13 patients—two of whom had suffered pain for 13 and 19 years, respectively—were nearly or fully relieved by taking 1200 to 1600 I.U. of vitamin E daily for six months. The remaining four were slightly or moderately improved.[5]

Another vitamin E experiment, this one with lower potencies and only eight patients—six women between ages 56 and 73 and two men from age 60 to 64—brought no improvement in severity or frequency of pain.[6] These individuals were started with 400 I.U. daily of alpha tocopherol acetate each day before meals, then, after two weeks, were upped to 800 I.U. daily for two weeks, followed by 1,600 I.U. daily for six weeks. This experiment was reported in the Archives of Dermatology.

However, researchers who conducted a study using far higher potencies, wrote a letter to the editors of the Archives of Dermatology, accenting the fact that from 1200 to 1600 I.U. of D-alpha tocopheryl acetate or succinate had to be taken for no less than six months to show relief from pain.[7]

Further, they stressed the need to avoid medications and estrogens—as well as white flour, vitamin-enriched cereals and mixed vitamins containing inorganic iron.[8]

Nutritional therapies reported here show clearly that shingles and its frequent successor, post-herpetic neuralgia—although tough and stubborn disorders—can be handled successfully.

Green Salad

1 c. Red Cabbage, Shredded	2 c. Iceberg Lettuce
1 c. Broccoli, Cut Up	4 Green Onions, Sliced

Dressing

1 t. Liquid Garlic
4 T. Lemon Juice
4 T. Sesame Oil

2 Large Cloves of Garlic
1 t. Celery Seed
1 t. Cayenne Pepper

Egg Nog

1 c. Raw Certified Milk
1 Raw Egg

1 T. Fructose
1 t. Nutmeg

Mix in blender.

CHAPTER 91

Skin Irritations, Abrasions, Stings

Don't look in your medicine chest for one of the best folk remedies for skin irritations and scrapes, because it isn't there. Of all places, you will find it in the fruit bowl. I'm talking about that golden delight called the banana.

The banana skin certainly helped me out when I was visiting with the Masai tribe of East Africa. A food allergy irritation broke out on my arms, and they itched mercilessly. Lost without my home fruit and vegetable medicine chest, I suddenly realized that bananas were plentiful with the Masai.

I hurriedly peeled several and applied the moist inside skin to my arms, and — presto! — the itch went away. Within a few hours, the irritation disappeared, to the amazement of the Masai.

No Secret Anymore

Another of my folk medicines for skin irritation is the potato. I don't know what I'd do without it. One day my hair stylist, Karl Rolfes, drove down the Peninsula from his San Francisco salon to do my hair before a telecast. A premier artist in his field, Karl pointed out an irritation above his right eye.

"I hate to appear before my clients looking like this," he said. "Do you have something to clear it up?"

"Yes, it's in the vegetable bin behind you."

At first he thought I had lost my mind. Then, having known me for years, he asked, "All right, which one?"

"The red potato."

I peeled it for him and cut a slice thin enough to be pliable, telling him to press it against his right eyelid. He did, and I secured it in place with some adhesive tape. The first phone call of the next day came far too early in the morning, before I had had time to brush the cobwebs out of my eyes and regain consciousness. It was Karl.

"Maureen, it's gone!" he shouted.

"What's gone?"

"That irritation above my eye."

"Hooray," I cried out. "The lowly potato scores again!"

Under the Section of this book called Frostbite, you will find an item about my friends Ronn and Connie Haus, who head Family Christian Broadcasting. They used banana skins successfully to promote healing of Ronn's frostbite.

Still another close friend benefitted by an old folk remedy. Gene Arceri, the writer of best-selling books about celebrities (Elizabeth Taylor and Susan Hayward, among them), had been sunning himself on my patio, had dozed off, and sustained a moderate sunburn. Not wanting his face to smart or peel, he asked me for some sunburn lotion.

Because there was none in the house, I recommended that he dab his face lightly with a cut strawberry or two. Gene followed my suggestion and, although he looked as if he were bleeding, he experienced no discomfort or peeling.

From Bananas To Burnt Toast

Far removed from strawberries or banana peels is another folk remedy for the skin: charcoal. If your spouse should happen to burn the toast black, don't be unhappy. Maybe it isn't edible, but it could turn out to be an excellent home remedy for insect and spider stings or bites.

It did for me while I lived with the Masai tribe. One enemy of these nomadic people living in the wild is the poisonous, brown recluse spider. A child had been bitten by one of these spiders the week before and had died in agony.

The same kind of spider struck again, and a child came running to a group of us around the fire, crying out in pain, holding the injured hand. I told the father to take a handful of cold charcoal from the edge of the fire, mix it with a little water and pack the wound in a piece of natural cloth, which he hurriedly did. The poultice was changed every ½ hr. Within two hours, the pain subsided. The child suffered a raging, high fever that night, but the next day he seemed normal. Again, the father packed the wound with charcoal. Before I left for home a few days later, the wound was almost healed, and the child was again in good health, although more wary of brown recluse spiders.

I have used charcoal from burned pinecones whizzed in the blender or burnt toast on mosquito bites and they have healed faster than usual. Honestly, I don't know what I would do without banana skins, potato slices and charcoal.

Folk medicine wouldn't be the same without them! Neither would I.

Burnt Toast

2 slices of whole wheat bread

Place bread in toaster and turn up to highest dial on toaster. Push down handle and wait for burnt toast to pop up.

6 pine cones burned and whizzed in blender.

CHAPTER 92

Sleeplessness (Insomnia)

A former comedian had what he called a perfect remedy for falling asleep. He advised people to sleep near the edge of the bed. "Then you're sure to drop off."

It's easy to see why he is a former comedian.

Sleeplessness is no laughing matter to those so desperate that they will try anything. So we have made an in-depth study of sleep-inducing methods that seem to work. We want you to sleep soundly, but—please! —not while you're reading this book.

Doing What Comes Naturally

Various foods have been tried to lure sleep. Folklore says that bananas, tomatoes, walnuts and honey are effective.

Modern biochemistry tells us why. They contribute to the making of serotonin, a brain neurotransmitter which produces a calming effect. Many viewers of my national "Accent on Health" TV program write to say that honey puts them to sleep. (They generally take a tablespoonful about an hour before bedtime.) "Honey calms me down, relaxes me, and I'm asleep in minutes," writes one of them.

WARNING: Honey is not for infants, cautions the Centers for Disease Control. Spores of botulism bacteria sometimes found in honey can colonize in the baby's not-yet-fully developed intestine and create a deadly poison.

Lettuce Fall Asleep With Milk

Some people I know follow the folklore method of luring sleep by eating lettuce. One friend puts a whole head of lettuce at her bedside and tears off chunks to nibble on. Soon she is fast sleep. If she wakes up during the night, she eats more lettuce and usually gets desired results.

Good old milk is the center of controversy again. This time the issue is: does a warm glass of milk make one sleep or not? Although I have never done a personal Gallup Poll with my televiewers, I feel that the vote runs about two to one that milk lives up to its folklore reputation.

Nothing works for everybody. My viewers tell me that very hot milk overheats them and makes sleep impossible. However, warm milk usually puts them to sleep. Some biochemists, speaking off the cuff, say that the tryptophan content of milk acts as a sedative.

This is hard to believe, because milk's tryptophan content is only a small fraction of the amount found in experiments to be sleep-inducing.

The late Carlton Fredericks, Ph.D, one of the all-time great nutritionists, agreed. He once told me he felt that calcium was the main sleep-inducing ingredient in milk, because it soothes neuromuscular irritability, acting as one of nature's tranquilizers. Our vote goes with Dr. Fredericks.

Down With Sleeping Pills!

Many authorities frown on sleeping pills, which, over the long run, work less and less well, may have side effects and could become habituating. Most of them favor taking a wholesome nutrient such as tryptophan or inositol.

Carlton Fredericks used to tell audiences that his pet way of falling asleep was taking 500 mg of the amino acid tryptophan early in the evening. Tryptophan converts into serotonin, a neurotransmitter which calms the brain. However, experiments by Dr. Richard Wurtman, of M.I.T., noted for his brain research, prove that tryptophan requires the intake of a carbohydrate food — cereal, fruit, or vegetable — to get into the brain.[1] A banana works fine.

Many research studies show that tryptophan makes an excellent sleepmate.

One gram (1000 mg) before bedtime reduced falling-asleep time by 50 percent for normal individuals tested.[2]

Although some persons who had trouble falling asleep did so readily with one gram of tryptophan, extreme insomniacs got desired results from higher amounts. Side effects are rare at potencies used in these studies. Researchers tested 400 patients at doses up to 15 grams and found side effects negligible, even at this stratospheric level.[3]

Better Than Tranquilizers

Carl C. Pfeiffer, Ph.D, M.D., director of Princeton's Brain Bio Center, has discovered that inositol, one of the B vitamins, is a harmless, yet excellent, sedative which works as well as the most popular tranquilizers, calming a person for sleep. Usually 1,000 mg of inositol in the morning and an hour before bedtime at night have proven sleep-effective.[4]

Enemies of Sleep

Numerous studies show that caffeine-containing soft drinks, coffee, chocolate, smoking and alcohol combine to keep people awake. Many authorities cite caffeine and coffee as major sleep assassins to be avoided or not used after mid-afternoon, because they make falling asleep difficult, lower the quality of sleep, and cause frequent wake-ups.

Rarely do orthodox doctors tell us that 65 prescription drugs and more than 100 over-the-counter medicines contain sleep-discouraging caffeine — something to remember, or we'll have to count sheep until the cows come home.

Teas That Make For ZZZs

One of my favorite ways to lure sleep is through sipping a warm cup of tea—with or without a tablespoon of honey. Camomile and Sleepytime tea usually bring me a good night's sleep.

However, nothing works if we put our brain in gear with a creative project before bedtime. A super-active mind chases away sleep. Worries and fears are also poor bedfellows. "Who by taking thought addeth a cubit to his stature?"

I often read the Bible to remember God's promises. In Psalms, I find that King David spent many an hour twisting and turning with insomnia, concerned about his enemies. He finds relief in Psalms 4:8: "I will both lay me down in peace, and sleep. For thou, Lord, only makest me dwell in safety."

Another of my favorite methods for falling asleep is reciting the 23rd Psalm, and, soon, the peace that passes all understanding settles over me, and I am gone.

On other occasions, all I have to do is remind myself of the scripture " . . . underneath are the everlasting arms," and, as a child of God, I fall asleep, knowing I have a tender, loving father holding and watching over me.

Here's to a sound, happy and health-restoring sleep for you!

Banana Delight

2 ripe bananas	1 T. honey
1 T. lemon juice	1 t. sunflower seeds

Mash bananas with fork in a blender. Add lemon juice and honey. Put in a dessert dish and sprinkle with sunflower seeds. Serves 1.

CHAPTER 93

Smell And Taste Loss

Some individuals regard loss of the sense of smell as a trivial ailment. It is anything but that.

So says Robert I. Henkin, M.D., of Georgetown University Medical Center's Center for Molecular Nutrition and Sensory Disorders.

It could be a matter of life or death for the simple reason that without the ability to smell, individuals would not be able to detect warning odors: gas escaping from a stove or heater, fumes from an auto's leaky fuel line, smoke from a fire, the odor of spoiled food.[1]

Over and above the risk, the smell-impaired individual, handicapped in not being able to savor tempting food aromas, often loses the desire to eat (followed by the loss of excessive weight) and also the ability to taste.[2]

Revealing Studies

Knowing that inefficiency in zinc metabolism is usually related to these sensory losses, Henkin and associates discovered that 25 percent of individuals with impaired smell and taste absorb zinc poorly.[3] Given daily zinc supplementation, they showed marked improvement in three to four months.

In another study, reported in the British magazine Nature, animals on a carotenoid-free diet developed an impaired ability to smell.[4] Carotenoids are the coloring matter in carotenes, a vitamin A precursor derived from vegetables and fruit which have orange, yellow, red or purple coloring.

Areas of the nose where smelling is done—the soft membranes—are yellow and known to contain carotenoids. Experiments show that carotenoids can be released from protein in which they are captives.[5]

Test subjects treated with vitamin A regained their sense of smell, probably because of the interaction between carotenes and carotenoids with vitamin A in the soft membrane area. Large amounts of vitamin A given intramuscularly returned the ability to smell to 48 of 53 patients.[6]

Lost Sense of Taste Responds To Zinc And More

As with the closely related sense of smell, the lost ability to taste often responds to supplementation with zinc. Although a deficiency of zinc is the major contributor to an impaired sense of taste, other vitamins and minerals are involved, too, says Dr. Henkin: vitamin A, vitamin B-6 and B-12 and copper.[7]

A proposed 50 mg of zinc daily for three to four weeks would probably be a proper test to find out whether or not zinc is the deficient nutrient, he indicates.[8]

Looking at the problem from the opposite pole, researchers have found that a zinc deficiency usually accompanies an impaired or absent sense of taste and that zinc supplementation corrects the deficiency.

One hundred thirty-two Denver children and youths—ages four to 17 —were tested for ability to taste and also for amount of zinc concentrated in their hair. Ten were found to be zinc-deficient and taste-impaired. Supplementation with zinc for one to three months corrected the taste problem.[9]

Ability To Taste

Another experiment demonstrated the importance of zinc to ability to taste. Young women were tested for zinc status by analysis of blood, diet, hair and saliva and found to be normal. Then they were given various potencies of zinc supplement, but showed no difference in ability to detect bitterness, saltiness and sourness. However, test subjects in the group taking 30 mg of zinc daily, revealed a significantly increased ability to taste sweetness.[10]

In still another experiment, ten individuals with a healthy sense of taste were given 15 mg of zinc daily for five weeks to see what would happen.[11] As in the previous study, they all improved markedly in ability to taste sweetness. They also registered a slight improvement in ability to taste bitterness.

Then supplementary zinc was cut off and, with it, the group's new more acute sensitivity to sweet tastes. Clearly zinc improved their ability to experience the taste spectrum at full intensity.[12]

An interesting observation came out of these experiments. Inasmuch as zinc increased the sensitivity to the full intensity of sweet taste, less sugar could probably satisfy the person. In other words, sufficient zinc might well discourage the sweet tooth. Also, the prevalent deficiency of zinc in the nation's soils and in people may be contributing to steadily increasing sugar use.

Foods For Better Smelling And Tasting!

Following are zinc-rich foods and supplements in milligrams per less than four ounce units: herring, 160; wheat germ, 14; sesame seeds, 10; torula yeast, 9.9; blackstrap molasses, 8.3; maple syrup, 7.5; liver, 7.0; soybeans, 6.7; sunflower seeds, 6.6; egg yolk, 5.5; lamb, 5.4; chicken, 4.8; brewer's yeast, 3.9; oats, 3.7; bone meal, 3.6; rye, 3.4; whole wheat, 3.2; corn, 3.1; coconut and beef, 3.0; beets, turkey and walnuts; barley, 2.7; beans and avocados, 2.4; peas, 2.3; bleu cheese, 2.2; buckwheat, 2.0; mangoes, 1.9; millet, rice and almonds, 1.5 and salmon, 1.4.

Best food and supplement sources of vitamin A and its precursor in International Units per less than four ounce servings are: cod liver oil, 200,000; sheep liver, 45,000; beef liver, 44,000; calf's liver, 22,000; dandelion greens, 14,000; carrots, 11,000; yams, 9,000; kale, 8,900; parsley and turnip greens, 8,500; spinach, 8,100; collard greens and chard, 6,500; watercress, 5,000; red peppers, 4,400; winter squash, 4,000; egg yolk and cantaloupe, 3,400; endive, 3,300; persimmons and apricots, 2,700; broccoli, 2,500; pimentos, 2,300; swordfish, 2,100; whitefish, 2,000; romaine, 1,900; mangos, 1,800; papayas, 1,700 and nectarines and pumpkins.

Richest food and supplement sources of vitamin B-6 in milligrams per less than four ounce units are: brewer's yeast, 4.0; brown rice, 3.6; whole wheat, 2.9; royal jelly, 2.4; soybeans, 2.0; rye, 1.8; lentils, 1.7; sunflower seeds and hazelnuts, 1.1; alfalfa, 1.00; salmon, 0.98; wheat germ, 0.92;

tuna, 0.90; bran, 0.85; walnuts, 0.73; peas and liver, 0.67; avocados, 0.60; beans, 0.57; cashews, peanuts, turkey, oats, chicken and beef, 0.40; halibut, 0.34; lamb, 0.32: banana, 0.32; blackstrap molasses, 0.31 and corn and egg yolk, 0.30.

Best food and supplement sources of vitamin B-12 in milligrams per less than four ounce units are: liver, 0.086; sardines, 0.034; mackerel and herring, 0.0100; red snapper, 0.0088; flounder, 0.0064; salmon, 0.0047; lamb, 0.0031; swiss cheese, 0.0021; eggs, 0.0020; haddock, 0.0017; muenster cheese, 0.0016; swordfish and beef, 0.0015; bleu cheese, 0.0014 and halibut and bass, 0.0013.

Richest food and supplement sources of copper in milligrams per less than four ounce units are: liver, 3.7; wheat germ, 2.9; thyme, 2.4; blackstrap molasses, 2.2; honey, 1.7; hazelnuts, 1.4; brazil nuts, 1.1; walnuts, 0.90; kelp and salmon, 0.80; cashews, 0.76; ginseng, 0.75; oats; 0.74; lentils, 0.71; barley, 0.70; almonds, 0.68; bananas, 0.51; tuna, 0.50; avocado and coconut, 0.39; brown rice, 0.36; bee pollen, 0.32; eggplant, 0.30; kale, 0.30 and chicken, 0.28.

PLEASE NOTE! It is not necessary to strive for the highest milligram foods in copper. Only a small amount is needed daily. The RDA is approximately 5 mg. More than that could be hazardous.

Lillian's Lamb Stew

3 onions, sliced
4 T. liquid garlic
4 potatoes, chunked
4 celery stalks, sliced
6 carrots, sliced
2 zucchini, chunked (optional)
2 t. wheatgerm
½ T. pimentos
⅛ t. thyme
1 broccoli stalk, sliced

1 large can tomatoes
2 T. Black Strap Molasses
2 T. parsley, chopped
2 t. dill weed
3 T. arrowroot
2 T. olive oil
2½ lbs. lean lamb,
    squared in 1-inch chunks
½ c. spring water

Saute lamb lightly in large skillet with olive oil until brown. Put spring water in large pot, add onions, garlic, potatoes, celery and carrots. Saute about 15 minutes. Add broccoli, lamb and wheat germ. Cover and steam about about 10 minutes. Add tomatoes, molasses, parsley, dill and zucchini. Cover and simmer over very low heat about 25 minutes longer. Serves 9.

Marinated Broccoli Salad

1 bunch broccoli, broken into
  small flowerets (discard stems)
Boiling sea salted water
½ c. oil

½ c. lemon juice
Sea salt to taste
Black pepper to taste, freshly ground
1 garlic clove, finely chopped

Put broccoli in large skillet and add boiling water to cover the bottom of pan to depth of one-half inch. Cover and simmer until broccoli is crisp-tender, about eight minutes. Drain. Meanwhile, beat together remaining ingredients. Pour dressing over hot broccoli. Chill well before serving. Serves six to eight.

CHAPTER 94

Smoking (Self-Protection, Coping, Quitting)

Not long ago at a delightful Brown Bag noonday concert in Menlo Park, California, Anne Regel, a non-smoking friend and I had just spread a Scotch plaid blanket on the grass at the edge of the crowd for as much privacy as you can get in a public place.

Who should plop down near us but a beefy, breathless, ruddy-faced man, puffing on a limp cigarette, grey ashes cascading down the front of his gravy-stained navy blue T-shirt.

Our faces must have registered disapproval, because he glanced sharply at us and asked, "Mind if I sit here?"

"Not at all," replied Anne.

Then he suddenly got our unspoken message.

"Oh, it's my cigarette," he grinned, taking one long last drag and snuffing out the cigarette in the grass. "A little second-hand smoke won't hurt you," he commented.

"Sorry, but you're wrong," I said. "Apparently you haven't read recent studies on the subject . . ."

Anne's sudden, firm and obvious grip on my elbow hushed me up.

"Let's change the subject!" she urged, smiling sweetly at the man and me. "Otherwise I'll have to bind and gag Maureen to keep her from giving a five-hour lecture on the evils of cigarette smoking."

Red Flags From The U.S. Surgeon General

We all laughed and settled down to enjoy the concert. But I couldn't help thinking about passive smoke and how really active it is. I remember U.S. Surgeon General C. Everett Koop saying that exhaled cigarette smoke is a lethal weapon against non-smokers, and that it leads to disease and death, with children particularly vulnerable.

At least 80 studies disclose that children of smokers are more inclined to bronchitis, pneumonia, hospitalizations and missed school days than other children. Worse than that, he indicated, is the fact that smoking of parents helps introduce children to the habit. Parents who love their kids and are interested in their welfare will stop smoking, he said, disclosing how his father kicked the habit when he overheard young Everett saying, "My pop hasn't got the guts to quit smoking."

The Evil That Men Do (And Women) Lives After Them

There's no question second-hand smoke is harmful. One study shows that the spouse of a heavy smoker is 3 1/2 times more prone to develop lung cancer than the spouse of a non-smoker.[1] The smoking issue is causing an increasing number of divorces, making it seem wise to resolve this question before marriage. Kathleen Stone, a researcher at Ohio State University, found that passive smoke causes a higher risk for pregnant women and their fetuses in that fetuses may pull away from the placenta wall prematurely.[2] In addition, smoke-exposed infants less than a year old are afflicted with more colds and pneumonia, she has found.

Actually, passive smoke can be a killer. Researcher Helmut Sinzinger and associates at the University of Vienna Medical School have discovered that second-hand smoke can increase chances of strokes and heart attacks.[3]

Fifteen minutes after subjecting nine non-smokers to smoke from 30 cigarettes in a closed room, they tested the blood of volunteers and found a dramatic change: platelets, tiny discs essential to blood clotting, became 75 percent less sensitive to prostaglandins, substances which prevent platelets from sticking together too readily and causing blood clots that could be fatal.[4]

Even an hour after the tested individuals left the smoky room, the platelets still remained far less sensitive than normal. Smokers put into the same room for 15 minutes showed only a slight reaction, because their platelet sensitivity had already been reduced 50 percent by smoking regularly.[5]

Sinzinger warns that smoke-filled rooms can make non-smokers as vulnerable to stroke and heart attack as persons who burn a package of cigarettes daily, because non-snokers have a far lower tolerance to cigarette smoke. Therefore, even small amounts of smoke can be far more hazardous to them than previously believed. Tell this to relatives and friends who smoke or are constantly exposed to smoke.[6]

Removing The Smokescreen

It's old news that cigarette smoking can contribute to heart and artery ailments and cancer. However, it's new news, thanks to sophisticated measuring instruments and computers, that we can now tell with greater precision how much cigarettes can shorten a smoker's life.[7]

Writing in the Journal of the American Medical Association, T.L. Petty claims that each cigarette shortens a person's life by five and a half minutes. Those who smoke regularly are slashing their lifespan by about seven years![8]

Another study— this by Gus Miller, a mathematics professor at the Indiana University of Pennsylvania, and Dean Gerstein, a National Research Council study director — tells us that men have shorter life expectancy than women, mainly because so many of them smoke.[9]

However, the 7.6 years of greater life expectancy for women may soon burn out, due to the sharp increase in smoking by teen-age girls, who have passed the boys in percentage of smokers. Unless drastic changes are made, the longevity advantage of women is about to go up in smoke.[10]

Anti-Smoking Strategy For Kids

All right, how best can parents and teachers discourage kids from starting a habit that's as hard to kick as alcoholism and cocaine-addiction? Will scare tactics work, the prospect of heart disease, emphysema and/or lung cancer?[11]

No. Try again. This obvious way is not the best way. Researchers at the University of Minnesota decided to go right to junior high school kids to find out just what can turn them off about smoking. And they found out. They ran an effectiveness study of smoking prevention programs with seventh graders at eight Minneapolis-St. Paul schools.[12]

One part of the program stressed the possible long-term health consequences. The second accented the socially negative effects of smoking: bad breath, yellowed fingers and teeth and being barred from many public places.

When the researchers evaluated the relative effectiveness of their programs a year later, they found that best results, by far, were scored with social consequences of smoking: negative physical appearance and less social acceptance — especially with children who hadn't tried smoking.[13]

This approach achieved desired results because youngsters are much concerned about physical appearance and being accepted by their peers, states David Murray, one of the researchers. Pointing out the dismal prospect of serious diseases was much less effective, because health consequences were too long-term, too far in the future for them to visualize and apply to themselves.[14]

Counteracting The Bad Effects

Those of us with more than a few miles on our age odometer can more easily visualize the serious health consequences and want to do something to protect ourselves, spouses, family members and friends from the damage of first and second-hand smoke.

You can do it nutritionally. I can hear you protest, 'But won't this destroy a smoker's motive to quit?' Not if you set out the vitamins and minerals — along with others — as part of that person's general health program. Not if you plan meals including foods that contain these supplements. Meanwhile, you try various motivations.

The same motivation that worked for the junior high school kids — negative social aspects of smoking — has helped me get numerous adults to kick the nicotine habit. Prayer is another powerful weapon that often works miracles. People who have repeatedly failed to break the habit — who are so discouraged they want to quit quitting — have experienced cold turkey release from their addiction. Prayer teams in many churches are available to help effect a miracle.

Nutrients That Protect

Following are vitamins and minerals which protect the smoker to some extent against the usual consequences of smoking. Much sound research underlies the nutrients mentioned.

A daily intake of five thousand to 10,000 International units daily of vitamin A, noted for promoting health of mucous membranes, has been shown to offer some protection for the respiratory tract. It is easy to reach this level with the natural foods mentioned below.[15]

Vitamin E cooperates with vitamin A, protecting it from destructive oxidation in the lungs and other mucous membranes.[16] Additionally, vitamin E on its own has been shown by researchers at four major universities to protect lung tissue from nitrogen oxide and ozone in smoggy areas and, yes, from cigarette smoke, too.[17]

San Diego area biochemist-nutritionist Karen Owens, who has made in-depth studies of vitamin E experiments, states that the average American takes in only about seven international units of Vitamin E daily. One experiment cited by her reveals that as much as 800 I.U. of vitamin E taken daily for three years caused no ill effects in human test subjects. A St. Louis University study discloses that the body best utilizes natural vitamin E (d-Alpha tocopherol), rather than the cheaper synthetic (dl-Alpha tocopherol), she says.[18]

Vitamin C (1,500 mg or more daily) has been shown to guard the bladder against cancer from smoking — (See the Section on Bladder Cancer) and from a wide range of toxic pollutants in tobacco smoke.[19]

Fifteen to 30 mg of zinc, needed for prostate gland function and to help prevent prostate enlargement, assists in keeping the immune system strong to resist pollutants from smoking. (See the Section on the Immune System).[20]

How To Break The Habit

Many systems seem to work for some to break the smoking habit: just quitting cold turkey; quitting and resisting one minute at a time; breaking the habit for someone you love; substituting something for cigarettes — for instance, sugarless chewing gum or coffee substitutes made from various grains and sold in health food stores (not decaffeinated coffee); substituting a favorite exercise, hobby or recreation when the urge to smoke comes on; the Buddy system, getting a relative, friend, or workplace associate to quit with you and offering support to one another and prayer (as mentioned earlier).

When I made a lecture tour of Australia, I met Hans Wagner, television nutritionist, who told me about a system for quitting smoking which works for many people.[21] It involves rolling one's own and mixing a little of the dried and granulated leaves of the herb colt's foot with tobacco and smoking it. (Colt's foot is a plant with clustered yellow flowers and leaves in the shape of a colt's foot and can be bought at health food stores.)

The strategy is to add a bit more colt's foot to the mixture with each smoking. This herb is said to purge the system of poisons from tobacco and gradually to make the taste and aroma of tobacco objectionable. Hans tells me results are amazing, and that colt's foot kills the craving for tobacco.[22]

I hope so.

Protective Nutrients

Meanwhile, following are natural foods which contain noteworthy amounts of nutrients said to offer protection against first and second-hand smoke.

First, let's look at a list of Vitamin A-rich supplements and foods in terms of international units per unit of less than four ounces: (It is easy to meet the daily quota of 5,000 to 10,000 I.U.): cod liver oil, 200,000; sheep liver, 45,000; beef liver, 44,000; calf's liver, 22,000; dandelion greens, 14,000; carrots, 11,000; yams, 9,000; kale, 8,900; parsley and turnip greens, 8,500; spinach, 8,100; collard greens and chard, 6,500; watercress, 5,000; red peppers, 4,400; winter squash, 4,000; egg yolk and cantaloupe, 3,400; endive, 3,300; persimmons and apricots, 2700; broccoli, 2,500; pimentos, 2,300; swordfish, 2,100; whitefish. 2,000; romaine, 1,900; mangos, 1,800; papayas, 1,700; nectarines and pumpkin, 1,600; peaches and cheese, 1,300; eggs, 1,200; cherries, lettuce and cream, 1,000; tomatoes and asparagus, 900; halibut, 850; soybeans, 700; kumquats, 600; watermelon, 590; okra, 520 and mackerel, 450.

Here are supplements and foods with highest amounts of vitamin C in milligrams per units of less than four ounces: rose hips, 3,000; acerola cherries, 1,100; guavas, 240; black currants, 200; parsley, 170; green peppers, 110; watercress, 80; chives, 70; strawberries, 57; persimmons, 52; spinach, 51; oranges, 50; cabbage, 38; papaya, 37; elderberries and kumquats, 36; dandelion greens and lemons, 35; cantaloupe, 33; green onions, 32; limes, 31; mangos, 27; loganberries, 25; tangerines and tomatoes, 23; squash, 22; and romaine lettuce and raspberries.

Following are supplements and foods richest in vitamin E in milligrams per units of less than four ounces: wheat germ, 160; safflower nuts, 35; sunflower seeds, 31; wholewheat, 30; sesame oil, 26; walnuts, 22; corn oil and hazelnuts, 21; soy oil and peanut oil, 16; almonds, 15; olive oil, 14; cabbage, 7.8; brazil nuts and peanuts, 6.5; cod liver oil, 5.4; cashews, 5.1; soy lecithin, 4.8; spinach, 2.9; asparagus, 2.5; broccoli, 2.0; butter, 1.9; parsley, 1.8; oats, barley and corn, 1.7 and avocados and pecans, 1.5.

Highest amounts of zinc in terms of milligrams per units of less than four ounces are in the following foods and supplements: herring, 110; wheat germ, 14; sesame seeds, 10; torula yeast, 9.9; blackstrap molasses, 8.3; maple syrup, 7.5; liver, 7.0; soybeans, 6.7; sunflower seeds, 6.6; egg yolk, 5.5; lamb, 5.4; chicken, 4.8; regular molasses, 4.6; brewer's yeast, 3.9; oats, 3.7; bone meal, 3.6; rye, 3.4; whole wheat, 3.2; corn, 3.1; coconut and beef, 3.0; beets, turkey, and walnuts, 2.7; beans and avocados, 2.4; peas, 2.3; bleu cheese, 2.2; buckwheat, 2.0; mangoes, 1.9 and millet, brown rice and almonds, 1.5.

Sousa's Cocktail

4 heaping T. fresh brewers yeast   1 t. honey
1 glass papaya juice   1 t. rose hips powder

Add brewers yeast to one glass of papaya juice. Fold in honey. Stir vigorously or use electric blender. Before drinking, sprinkle with rose hips powder. Drink minutes before your meal.

Pumpkin Pancakes

1⅓ c. whole raw, certified milk   1 T. wheat germ
½ c. plain yogurt   3 T. sunflower seeds, finely chopped
2 eggs, well beaten   1½ c. pumpkin, cooked and mashed
1 T. sesame oil   ¼ t. nutmeg
1 T. unsulfured molasses   ½ t. cinnamon
2 c. whole wheat flour

Combine milk, yogurt, eggs, oil, honey and molasses. Gently stir in flour, wheat germ and sunflower seeds. Fold in pumpkin, nutmeg and cinnamon. Stir until mixed. Spoon onto hot greased griddle. Yield: 10-16 pancakes.

CHAPTER 95

Snoring

Pity the poor snorer! Even more so, pity the poor person sentenced to sleep next to him or her, because that often proves next to impossible.

Some snoring is incredibly loud and powerful, the oddity lover's delight: enough to shatter a window, drown out a sawmill, or register a nine on the Richter scale.

Yet the snorer doesn't want to be a sound polluter, a prime candidate for divorce, or a social reject. If only one of the more than 300 anti-snoring devices on record at the U.S. Patent Office were practical, he would be the happiest ex-snorer in the world.

Well, at least one of them is. For instance, there's a collar that holds the head in a position that supposedly prevents snoring. The only minor problem is that their wearers start walking on all fours and barking at the mail-deliverer.

Silence Snoring

You probably wonder how foods that heal relate to preventing snoring. Frankly, so do I. But anti-snoring must be dealt with in one way or another for the preservation of marriages, sanity, and society. Not long ago, helpful advice was issued by the American Academy of Otolaryngology: (I'm glad I don't have to pronounce that word. It's hard enough to spell.) Exercise and improve muscle tone, and avoid alcohol, histamines, sleeping pills and tranquilizers right before bedtime. (You might want to avoid them, period.)

Before revealing this academy's best piece of advice and also mentioning how a natural food can contribute to a snoringless society, I must deal with a most serious subject: sleep apnea, a frequent problem of snorers, stopping breathing for anywhere from five or ten seconds to two minutes. This condition, caused by obstructed airways, could lead to cardiovascular complications.

Although surgery can correct sleep apnea, any surgery of this kind can be hazardous — particularly something with the suspect name of a "tracheostomy".

Now some Chicago researchers have come up with a device that the apnea sufferer wears in his mouth to retain his tongue in a forward position so that he doesn't block his airway. An article in the August 13, 1982 issue of the Journal of the American Medical Association describes the device, then in its experimental stage, saying that it reduces the number of apneic events and improves sleep, although it may be a bit uncomfortable.

Never having seen this device, I really have no idea how big, small or uncomfortable it is. However, somehow I feel wearing it would be like trying to sleep with a gopher trap in my mouth.

Meanwhile, back to the advice of the American Academy of Otolaryngology. Some of their authorities state that merely sleeping with head raised helps the cause. A mountain of pillows won't do the job. Bricks under the legs at the head of the bed could help. Better yet is a hospital bed, whose head can be raised.

Another of the otolaryngologist's ways to reduce or eliminate snoring, is for snorers to sleep on their side— one side or another— rather than on their back.

Yet how can a person monitor himself to sleep on his side all night?

Good question. Some genius came up with the idea of sewing a tennis ball into the back of the pajamas. It really works, sigh many grateful wives. Now, so far as foods that heal go, you simply use a substitute for the tennis ball: a small, firm, organically grown rutabaga!

CHAPTER 96

Stress

Stress manhandles those who don't know how to handle it.

And, until recent years, handling stress lacked know-how, imagination and positive results. Whenever possible, people avoided it. Whenever impossible, they faced the inevitable, gritted their teeth and took their lumps.

Consequently, stress left its cruel calling card in billions of human bodies and minds — every imaginable bacteria and virus-caused illness and degenerative disease and, in addition, emotional warping.

Now psychologists have shown us how to make a healthy adjustment to our daily stress without physical consequences. A brilliant study by Dr. Suzanne Kobasa and Salvatore Maddi revealed that it isn't excessive stress that makes people sick. It is the way they react to stress that makes them ill or keeps them well. [1]

Kobasa and Maddi studied 200 Illinois Bell Telephone Company executives who were going through a morale-devastating divestiture, during which departments were being consolidated, positions wiped out and long-time salaried personnel were walking a tightrope to stay with the company. [2]

A Logical Explanation

The psychologists directed their attention to 200 executives who had experienced many traumatic events during this daytime nightmare. One hundred of them had reported a succession of diagnosable illnesses. The other hundred had hardly been ill at all. Why the sharp contrast? [3]

In-depth interviews by Kobasa and Maddi revealed that the one group of executives stayed well due to a deep and continued dedication to their work and a healthy and positive outlook on the company transition. Change is neither good nor bad, they felt. It is a part of living, a challenge, a chance for growth, not a threat to security.[4]

While these individuals had no control over the divestiture— that was an objective reality— they could control their reactions to it. Their security seemed to come from faith in their ability or in God, or both.

The Kobasa team found virtually the same results in a study of male attorneys, the same psychological hardiness in those who stayed well through crisis living. Then they turned to a study of women gynecological outpatients going through numerous stressful experiences. Again, the psychologically hardy— with a strong sense of control, dedication to self, family and occupation and welcoming challenge— emerged with far fewer symptoms than a control group.[5]

These three studies left no doubt in the minds of Kobasa and associates that people can train themselves to increase their resistance to sickness by developing psychological hardiness toward stress.

An Effective Spiritual Route

My own way of lessening the power of stressors I cannot change is to rely in full faith on God. In that way, my immune system remains strong and my boundless good health and well-being stay intact.

The following scriptures always bolster my faith.

"Fear thou not; for I am with thee. Be not dismayed, for I am thy God. I will strength thee. Yea, I will help thee. I will uphold thee with the right hand of righteousness." Isaiah 41:10 (KJV).

"Come unto me, all ye that labor and are heavy laden, and I will give you rest." Matthew 11:28 (KJV).

The Bible is an endless source for timeless answers to today's stressors, giving "good measure, pressed down, shaken together and running over." I don't know what I would do without it.

A Wide Range Of Stressors

The range of stressors to which individuals react is broad: physical exhaustion, demanding deadlines, infections, long exposure to intense cold or heat, rarefied air, radiation or electric shock, chemotherapy, crash diets, fasting, major surgery, severe burns and, among others, a serious car accident.

Among the more prominent emotional stressors are: the death of a loved one, unrelenting frustration, depression, mental illness, imprisonment, being fired from a job or position, retirement, extended illness of self or a loved one, pregnancy, acute sexual problems, anxiety, fear, and hatred.

Again, the key here is the reaction of the stressed one, rather than just the intensity or repetition of the stress. ·

Selye Needs An Updating

Dr. Hans Selye's theory is that stress causes disease due to the fact that extreme pressure on a person activates the outer covering of the adrenal glands (cortex) to discharge high levels of hormones. These hormones, intended to help us survive the stress, do so at a cost: lowering of immune system efficiency and body resistance, leading to organ damage and disease.

Excessive and continuous discharge of these hormones apparently does what Selye indicates. However, the question is: is it only the stress that sets off this high production of hormones or is it the person's response to that stress?

Recent research indicates it is also the latter. A study of 117 college students by Harvard psychiatrist Steven Locke and associates reveals that anxious and depressed students had low natural killer (NK) cell activity, a part of the immune system defense. However, the psychologically hardy triggered the release of less adrenal hormones, so NK cell activity was markedly higher than in the other students.[6]

Foods For Stress

Of course, when individuals react negatively to physical or emotional stress, the metabolic rate steps up, and more key nutrients are burned up quickly. Stress increases the requirement for various nutrients: protein, vitamin A, pantothenic acid— a B vitamin— vitamin C and magnesium.

Best protein sources are eggs, milk products, meat, fish, soy, nuts and seeds.

Richest supplement and food sources of vitamin A and its beta carotene precursor in International Units per portion of less than four ounces are: cod liver oil, 200,000; sheep liver, 45,000; beef liver, 44,000; calf's liver, 22,000; dandelion greens, 14,000; carrots, 11,000; yams, 9,000; kale, 8,900; parsley and turnip greens, 8,500; spinach, 8,100; collard green and chards, 6,500; watercress, 5,000; red peppers, 4,400; squash, 4,000; egg yolk and cantaloupe, 3,400; endive, 3,300; persimmons and apricots, 2,700; broccoli, 2,500, pimentos, 2,300; swordfish, 2,100; whitefish, 2,000; romaine lettuce, 1,900, mangoes, 1,800; papayas, 1,700; nectarines and pumpkins, 1,600; peaches and cheeses, 1,300; eggs, 1,200; cherries, lettuce, and cream, 1,000.

Here are the highest content supplements and foods in pantothenic acid in milligrams, per units of less than four ounces: royal jelly, 35; brewer's yeast, 11; torula yeast, 10; brown rice, 8.9; sunflower seeds, 5.5; soybeans, 5.2; corn, 5.0; lentils, 4.8; egg yolk, 4.8; peas, 3.6; alfalfa, 3.3; whole wheat, 3.2; peanuts, 2.8; rye, 2.6; eggs, 2.3; bee pollen and wheat germ, 2.2; bleu cheese, 1.8; cashews, 1.3; chickpeas, 1.2; avocado, 1.1 and chicken, sardines, turkey and walnuts, 0.90.

Richest supplement and food sources of vitamin C in milligrams per units of less than four ounces: rose hips, 3,000; acerola cherries, 1,100; guavas, 240; black currants, 200; parsley, 170; green peppers, 110; watercress, 80; chives, 70; strawberries, 57; persimmons, 52; spinach, 51; oranges, 50; cabbage, 47; grapefruit, 38; papaya, 37; elderberries and kumquats, 36; dandelion greens and lemons, 35; cantaloupe, 33; green onions, 32; limes, 31; mangoes, 27; loganberries, 24; tangerines and tomatoes, 23; squash, 22; raspberries and romaine lettuce, 18.

Following are the best supplement and food sources of magnesium in terms of milligrams per units of less than four ounces: dolomite, 13,000; kelp, 740; blackstrap molasses, 410; sunflower seeds, 350; wheat germ, 320; almonds, 270; soybeans, 240; brazil nuts, 220; bone meal, 170; pistachios and soy lecithin, 160; hazelnuts, 150; pecans and oats, 140; walnuts, 130; brown rice, 120; regular molasses, 81; chard, 65; spinach, 57; barley, 55; coconut, 44; salmon, 40; corn, 38; avocados, 37; bananas, 31, cheese, 30 and tuna, 29.

Fruited Pot Roast

3 T. sesame oil
1 red pepper, chopped
4 to 5 lbs. rump or chuck roast
(trimmed of fat)
3 medium onions, coarsely chopped
¼ t. cloves, ground

2 c. apple juice or cider
10 ounces dried prunes, pitted (1½ c.)
½ lb. dried apricots (1½ c.)
2 to 4 T. cornstarch
(dissolved in ¼ c. cold spring water)
½ c. sesame seeds

Heat oil in a dutch oven or roasting pan and brown meat on all sides. Add onions, cloves and apple juice. Cover tightly, reduce heat and simmer for 2 hours, or until nearly tender. (Or cover and bake at 350 degrees for 2½ hours.) Add prunes and apricots and continue to cook or bake 30 minutes longer. If desired, thicken liquid in pot by removing meat and adding cornstarch mixture. Cook until thickened, stirring constantly. Serve over meat and fruit. Makes 10 Servings.

Banana Pineapple Shake

2 bananas, sliced
1 c. fresh cut pineapple
1 c. coconut pineapple juice
(unsweetened)

1 t. vanilla
½ c. spring water
crushed ice

Peel bananas and freeze. Combine all ingredients in blender, except for bananas. Add bananas slowly until shake becomes thick. The more bananas used, the thicker the shake. Serve with half pineapple wedge and straw.

Hearty Tangerine Chicken Salad

3 c. cooked chicken, diced
6 tangerines, peeled, separated into
segments, seeded
½ c. slivered toasted almonds
½ c. celery, chopped
½ c. green pepper, chopped

⅓ c. mayonnaise (home-made)
⅓ c. dairy sour cream (raw certified)
2 T. candied ginger, finely chopped
Salad greens
1 T. brewers yeast

In large bowl, combine chicken, tangerine segments, almonds, yeast, celery and green pepper. Thoroughly combine mayonnaise, sour cream and ginger. Pour over salad. Toss lightly to mix well. Chill at least one hour before serving on crisp salad greens. Serves 5 to 6.

CHAPTER 97

Stretch Marks

Once upon a time, stretch marks— scarring or seam-like blemishes on the skin of the belly, breasts, hips, shoulder girdle or thighs — were considered exclusive to women who had lost a lot of weight or who had just delivered babies.

More and more, these markings are appearing on young women and, now, even on men.

About the latter, Carl C. Pfeiffer, Ph.D, M.D., director of Princeton's Brain Bio Center, mentions such a case in his book, Mental And Elemental Nutrients (Keats Publishing).

An out-of-condition young man in a YMCA weight-lifting class stated that he was the only one out of 25 who developed stretch marks (also called striae) in the skin of the shoulder girdle. As he lifted weights, he could actually feel the skin under the epidermis breaking.

More Subtle With Women

Increasingly, young women come to doctors with embarrassing stretch marks that keep them from wearing bikinis. Alternative physicians tell me that this condition results from poor nutrition, little physical exercise and too much exposure to sun, which diminishes skin elasticity.

How can most women go through a number of pregnancies with so much stress on the under-surface skin and not develop stretch marks? How can many obese individuals whose dermis is well stretched lose weight without any sign of striae? Due to inherited factors, says Dr. Pfeiffer.

Those most prone to develop stretch marks— breaks in connective tissue — are diabetics and persons who secrete too much cortisone. Actually, any women can develop them due to deficiencies in diet— insufficient protein, pantothenic acid, vitamin C, vitamin E and zinc— particularly pregnant women and those on low-calorie weight reduction diets.[1]

Reversal Of Stretch Marks?

In most instances, stretch marks cannot be reversed. However, what happened to one of my acquaintances may be encouraging. This woman gave birth to a normal size baby and emerged with obvious belly stretch marks.

She had read that high protein, 300 mg of pantothenic acid, 1000 mg of vitamin C and 600 I.U. of vitamin E and 15 to 25 mg of zinc daily, plus vigorous walking, could help and followed this regimen. Nothing promising happened after five months, but then she soon found herself pregnant once more. She stayed with the program for most of her pregnancy and then gave birth to an oversize baby.

Overjoyed about the good health of her son, she looked at her now flattened belly and almost cried out with happiness. The stretch marks from the first pregnancy were gone— and there were no new ones!

Of paramount importance in preventing striae are protein— in eggs, dairy products, meat, fish, legumes, nuts and whole grains and food supplements— pantothenic acid, vitamin C, vitamin E and zinc.[2]

Treasure Houses Of The Proper Nutrients

Best supplement and food sources of pantothenic acid in milligrams per less than four ounce servings are: royal jelly, 35; brewer's yeast, 11; torula yeast, 10; brown rice, 8.9; sunflower seeds, 5.5; soybeans, 5.2; corn, 5.0; lentils, 4.8; egg yolk, 4.2; peas, 3.6; alfalfa, 3.3; whole wheat, 3.2; peanuts, 2.8; rye, 2.6; eggs, 2.3; bee pollen and wheat germ, 2.2; bleu cheese, 1.8; cashews, 1.3; chickpeas, 1.2; avocado, 1.1; chicken, sardines, turkey and walnuts, 0.90; perch and salmon, 0.80 and lamb, 0.60.

Supplements and foods richest in vitamin C in milligrams per less than four ounce units are: rose hips, 3,000; acerola cherries, 1,000; guavas, 240; black currants, 200; parsley, 170; green peppers, 110; watercress, 80; chives, 70; strawberries, 57; persimmons, 52; spinach, 51; oranges, 50;

cabbage, 47; grapefruit, 38; papaya, 37; elderberries and kumquats, 36; dandelion greens and lemons, 35; cantaloupe, 33; green onions, 32; limes, 31; mangoes, 27; loganberries, 24; tangerines and tomatoes, 23; squash, 22; raspberries and romaine lettuce, 18 and pineapple, 17.

Food supplements and foods highest in content of vitamin E in International Units per less than four ounce portions are: wheat germ, 160; safflower nuts, 35; sunflower seeds, 31; whole wheat, 30; sesame oil, 26; walnuts, 22; corn oil and hazelnuts, 21; soy oil and peanut oil, 16; almonds, 15; olive oil, 14; cabbage, 7.8; brazil nuts and peanuts, 6.5; cod liver oil, 5.4; cashews, 5.1; soy lecithin, 4.8; spinach, 2.9; asparagus, 2.5; broccoli, 2.0; butter, 1.9; parsley, 1.8; oats, barley and corn, 1.7; avocados and pecans, 1.5.

Richest food sources of zinc in milligrams per less than a four ounce serving are: herring, 110; wheat germ, 14; sesame seeds, 10; torula yeast, 9.9; blackstrap molasses, 8.3; maple syrup, 7.5; liver, 7.0; soybeans, 6.7; sunflower seeds, 6.6; egg yolk, 5.5; lamb, 5.4; chicken, 4.8; brewer's yeast, 3.9; oats, 3.7; rye, 3.4; whole wheat, 3.2; corn, 3.1; coconut and beef, 3.0; beets, turkey and walnuts, 2.8; barley, 2.7; beans and avocados, 2.4; peas, 2.3; bleu cheese, 2.2; eggs, 2.1; buckwheat, 2.0; mangoes, 1.9 and millet, rice and almonds, 1.5.

Maureen's Dilled Cucumbers and Avocado

½ c. vinegar
½ c. sesame oil
1½ t. dill weed
¼ t. onion salt
Dash pepper
2 garlic cloves, minced

2 medium cucumbers,
    pared and thinly sliced
3 or 4 avocados,
    unpeeled and cut in half
Salad greens

Combine vinegar, oil and seasonings. Pour over cucumbers in shallow dish. Chill several hours, or overnight, turning occasionally. Arrange avocado halves, shells, on salad greens. Fill with cucumbers. Sprinkle with wheat germ. Serves six to eight.

CHAPTER 98

Teeth, Grinding (Bruxism)

Habitually grinding the teeth or pressing them against one another (bruxism) may seem like a harmless practice.

But don't you believe it! Bruxism can cause loosening of teeth in their sockets, loss of teeth and gum recession. If ignored, it won't go away. It will only get worse.

A stealthy disorder, bruxism, like most burglars, operates mainly at night, stealing your dental health while you sleep. You may not become aware that you are grinding or clenching your teeth unless someone else tells you about it.

Occasionally bruxism becomes a way of life so that you may even carry on the practice by day and suddenly realize that you are damaging your teeth, their substructure, the jaw joint and the gums.

Fortunately, if you are a solo sleeper, certain symptoms that are sensed by day can alert you to your teeth-grinding in time to prevent serious dental damage: sore jaw muscles and joints and the start of loose teeth and damaged gums.

Not a Psychological Problem

Present in children as frequently as in adults, bruxism is often considered to be the outward sign of a deep-seated emotional problem.

Is this fact or fiction?

"Fiction," say two University of Chicago researchers, George R. Reding, Ph.D, assistant professor of psychiatry, and John E. Robinson, Jr., M.D., associate professor in that university's Walter T. Zoller Dental Memorial Clinic, who made an in-depth study of teeth-grinders through dental exams, interviews and observation with numerous sleep lab and instruments.[1]

Victims of bruxism are not any more emotionally disturbed than persons who don't grind their teeth.

A Double- Headed Nutritional Deficiency

So, what's the answer? Dental investigators Emanuel Cheraskin, M.D., D.M.D. and W. Marshall Ringsdorf, Jr., D.M.D., studied bruxism and nutrient intake of dentists and their wives for a year and discovered that bruxists need additional pantothenic acid (a member of the vitamin B family) and calcium.

Why these nutrients? Participants in this study stopped grinding their teeth when given more pantothenic acid and calcium. A deficiency of pantothenic acid, an anti-stress vitamin, reduces the working of the adrenal glands and production of their hormones.

So far as our daily stress is concerned, the adrenal glands have first rights to available pantothenic acid, short-changing the biochemical means of making acetylcholine, a neuro-transmitter that sends signals for controlling motor activity. Bruxism is a sign that motor activity is not under control.[3]

Like pantothenic acid, calcium has to be liberally supplied so that nerve impulses can travel with efficiency and lightning speed from one part of the body to the other, as discovered by Sir Bernard Katz, a Nobel prize winner.[4]

A deficiency of calcium can bring on cramps, convulsions and involuntary movement. In this instance, the involuntary movement is in the mouth muscles: the grinding of teeth.

The Right Foods Can Help

Following are the most pantothenic acid-rich foods and supplements in terms of milligrams per less than four-ounce portion: royal jelly, 35; brewer's yeast, 11; torula yeast, 10; brown rice, 8.9; sunflower seeds, 5.5; soybeans, 5.2; corn, 5.0; lentils, 4.8; egg yolk, 4.2; peas, 3.6; alfalfa, 3.3; whole wheat, 3.2; peanuts, 2.8; rye, 2.6, eggs, 2.3; bee pollen and wheat germ, 2.2; bleu cheese, 1.8; cashews, 1.3; chickpeas, 1.2 and avocado, 1.1.

Most calcium-rich foods are: sesame seeds, 1,200; kelp, 1,100; cheeses, 700; (see Section on Milk Intolerance); brewer's yeast, 420; sardines and carob, 350; caviar, 280; soybeans and almonds, 230; torula yeast, 220; parsley, 200; brazil nuts, 190; watercress, chickpeas and salmon, 150; egg yolk, beans, pistachios, lentils and kale, 130; sunflower seeds and cow's milk, 120; buckwheat, 110; maple syrup, cream and chard, 100.

CHAPTER 99

Tooth Decay

Most of us believe that sugar-laden foods are the greatest promoters of tooth decay ever to enter our mouths.

"Tain't so!" states Frank De Fazio, D.D.S., veteran dental researcher.[1]

"Nibbling on a chocolate bar may do less damage to your teeth than snacking on bread sticks," he writes, based on experiments reported in the Journal of the American Dental Association. "High sugar content foods produce less acid than high starch snacks with less sugar."

Decaying of teeth is an involved process. Plaque, a sticky, colorless bacterial film collects at the base of the teeth and combines with sugars and starches from the diet. Bacteria then digest sugars and starches and produce acids which dissolve tooth enamel.

How long food lingers in your mouth could be just as significant in cavity-causing potential as the amount of acid it generates. Foods with high sugar content leave the mouth quickly in most instances. However, high starch foods such as white bread, bread sticks and pretzels stay longer in the mouth, making for more acid production.

"An acid attack, may last 30 minutes or more," explains De Fazio.

Okay, so how can you counter acid attacks from between-meal snacks, over and above the usual water gargling? Here are the De Fazio guidelines:

1. Try to exclude sticky foods that cling obstinately to the teeth: bananas, chewy candy, dates or raisins. (Or brush teeth pronto.)

2. Skip hard candies or breath mints that stay in the mouth long.

3. Avoid soft drinks, but, if you don't, choose those without sugar.

4. Substitute cheese, meat, nuts, olives and yogurt for starchy or sugary snacks.

Semper's Salmon Steak Dinner

4 salmon steaks	4 T. Alta Dena butter
¼ c. capers	1 t. parsley, chopped
1½ T. lemon juice	4 garlic cloves, minced

Heat butter in saucepan until liquidy. Add capers, lemon juice, parsley and garlic. Place salmon on cookie sheet with sauce poured over it. Cover with foil with sides of foil up. Broil for 5 to 12 minutes.

"C" Fruit Salad

Salad greens	1 c. strawberries, hulled and washed
1 avocado, cut in lengthwise strips	8 ounces cheddar cheese, cut in strips
3 cantaloupe balls	Honey-Nut Dressing
1 c. fresh pineapple, cubed	½ c. fresh papaya, cubed

Line a shallow salad bowl with salad greens. Sprinkle sliced avocado with lemon juice. Combine cantaloupe, pineapple and berries and fill bowl. Garnish with cheese and avocado. Serve with dressing. Serves 6.

Honey-Nut Dressing:

Mix 1 cup home-made mayonnaise, 2 tablespoons honey and 2 tablespoons slivered almonds.

Home-Made Mayonnaise

2 eggs	¾ c. cold-pressed olive oil
2 T. fresh lemon juice	¾ t. fine mixed herbs

Place eggs, herbs and lemon juice in blender. Add oil very slowly as you blend. Chill in refrigerator until ready to serve. Delightful on either a cold vegetable salad or on hot steamed vegetables.

CHAPTER 100

Tooth, Knocked Out

"A knocked-out permanent tooth is lost forever!"

This often-expressed opinion is a myth. If a knocked-out tooth is handled properly, it can be implanted successfully in the mouth of a child — sometimes even in that of an adult.[1]

The words "handled properly" are the keys. "Properly" means several things: (1) rushing the child and his or her tooth to the dentist for emergency treatment; (2) carrying the tooth in a cup of milk or water, not in the hand or wrapped in a piece of tissue and (3) keeping the tooth in milk, if the accident occurred in a remote place or dentists' offices are all closed.[2]

Research Findings

This is the advice of Dr. Frank Courts, assistant professor of pediatric dentistry at the University of Florida, based on a study which he made.

"Dentists usually recommend washing the tooth and placing it in water or back in the mouth where it can be bathed in saliva," says Dr. Courts.[3] I have heard of a kid swallowing a tooth held in his mouth to keep it bathed in saliva.

Anyhow, in-the-mouth is not Dr. Courts' first choice for storing the tooth until a dentist is available.

"Milk was found to be 80 percent better than water and 50 percent better than saliva," states Dr. Courts. "Because of the nature of supporting structure of teeth in pre-adolescents (ages 6-12), the tooth usually will be completely knocked out after an accident, instead of being fractured."[4]

Other Sources Of Advice

Other dentists recommend persistency in finding a dentist after office hours, because a knocked out tooth is definitely an emergency. Enlist help of the dentist's answering service, either to track him or her down or to get a referral. Sometimes the emergency service of a hospital can help.

In any event, remember that the quicker the implanting can be done, the greater the chances of success. However, authorities advise not to give up— even if no dentist is immediately available. Just remember to keep the tooth bathed in milk.

All of them warn against the parent trying to reinsert the tooth. It won't work, and it may cause infection, complicate the dentist's job later, and diminish chances of a successful implant.

Adults sometimes can have their own knocked-out tooth successfully implanted, but only if the tooth has come out cleanly and unfractured and he or she can see a dentist soon after the accident.

Super-Nutrition Boosts Chances Of Success

Alternative dentists faced with an implantation problem usually recommend a stepping up of vitamins and minerals which are essential to forming and maintaining teeth: vitamin C, which contributes to the making of connective tissue in gums and the teeth, as well; vitamin D, to help the absorption of calcium and magnesium, and, of course, zinc to speed wound healing.

Richest sources of vitamin C in milligrams per less than four ounce servings are: rose hips, 3,000; acerola cherries, 1,100; guavas, 240; black currants, 200 parsley, 170; green peppers, 110; watercress, 80; chives, 70; strawberries, 57; persimmons, 52; spinach, 51; oranges, 50; cabbage, 47; grapefruit, 38; papaya, 37; elderberries and kumquats, 36; dandelion greens and lemons, 35; cantaloupe, 33; green onions, 32; limes, 31; mangoes, 27; loganberries, 24; tangerines and tomatoes, 23; squash, 22; raspberries and romaine lettuce, 18; pineapple, 17 and tangelos and royal jelly, 16.

Best supplement and food sources of vitamin D in International Units per less than four ounce portions are: cod liver oil, 20,000; sardines,

500; salmon, 400; tuna, 250; egg yolk, 160; sunflower seeds, 92; eggs, 48; butter, 40; cheeses, 30; cream, 15; corn oil, 9.0; mother's milk, 6.0; cottage cheese and cow's milk, 4.0; bee pollen, 1.6 and bass. 1.0.

Calcium-richest food and supplement sources in milligrams per less than four ounce units are: sesame seeds, 1,200; kelp, 1,100; cheeses, 700; brewer's yeast, 420; sardines and carob, 350; caviar, 280; soybeans and almonds, 230; torula yeast, 220; parsley, 200; brazil nuts, 190; watercress, salmon and chickpeas, 150; egg yolk, beans, pistachios, lentils, and kale, 130; sunflower seeds and cow's milk, 120; buckwheat, 100; maple syrup, cream and chard, 100; walnuts, 99; spinach. 93; endive, 81; pecans, 73; wheat germ, 72; peas, 70; peanuts, 69; eggs, 54 and oats, 52.

Supplements and foods with the highest content of magnesium in milligrams per less than four ounce units are: kelp, 740; blackstrap molasses, 410; sunflower seeds, 350; wheat germ, 320; almonds, 270; soybeans, 240; brazil nuts, 220; bone meal, 170; pistachios and soy lecithin, 160; pecans and oats, 140; walnuts, 130; brown rice, 120; chard, 65; spinach, 57; barley, 55; coconut, 44; salmon, 40; corn, 38; avocados, 37; bananas, 31; cheeses, 30; tuna, 29; potatoes, 27 and cashews, 27.

Richest food and supplement sources of zinc in milligrams per less than four ounce units are: herring, 110; wheat germ, 14; sesame seeds, 10; torula yeast, 9.9; blackstrap molasses, 8.3; maple syrup, 7.5; liver, 7.0; soybeans, 6.7; sunflower seeds, 6.6; egg yolk, 5.5; lamb, 5.4; chicken, 4.8; brewer's yeast, 3.9; oats, 3.7; bone meal, 3.6; rye, 3.4; whole wheat, 3.2; corn, 3.1; coconut and beef, 3.0; beets, turkey, and walnuts, 2.8; barley, 2.7; beans and avocados, 2.4; peas, 2.3; bleu cheese, 2.2; eggs, 2.1; buckwheat, 2.0; mangoes, 1.9; millet, rice and almonds, 1.5.

CHAPTER 101

Thyroid Function (High) Hyperthyroidism

All systems of the body seem to race in high gear in the ailment called high thyroid function (hyperthyroidism), in which the thyroid gland secretes too much hormone. Heartbeat revs up, blood pressure rises, blood volume swells, the patient is overheated, sometimes to the point of low fever, perspires easily and profusely, is jittery, often sleepless, and may have diarrhea.

Many hyperthyroids have a feeling of driving desperation and are so wound up and super-nervous that they want to jump out of their skin.

As related in the section Thyroid Function, Low (Hypothyroidism), sometimes there is a condition which seems to be true hyperthyroidism but actually isn't: a deficiency of vitamin C and/or vitamin E that brings on the same symptoms. This is why it pays to see a nutrition-oriented physician familiar with the writings of Isobel Jennings, author of "Vitamins in Endocrinology," an in-depth volume which includes the numerous nutrients that influence the work of the thyroid gland.[1]

True or False? It Makes A Difference

Whether the condition is a false form of hyperthyroidism or the true form, the results are the same, except that the false form is sometimes correctable with high vitamin C and E foods or supplements. In deficiencies of either of these vitamins over a long period, normal (not malignant) cells of the thyroid gland multiply abnormally — a condition called hyperplasia — and then secrete too much hormone.

Danger lies in being diagnosed as a real hyperthyroid when you may be a false hyperthyroid. Orthodox medical treatment for thyroid overactivity is usually to remove part of this gland by surgery or by radiation or to prescribe chemicals such as thiouracil or thiourea to reduce over-production of thyroid hormone.

Physicians who are not nutrition-wise don't always understand that these medicines are strong thyroid antagonists, which prevent the con-verting of carotene to usable vitamin A, as emphasized by Jennings.[1]

The Proper Route For Vegetarians

If, under this circumstance, the vegetarian fails to take preformed vitamin A—not carotene—he or she soon runs out of vitamin A stored in the liver and kidneys. Without vitamin A, protein in the diet can't be properly used, and the patient gradually becomes malnourished.[2]

Jennings states that if the physician prescribes a thyroid supplement to neutralize the vitamin antagonists, carotene again can be turned into vitamin A and assimilated, making it possible to absorb protein once more.[3]

Nutrition To Cope With Hyperthyroidism

An overactive thyroid literally devours vitamin B-1, making it necessary to take as much as 100 mg daily—preferably in a B-complex supplement so that all members of the B family stay in proper relations for biochemical harmony.[4]

Hyperthyroidism and eating a liberal amount of protein demand a high intake of vitamin B-6, preferably in a B-complex supplement including 100 mg of vitamin B-6.[5] Sometimes the drain on vitamin B-6 in the usual diet is so great that nutrition-oriented doctors give a daily injection of this vitamin to prevent muscle weakness.

In hyperthyroidism, other vitamins—C and E and the mineral calcium—are literally pulled from the tissues and blood. Alternative physicians tell me that they recommend supplements of 1,000 mg of vitamin C daily in such cases and at least 400 I.U. each of vitamins E and D. The latter vitamin usually restores the blood level of calcium to normal.

Essential fatty acids (EFAs) are also burned up quickly by hyper-thyroidism. Two tablespoonsful of safflower or sesame seed oil in addition to the EFAs in the usual daily diet appear to satisfy the thyroid enough for it to function normally, nutrition-oriented doctors inform me.

When rats were deprived of EFAs, their thyroid hormone production increased, and they became hyperactive, for reasons which researchers do not as yet understand.[6]

The Barnes Method of Coping With Hyperthyroidism

On several occasions, the eminent thyroidologist Broda O. Barnes, M.D., Ph.D, told me that he manages to reduce secretion of an overactive thyroid by prescribing one, two or three grains of natural, desiccated, oral thyroid tablets daily.

With so much thyroid hormone in the bloodstream, the thyroid gland tends to slow down, he explained. Is it possible to feed the thyroid properly with all the vitamins mentioned above from food alone?

Only with vitamin D, because the daily requirement is low: 400 I.U. However, it is important to have a natural food base for all supplements to be most effective. So let's review the natural foods which are richest in vitamins B-1, B-6, C, D, and E and the essential fatty acids. These foods will be listed in milligrams per less than four ounce servings, except for vitamins D and E, which will be rated in International Units:

VITAMIN B-1: soybeans, 1.10; sesame seeds, 0.98; brazil nuts, 0.96; bee pollen, 0.93; pecans, 0.86; alfalfa and peas, 0.80; millet, 0.73; beans, 0.68; buckwheat and oats, 0.60; whole wheat, 0.57; hazelnuts, 0.46; whole rye, 0.43; lentils and corn, 0.37; brown rice, 0.34; walnuts, 0.32; egg yolk, 0.32; chickpeas, 0.31; liver, 0.25; almonds, 0.24; barley and salmon, 0.21 and eggs, 0.17.

VITAMIN B-6: brewer's yeast, 4.0; brown rice, 3.6; whole wheat, 2.9; royal jelly, 2.4; soybeans, 2.0; rye, 1.8; lentils, 1.7, sunflower seeds and hazelnuts, 1.1; alfalfa, 1.0; salmon, 0.98; wheat germ, 0.92; tuna, 0.90; bran, 0.85; walnuts, 0.73; peas and liver, 0.67; avocados, 0.60; beans, 0.57; cashews, peanuts, turkey, oats, chicken, and beef, 0.40; halibut, 0.34; and lamb and bananas, 0.32.

VITAMIN C: Acerola cherries, 1,100; guavas, 240; black currants, 200; parsley, 170; green pepper. 110; watercress, 80; chives, 70; strawberries, 57; persimmons, 52; spinach, 51; oranges, 50; cabbage, 47; grapefruit,

38; papaya, 37; elderberries and kumquats, 36; lemons, 35; cantaloupe, 33, green onions, 32; limes, 31; mangos, 27; loganberries, 24 and tangerines and tomatoes, 23.

VITAMIN D: sardines, 500; salmon, 400; tuna, 250; egg yolk, 160; sunflower seeds, 92; liver, 50; eggs, 48; butter, 40; cheeses, 30; cream, 15; human milk, 6.0 and cottage cheese and cow's milk, 4. (Although we don't recommend pasteurized and homogenized milk, that is all that's available in most areas, and each quart has approximately 40 I.U. of vitamin D added. A quart of milk also brings about 1,000 mg of calcium to the diet.)

VITAMIN E: wheat germ, 160; safflower nuts, 35; sunflower seeds, 31; whole wheat, 30; sesame oil, 26; walnuts, 22; corn oil and hazelnuts, 21; soy and peanut oil, 16; almonds, 15; olive oil, 14; cabbage, 7.8; brazil nuts and peanuts, 6.5; cod liver oil, 5.4; cashews, 5.1 and soy lecithin, 4.8.

ESSENTIAL FATTY ACID (Linoleic acid): safflower oil, 77,000; sunflower oil, 60,000; corn oil; 54,000; soy oil, 52,000; wheat germ oil, 44,000; sesame oil, 42,000; sunflower seeds, 30.000; walnuts, 29,000; peanut oil, 25,000, brazil nuts, 23,000, sesame seeds, 20.000; pecans, 14.000; peanuts, 12.000; almonds, 11,000; olive oil, 10,000; hazelnuts, 9,300; wheat germ, 4,400; cashews, 3,200; butter, 2,700; oats, 2,600 and olives, 2.200.

The natural foods regime often can control the symptoms of hyperthyroidism and—in instances of false high thyroid function—even reverse the condition.

Chicken Rice Soup

2 Cans (1 lb. each) Tomatoes	½ c. Uncooked Brown Rice
1 Potato, Diced	1 T. Sea Salt
1 Onion, Diced	½ t. Pepper
1 Green Pepper, Diced	2½ c. Cooked Chicken, Diced
2 Carrots, Diced	4 c. Chicken Broth

Place chicken broth, tomatoes, potato, onion, green pepper, carrots, rice, salt and pepper in heavy saucepan. Simmer covered for 45 minutes. Add chicken and cook 25 minutes longer, or until vegetables and rice are tender.

CHAPTER 102

Thyroid Function, Low

One of the most widely suffered and least-detected illnesses— a silent saboteur of health and morale— is low thyroid function (hypothyroidism). Why?

Because laboratory tests are not sensitive enough to reveal this condition and orthodox doctors depend almost entirely on them.

So says Broda O. Barnes, M.D., Ph.D, world-renowned authority on the thyroid gland who has had more than 100 papers on this subject published in leading medical journals.

Another respected authority, A.S. Jackson, M.D., who specializes in disorders of the thyroid gland, states that low thyroid function is the most common ailment entering the doctor's office and the "diagnosis most missed." Many other authorities at the forefront of information in this field agree.

Why So Much Hidden Hypothyroidism?

What are the answers? After many years of studying the literature and practicing medicine, Dr. Barnes found that if metabolism— the "burning" of food in the cells— is low, body temperature is also low. So temperature tells better than any other indicator how well the thyroid is working.

Normal function of the thyroid gland depends on quite a few factors — mainly on taking in enough of its principal nutrient, iodine. Although only a tiny amount of iodine is needed, this is hard to get, because soils of the United States are notoriously deficient in iodine and many other trace minerals. Mountains and areas near them, as well as the plains of the nation's central states, are dangerously low in iodine.

Therefore, plants grown in mountainous regions and on plains cannot fully support animal and human life. Iodized salt offers just enough iodine to prevent goiters but not enough to prevent other symptoms of hypothyroidism.

The Worst And Most Common Symptoms

Here are the top 25 symptoms of low thyroid function, some of which most hypothyroids experience: (1) coldness while others are comfortable — cold hands and feet; (2) tiredness, even exhaustion; (3) constipation; (4) heart palpitation; (5) nervousness; (6) dry coarse skin; (7) slow speech; (8) swelling of face and eyelids; (9) thick tongue; (10) coarse hair; (11) loss of hair; (12) pale skin; (13) gain of weight; (14) labored, difficult breathing; (15) swollen feet; (16) loss of appetite; (17) hoarseness; (18) menstrual problems of any or every sort; (19); brittle nails; (20) slow movement; (21) poor memory; (22) inability to think clearly; (23) depression; (24) frequent headaches and (25) loss of interest in sex.[1]

If one secretes too little thyroid hormone, the biochemical "motor" in our trillions of cells runs sluggishly. Heartbeat rate slows down. Blood pressure drops. Circulation becomes weak, (making for being cold and having cold hands and feet.) Energy and endurance run low. Digestion slows down. Constipation is likely. Headaches occur. Hair becomes lifeless and falls out more easily. Wounds heal slowly. Thinking is sluggish and memory faulty. Sex urge is weak or asleep.

The Reliable Do-It-Yourself Test

So much for symptoms which help make a diagnosis possible. If lab tests are not always reliable, how can one get further evidence that he or she is hypothyroid? By means of the do-it-yourself Barnes Basal Temperature Test. Here's how to perform it.[2]

Before going to sleep at night, shake down a thermometer and place it on the nightstand near the bed. Upon awakening— no later!— stay in bed and tuck the thermometer snugly in the armpit for ten minutes.

"If your temperature is in the range of 97.8 to 98.2 F, your thyroid function is probably normal," informs Dr. Barnes. "If it is below 97.8

— even a fraction of a degree— there's a good chance you are hypothyroid."

Perform the test two days in a row. Pre-menopausal women should take the test when not menstruating or on the second and third day of the menstrual cycle. Stephen Langer, M.D. of Berkeley, California, a disciple of Dr. Barnes, says: "If you are a first generation hypothyroid, you can usually compensate by taking one kelp capsule daily (for its iodine). Second generation hypothyroids and beyond will need to take thyroid tablets prescribed by a physician."

Most alternative medical doctors know about the Barnes Basal Temperature Test and accept its results. See the list of alternative doctors in the back of this book. If there's none listed in your area, try the National Health Federation at 212 W. Foothill Boulevard, Monrovia, CA 91016, Phone: (818) 357-2181 or your local health food store.

Best Food Sources Of Iodine

Due to the great amounts of iodine in seawater, ocean plants and seafood are the richest sources of iodine. Steadily decreasing amounts of iodine in soils of the United States make land-grown food sources inferior.

Kelp is the king of sea sources of iodine with 180 mg per less than four ounces. Then come seaweeds with a rating of 62 and cod liver oil, 0.84; haddock, 0.31; codfish, 0.14; perch, 0.074; herring, 0.052 and halibut, 0.046.

Land-grown foods are commoners with a modest iodine content: chard and beans with a 0.10 rating; sunflower seeds, 0.070; turnip greens, 0.047; vegetable oils, 0.024; peanuts and cantaloupe, 0.020 and soybeans, 0.017.

Don't Short-Change Your Thyroid On Other Key Nutrients!

In a classic book which shows how nutrients influence thyroid health and function, "Vitamins In Endocrine Metabolism," (Charles C. Thomas), Isobel Jennings of the University College, University of Cambridge, England writes that deficiencies of the following vitamins can cause serious thyroid problems: vitamins A, B-2, niacin (B-3); B-6, B-12, C and E.[4]

VITAMIN A: The liver's ability to translate the vitamin A precursor carotene (found in vegetables and fruits) into vitamin A is restricted or blocked when the supply of thyroid hormone is limited.[5] In animal experiments, the pituitary gland, which makes thyroid-stimulating hormone, often deteriorates if there is a vitamin A deficiency.[6] Without enough vitamin A, the thyroid gland cannot absorb iodine properly and, therefore, secretes too little thyroid hormone.

VITAMIN B-2: In a deficiency of vitamin B-2, working of the thyroid gland, the ovaries and testes becomes depressed, and they fail to secrete their hormones properly.[7]

NIACIN: Efficiency of the thyroid gland and other glands, organs and cells is reduced when niacin is scarce.[8]

VITAMIN B-6: Unless vitamin B-6 is liberally supplied, the thyroid gland cannot use its iodine effectively in producing hormones which can make the difference between illness and well-being.[9]

VITAMIN B-12: Animal experiments show that vitamin B-12, the hard-to-absorb nutrient, resists absorption if the thyroid gland is not working properly, contributing to pernicious anemia— see the section on Anemia — and these neurological disorders: bursitis, neuralgia and neuritis.[10]

VITAMIN C: Guinea pig experiments revealed that, in long-standing vitamin C deficiencies, capillaries in the thyroid gland bleed, normal thyroid gland cells multiply at an abnormal rate (hyperplasia) and secrete too much hormone. (These negative conditions disappeared when the animals were given enough vitamin C.[11]

VITAMIN E: In extreme deficiencies of vitamin E, animals (rabbits) made too little thyroid-stimulating hormone in the pituitary gland, showed unnatural and rapid multiplication of normal thyroid gland cells (hyperplasia) and transmitted this tendency to litters born to them.[12]

It is tragic that from the turn of the century to the late 1950s, overproduction of thyroid hormone due to hyperplasia caused by too little intake of vitamins C or E was often interpreted as hyperthyroidism (an overactive thyroid) and usually led to surgical removal of the thyroid gland. (See the section Thyroid Function, High, Hyperthyroidism).

Richest Sources Of These Critical Vitamins

In less than a four ounce serving, the following foods are the richest in terms of milligrams for all nutrients but vitamins A and E, which are listed in terms of International Units:

VITAMIN A: Cod liver oil, 200,000; sheep liver, 45,000; beef liver, 44,000; calf's liver, 22,000; dandelion greens, 14,000; carrots, 11,000; yams, 9,000; kale, 8,900; parsley and turnip greens, 8,500; spinach, 8,100; collard greens and chard, 6,500; watercress, 5,000; red peppers, 4,400; winter squash, 4,000; egg yolk and cantaloupe, 3,400; endive, 3,300; persimmons and apricots, 2,700; broccoli, 2,500, pimentos, 2,300; swordfish, 2,100; whitefish, 2,000; romaine, 1,900; mangoes, 1,800; papayas, 1,700; nectarines and pumpkin, 1,600; peaches and cheeses, 1,300; eggs, 1,200; cherries, lettuce and cream, 1,000. (A reminder: fruits and vegetables offer carotene, the vitamin A precursor, which has to be translated into vitamin A by the liver. Animal sources offer vitamin A that doesn't have to be translated by the liver, which often operates sluggishly in hypothyroids.)

VITAMIN B-2: torula yeast, 16; brewer's yeast, 4.2; liver, 4.1; royal jelly, 1.9; alfalfa, 1.8; bee pollen, 1.7; almonds, 0.92; wheat germ, 0.68; mustard greens, 0.64; egg yolk, 0.52; cheeses, 0.46; human milk, 0.40, millet, 0.38; chicken, 0.36; soybeans and veal, 0.31; eggs and sunflower seeds, 0.28; lamb, 0.27; peas, blackstrap molasses, and parsley and cottage cheese, 0.25.

NIACIN: torula yeast, 100; brewer's yeast, 38; bee pollen, 19; peanuts, 17; liver, 16; salmon, 13; chicken and tuna, 12; swordfish, turkey and rabbit, 11; halibut, 9.2; royal jelly, 8.2; veal, 7.8; sunflower seeds, 5.6, sardines and sesame seeds, 5.4 and beef and alfalfa, 5.

VITAMIN B-6: brewer's yeast, 4.0; brown rice, 3.6; whole wheat, 2.9; royal jelly, 2.4; soybeans, 2.0; whole rye, 1.8; lentils, 1.7; sunflower seeds and hazelnuts, 1.1; alfalfa, 1.00; salmon, 0.98; wheat germ, 0.92; tuna, 0.90; bran, 0.85; walnuts, 0.73; peas and liver, 0.67; avocados, 0.60 and beans, 0.57.

VITAMIN B-12: liver, 0.086; sardines, 0.034; herring and mackerel, 0.0100; red snapper, 0.0088; flounder, 0.0064; salmon, 0.0047; lamb,

0.0031; swiss cheese, 0.0021; eggs, 0.0020; haddock, 0.0017; muenster cheese, 0.0016, beef, 0.0015 and bleu cheese, 0.0014.

VITAMIN C: rose hips, 3,000; acerola cherries, 1,100; guavas, 240; black currants, 200; parsley, 170; green peppers, 110; watercress and chives, 80; strawberries, 57; persimmons, 52; spinach, 51; oranges, 50; cabbage, 47; grapefruit, 38; papaya, 37; elderberries and kumquats, 36; lemons, 35; cantaloupe, 33; green onions, 32; limes, 31; mangos, 29; loganberries, 24 and tangerines and tomatoes, 23.

VITAMIN E: wheat germ, 160; safflower nuts, 35; sunflower seeds, 31; whole wheat, 30; sesame oil, 26; walnuts, 22; corn oil and hazelnuts, 21; soy and peanut oil, 16; almonds, 15; olive oil, 14; cabbage, 7.8; almond oil, 7.5; brazil nuts and peanuts, 6.5; cod liver oil, 5.4; cashews, 5.1 and soy lecithin, 4.8.

Food And Drugs Which Supress The Thyroid Gland

Cabbage, rutabagas and turnips suppress the working of the thyroid gland— something for vegetarians to consider in planning daily menus. This, in turn, makes it difficult for the liver to convert carotene from vegetables and fruit into vitamin A. And, with too little vitamin A, protein use is blocked— still another blow to a weak thyroid.[13]

Milk and milk products, as well as eggs, can help supply vegetarians with vitamin B-12, which is poorly absorbed by hypothyroids.

Drugs and chemicals can also suppress the thyroid gland: sulfa drugs, antidiabetic agents, prednisone and estrogen in large doses (a vitally important factor for women taking birth control pills.[14] (See the section Birth Control.) These prescription items also interfere with the thyroid gland taking up iodine.

Two other factors can reduce thyroid efficiency[15]: thyocyanide in cigarette smoke— important to smokers and those exposed to secondhand smoke— and fluorides in municipal drinking water supplies, particularly where water is low in iodine. (See section on Wrinkles related to fluoridation.)

It is important to cooperate with your thyroid gland, if you want it to cooperate with you!

CHAPTER 103

Ulcers, Stomach

A peptic ulcer is an open sore on the lining of the stomach or duodenum, a horseshoe-shaped forepart of the small intestine extending downward from the valve of the stomach.

This is caused by stomach acid and pepsin, an enzyme which breaks down eaten protein, attacking the lining of the stomach or intestines when too little protective mucus insulation is formed.

Symptoms

Many, if not most, ulcer patients are only vaguely aware of stomach or intestinal discomfort, bloating or pain until bleeding is dramatically demonstrated in black, sticky stools or even red blood-stained bowel movements.

Natural Food Approaches

Cabbage juice, large tropical bananas called plantains, essential fatty acids (EFAs) from cold-pressed vegetable oils (safflower, sesame, sunflower seed, and, among others, soy), whole grain bread and cereals, and the juice of the aloe vera plant have shown an ability to help heal ulcers. Presumably they help to prevent them, too.

Cabbage Juice

Dr. Garnett Cheney, a professor at Stanford University's School of Medicine, fed thirteen ulcer patients one-fifth of a quart of freshly squeezed cabbage juice at intervals five times daily.[1]

All were healed within 7.3 to 10.4 days, as shown by X-ray evidence. The healing ingredient was called vitamin U, because of its action on ulcers. (Four to five pounds of cabbage will yield a day's supply of juice.)[2]

And, speaking of cabbage juice, I remember visiting my late mother-in-law in the hospital and warning her that the arthritis medicine she was taking might cause bleeding ulcers.

"Of course, cabbage juice can manage most cases of ulcers," I informed her. She looked at me as if I had lost my mind and pooh-poohed the idea as only she could pooh-pooh.

Just then her doctor came in and she told him my "ridiculous idea" about cabbage juice for ulcers.

"Oh, sure," he nodded knowingly. "Cabbage juice really works. It contains what is called vitamin U, because it helps to heal ulcers."

Other Sources Of Vitamin U

Celery and other fresh greens— cooking destroys this factor— raw egg yolks; unpasteurized milk and vegetable fats (in safflower, sesame, sunflower and soy oil) are the best additional sources of vitamin U.

Plantains

Two groups of associated researchers from India and England discovered the strange fact that rats which ate plantains had a third as many ulcers — also less severe ones— as those which didn't.[3]

Rats fed a powder made from unripe, green plantains — the most effective kind— resisted ulcers induced through a chemical injection by producing an observably thicker lining of stomach mucus.[4] Given this powder, human beings with ulcers usually healed, too. Plantains are available in many markets and in most produce stores.

Essential Fatty Acids

After an intake of essential fatty acids, there is a dramatic increase in prostaglandins, hormone-like substances which help to control body functions and, among other things, contribute to healing.

Prostaglandins have been shown at the University of California at Irvine and elsewhere to prevent ulcerations caused by aspirins, alcohol, bile acids and other irritants, states Dr. Daniel Hollander, professor of medicine and chief of gastroenterology at this university's College of Medicine.[5] Fatty acids appear to bolster the healing of existing ulcerations, as well as protect the stomach and intestinal tract from ulcers, he says.

"Until now, we've never had a rational reason to emphasize specific diets for ulcer patients," Hollander admits. "There's some evidence that maybe some people have peptic ulcer disease because they have a defect in their ability to make prostaglandins."[6]

Best Sources Of EFAs

Found in safflower, corn, sunflower seed, soybean and sesame seed oils, linoleic acid is needed to assure normal cells and normal metabolism (efficient changing of nutrients into energy).

Nutrition-oriented physicians usually recommend that their patients add two tablespoons of these EFAs to their daily diet — on salads.

Whole Grains

An experiment with 73 patients who had just recovered from duodenal ulcers, reported in "Lancet", revealed the preventive benefits in dietary fiber. The thirty-eight individuals who were told to eat a great deal of whole grain bread, cereals (from wheat, barley and oats) and vegetables had a 45 percent rate of return of ulcers, compared with 80 percent for the low fiber group.[7]

Aloe Vera Juice

History tells us that Alexander the Great conquered the island of Madagascar to make sure of a steady supply of aloe vera plants for use in healing the wounds of his soldiers. Aloe vera gel and juice were used for healing in India as long ago as 3,500 years. American Indians referred to it as "The Wand of Heaven."

In folklore, people have split the leaf of this plant and applied its gel to scratches, burns, cuts, and wounds to hurry up the healing process. Aloe vera juice has been used internally, too, for ulcers— four ounces of juice two times a day, supposedly with success.

Some years ago, Russian medical men built a small foundation of science under Aloe vera's folklore. An article in the "Journal of the American Osteopathic Association" (Vol. 62, April, 1963) reported research in which Aloe vera gel was used successfully to treat peptic ulcers.

The theory of some of the researchers was that Aloe Vera gel soothes and heals stomach ulcers by neutralizing hydrochloric acid. A theory I adhere to is shared by many biochemists with whom I talked. They think the gel serves to put a protective coating where stomach mucous does not cover.

Foods such as cabbage juice, plantains, cold-pressed vegetable oils— not the usual commercial supermarket brands— whole grain breads and cereals and Aloe vera juice seem to be helpful for preventing or coping with ulcers.

Carrot and Raisin Salad

¾ c. natural seedless raisins	2 T. instant fresh mayonnaise (see
½ c. fresh carrot juice	below)
4 medium carrots	4 large or small lettuce leaves
1 medium beet	½ c. alfalfa, sprouts

Soak rasins in carrot juice for approximately one hour, or until plump. Grate carrots and beet and and mix with soaked raisins. Place in refrigerator until cool. Mix in a dash of mayonnaise and serve on a bed of lettuce leaves. This is an excellent accompaniment to a fiber-rich main course meal.

Instant Fresh Mayonnaise:

2 Fresh Egg yolks	¾ c. Cold pressed sunflower seed oil
2 T. Fresh lemon juice	or sesame oil

Ulcer Drink

1 c. fresh carrot juice
1½ stalks celery
1½ c. cabbage, chopped
¼ c. alfalfa sprouts
½ c. cut broccoli spears

¼ c. radish tops
½ c. carrot tops
½ c. parsley
¼ c. sunflower seeds

Pour carrot juice into blender and gradually add other ingredients, blending between each addition. Blend until smooth. If too thick, add more juice. If too thin, add more greens. Will be pulpy, but extremely nutritious. Makes 3 servings.

CHAPTER 104

Vaginitis
(Inflammation of the Vagina)

Easy to develop and hard to clear up.

These words characterize vaginitis, inflammation of the vagina, which is quickly becoming one of the most common disorders seen by general practitioners and gynecologists.

A yeastlike fungus, Candida albicans, which thrives in warm and moist parts of the body, brings on many unpleasant symptoms: severe itching, a red and swollen vulva, a burning feeling when passing urine, white curdy discharges and discomfort or pain during sexual intercourse, due to irritation and involuntary muscle contraction to protect the sore vagina. However, this tightness worsens the problem.

As mentioned in the section on Candida albicans, this organism is caused by many modern developments: the introduction and widespread use of antibiotics since World War II, steadily increasing consumption of refined carbohydrates (mainly sugar), popularization of the Pill and utilization of far more cortisone.

Additional Causes

Antibiotics kill off good organisms along with the bad, particularly the ones which check overgrowth of the Candida yeast, which thrives on the sugary diets and multiplies almost out of control.

Pantyhose, tight underthings made of synthetic fabrics, reduce air circulation at the vagina, causing over-warmth and perspiration, conditions which encourage the Candida to multiply and flourish. One authority states that this could not have happened several generations ago when women wore long skirts and no panties, permitting better circulation of air and consequent greater dryness.

463

Dye in pantyhose and a residue of detergents can also contribute to an overgrowth of Candida— as can diabetes, pregnancy and strength-sapping illness.

This condition should be checked by an alternative medical doctor, because the fungus multiplies rapidly and can be a threat. Women feel frustrated and almost compelled to treat themselves, because medicines prescribed by orthodox physicians either fail to work or they must be used continually to keep the infection under control.

Folk Medicines Seem Best

Few ailments respond as well to folk medicines as Candida. Douching with yogurt is a well-known natural therapy in various European and Asian areas where yogurt has existed for many centuries. One study shows that physicians were able to clear up vaginal tract infections in 93 percent of the cases with injections of lactobacillus acidophilus derived from organisms in yogurt.

Some women mix potent lactobacillus culture bought at the health food store with yogurt, which is then delivered inside the vagina by means of an applicator. They also eat as much as a cup of yogurt at a time, three or four times daily.

Still another folk medicine contributes to conquering the Candida infection: raw garlic, two or three cloves a day. Because garlic can sting in the mouth and throat, some women dice a clove or two on bread and make a sandwich or take six or seven squirts of odorless garlic from its squeezable plastic container three times daily.

A third helpful folk remedy for stubborn and severe cases is the apple cider vinegar douche: two tablespoons in a quart of warm water, used two to three times daily. The tip of the douche should be inserted and then the hand should seal off the opening so that fluid can fill, stretch and clean the entire vagina.

Yet another douche from folklore is made up of a teaspoon of 3 percent hydrogen peroxide and a teaspoon of table salt in a quart of warm water.

External and topical applications appear to work better if accompanied by internal treatment: yogurt or acidophilus capsules or both, and garlic, plus refraining from use of sugar— even sugary fruit, as elaborated in the section on Candida albicans.

One final statement: beating vaginitis takes persistency, even stubbornness, for the enemies are both persistent and stubborn.

Cold Yogurt Soup

2 Large Cucumbers
2 c. Yogurt
1 T. Mint, Finely Chopped
1 T. Green Onion, Finely Chopped

2 t. Sea Salt
¼ t. Black Pepper
¼ c. Dried Currants or Raisins

Peel cucumbers and grate or chop very fine. Mix all ingredients together and chill in refrigerator. Just before serving, stir in a few ice cubes. Serve in bowls as you would soup. Serves 4.

CHAPTER 105

Vitiligo
(White Skin Patches)

A disorder characterized by loss of skin coloring, resulting in white patches, vitiligo is viewed by conventional medicine as one of those conditions "about which nothing can be done."

Research on this disorder is not abundant, but several studies indicate that perhaps "something can be done," because vitiligo appears to be a symptom of malnutrition.

H.W. Francis, M.D., who had this disorder, discovered that his stomach was deficient in free hydrochloric acid. Taking 15 cubic centimeters of hydrochloric acid with each meal for two years, he found that his white skin areas had vanished. This regime worked for three of his patients, too.[1]

Benjamin Sieve, M.D., a professor at Tufts Medical School, after reviewing the literature, found some promising therapies for vitiligo, one of them calling for additional hydrochloric acid, as in the Francis regime. Dr. Sieve concluded that the hydrochloric acid brought good results because it improved digestion, therefore, supplying more of the needed nutrients. (Hydrochloric acid, designated HCL, is an ingredient in most digestive enzymes.)[2]

Another therapy, a daily 100 mg tablet or capsule of PABA (para-aminobenzoic acid), one of the B vitamins, corrected vitiligo of the eyelids of a two-year-old child.[3]

Impressed, Sieve designed an experiment to test PABA on 25 female and 23 male vitiligo patients, ages 10 to 70, who had had this disorder for from two to 28 years. Almost all the test subjects presented the symptoms of a chronically deficient diet and a medical history of glandular imbalance.[4]

A physical exam revealed that many of the patients had symptoms of hypothyroidism (low thyroid function): cold hands and feet, fatigue, emotional instability, constipation, overweight, arthritis, headaches, brittle nails, and, among others, coarse and thickened skin.[5]

Thyroid authority Stephen E. Langer, M.D. of Berkeley, California, states that iodine in one kelp tablet often can correct low thyroid in first generation hypothyroids, but that a prescription item: thyroid hormone — preferably, Armour natural desiccated thyroid, rather than a synthetic, is necessary for second or third generation hypothyroids.[6]

Dr. Sieve had only moderate success with a combination of B vitamins, so twice daily— morning and evening— he began injecting PABA along with monoethanolamine to assure that the vitamin would remain in the blood for a longer time. A single 100 mg tablet of PABA was taken each morning and evening, as well.[7]

His success was phenomenal. Within four to eight weeks, the white patches began turning pink. Within six to 16 weeks, brown pigment began to form in the white areas and soon the white spots disappeared. After six or seven months, Dr. Sieve noted what he called "striking results," IN EVERY ONE OF THE 48 PATIENTS: COMPLETE DISAPPEARANCE OF THE WHITE SPOTS.[8]

Two other approaches undergirded with research have produced positive results: (1) a daily supplement of 150 to 300 mg of pantothenic acid; (2) 1,000 mg of PABA each day.

Carl C. Pfeiffer, Ph.D, M.D., director of Princeton's Brain Bio Center, in his book, Mental and Elemental Nutrients (Keats Publishing) reports that pantothenic acid and PABA supplements have been effective in managing vitiligo—particularly with "good amounts of zinc, manganese and vitamin B-6."[9]

Although it is almost impossible to eat enough food to take in the potencies of nutrients mentioned, alternative doctors usually like patients to eat foods which are rich in them as a base for supplements. Following are lists of foods high in PABA, pantothenic acid, zinc, manganese and vitamin B-6.

Supplements and foods with the largest amounts of PABA in milligrams per less than four ounce units are: sunflower seeds, 62; liver, 0.62; brewer's yeast, 0.49 and wheat germ, 0.037. Very few foods have been tested for PABA. Other good sources are rice bran, kidney, whole grains and molasses.

Best bets for pantothenic acid in milligrams per less than four ounce units are: royal jelly, 35; brewer's yeast, 11; torula yeast, 10; brown rice, 8.9; sunflower seeds, 5.5; soybeans, 5.2; corn, 5.0; lentils, 4.8; egg yolk, 4.2; peas, 3.6; alfalfa, 3.3; whole wheat, 3.2; peanuts, 2.8; rye, 2.6; eggs, 2.3, bee pollen, and wheat germ, 2.2; bleu cheese, 1.8; cashews. 1.3; chickpeas, 1.2; avocado, 1.1, chicken, sardines, turkey and walnuts, 0.90 and perch and salmon, 0.80.

Here are richest sources of zinc in milligrams per less than four ounce units: herring, 110; wheat germ, 14: sesame seeds, 10; torula yeast, 9.9; blackstrap molasses, 8.3; maple syrup, 7.5; liver, 7.0; soybeans, 6.7; sunflower seeds, 6.6; egg yolk, 5.5;T lamb, 5.4; chicken, 4.8; regular molasses, 4.6; brewer's yeast, 3.9; oats, 3.7; bone meal, 3.6; rye, 3.4; whole wheat, 3.2; corn, 3.1; coconut and beef, 3.0; beets, turkey and walnuts, 2.8; barley, 2.7; beans and avocados, 2.4 and peas, 2.3.

Top supplements and foods for manganese in milligrams per less than four ounce units are: tea leaves, 28; cloves, 26; ginger, 8.7; buckwheat, 5.1; oats, 4.9; hazelnuts, 4.2; chestnuts, 3.7; whole wheat, 3.6; pecans, 3.5; barley, 3.2; brazil nuts, 2.8; sunflower seeds, 2.5; ginseng, watercress, peas and beans, 2.0; almonds, 1.9; turnip greens and walnuts, 1.8; brown rice, 1.7; peanuts, 1.5; honey, 1.4, coconut, 1.3; pineapple, 1.1 and parsley, 0.94.

Best sources of vitamin B-6 in milligrams per less than four ounce portions are: brewer's yeast, 4.0; brown rice, 3.6; whole wheat, 2.9; soybeans, 2.0; rye, 1.8; lentils, 1.7; sunflower seeds and hazelnuts, 1.1; alfalfa, 1.00; salmon, 0.98; wheat germ, 0.92; tuna, 0.90, bran, 0.85; walnuts, 0.73; peas and liver, 0.67; avocados, 0.60; beans, 0.57; cashews, peanuts, turkey, oats, chicken and beef and halibut, 0.34.

Jack's Lemon Liver

1½ lbs. beef liver
¼ c. soy flour
¼ c. whole wheat flour
1 T. brewers yeast
¼ t. kelp

¼ t. paprika
⅛ t. thyme, crushed
1 t. sesame salt
2 T. sesame seeds

Marinate liver in juice of one lemon (or lime) for approximately one hour. Drain liver at least 30 minutes before cooking to prevent a mushy texture. Mix coating of all seasonings. In skillet, saute sliced onions just until they begin to turn limp. Remove, drain and save. Dip liver into flour mixture and brown quickly. It will only take about 3 minutes to get liver brown and crusty on the outside, and tender, moist and medium-well on the inside. So don't begin frying until everyone is ready to sit down and eat. The strong flavor often associated with liver comes from overcooking. Remove to serving platter and cover with onions and serve.

Banana Salmon Salad

2 c. cooked salmon
½ c. green pepper or celery, chopped

2 bananas
Salad greens

In large bowl, combine salmon and green pepper. Peel bananas and cut into slices. Add to salad. Add Curry Mayonnaise (see below) and mix well with salad greens. Makes 4 servings.

Curry Mayonnaise

¼ c. mayonnaise
¼ c. sour cream
½ t. curry powder
2 t. lemon juice

¼ t. sea salt
1 T. parsley, chopped
⅛ t. tabasco pepper sauce
1 t. sesame salt

CHAPTER 106

Warts

His was a tough problem for a seventh grader.

After his mother Carol had him show me his hands, covered with more warts than I had ever seen in two places, he had plunged them deep in the pockets of his jeans.

"Warts will never win a beauty contest," commented Phil, a trace of bitterness in his voice.

Several months before, Carol had had the warts burned off. Now there they were again — as big and unsightly as ever.

"Maureen, we're desperate," she said with a deep sigh. "Isn't there some folk medicine cure for warts?"

I told her and Phil that medical literature had mentioned two vitamins, proved over and over again: vitamins A and E. Each day test subjects in various studies had spread the contents of a 100 International Unit capsule of natural vitamin E (Alpha Tocopherol) on a clean Band-Aid to cover each wart. The warts had soon disappeared.

"The best Phil can do is wash his hands, then spread vitamin E over them and wear clean cotton gloves to hold the vitamin in place. The best time to do that is before bedtime."

Eager to try anything, Phil followed through. Four weeks later, he showed me that every wart was gone. Delighted, Phil hugged me, and said, "Maureen, if I were two feet taller, thirty years older, and wealthy, I'd ask you to marry me."

Unlike the warts, the wedding never came off!

More Than One Way To Beat Warts

The best existing information holds that viruses cause warts and that by building up the immune function, one can get rid of them most effectively.

In an article in the Southern Medical Journal, B.H. Kuhn, M.D. told about using 25,000 international units of vitamin A palmitate (water-dispersible form) each day for a week to six months for treating 79 patients with different types of warts.

Dr. Kuhn achieved a cure rate of 50 to 100 percent with no total failures. In another study, (Clinical Medicine, July, 1959) 119 medical doctors used a similar vitamin A palmitate regime in treating 228 patients with plantar warts, warts growing on the sole of the feet. In 208 of the 228 cases, patients received substantial benefits or total cures.

Daniel Hyman, M.D. of Roosevelt Hospital in New York City, stated that just three desiccated liver tablets three times a day successfully treated warts in hospitalized patients.[1]

Hyman believes that sulfur-containing amino acids in the liver tablets somehow interacted with the hypothalamus gland, responsible for stimulating antibodies, front-line soldiers in the immune system army. Further, this food supplement is rich in B-complex vitamins as well.[2]

Other Approaches

So far, I have covered clinical therapies which have worked. Now let me mention some real folk remedies for warts: the inner side of a banana skin, dandelion milk and juice from the aloe vera leaf.

The banana skin routine worked well on one of the very few warts I have ever had. I have not had enough warts to try the other two methods, but friends have, and they give me glowing reports such as, "Dandelion milk was the first thing that ever got rid of my warts— and it didn't cost me a cent." Other friends say aloe vera juice heals warts, too. One of them buys it at health food stores and refers to it as, "My First Aid Kit in a bottle."

Here's how I treated my wart. First I washed my hands thoroughly, then applied the inside skin from a freshly pealed banana to the wart, securing it in place with adhesive tape. I followed this routine daily, until the wart gave up and disappeared, never to return, thank heavens!

Another folk medicine cure for warts is Elmer's glue. (Yes directly from

Borden's Elsie) applied directly to warts. Scrape off with finger nail and reapply until they're gone. My theory for this was that oxygen deprivation seemed to dry the warts allowing them to sluff off. Connie Haus verified this for me by telling me she had seen warts come off an employee's finger after an interim of wearing rubber finger grips for filing.

Now, let's consider the foods richest in vitamins A and E, which may prevent warts from happening in the first place.

Vitamin A is one of the few vitamins obtainable in foods in high enough potencies to reach the levels used by medical doctors cited earlier to deal with warts. The RDA for women is 4,000 I.U. daily, and for men, 5,000. It may be risky to ingest 25,000 to 50,000 I.U. daily for a long period. Some individuals have made the mistake of eating polar bear liver, which contains 50,000,000 international units of vitamin A per less than four ounces. They did not live to have a second helping!

Common foods with the highest content of vitamin A in terms of International Units per less than a four ounce serving are: cod liver oil, 200,000; sheep liver, 45,000; beef liver, 44,000; calf's liver, 22,000; dandelion greens, 14,000; carrots, 11,000; yams, 9,000; kale, 8,900; parsley and turnip greens, 8,500; spinach, 8,100; collard greens and chard, 6,500; watercress, 5,000, red pepper, 4,400; winter squash, 4,000; egg yolk and cantaloupe, 3,400; endive, 3,300; persimmons and apricots, 2,700; broccoli, 2,500; pimentos, 2,300; swordfish, 2,100; whitefish, 2,000; romaine, 1,900; mangoes, 1,800; papayas, 1,700; nectarines and pumpkin, 1,600; peaches and cheeses, 1,300; eggs, 1,200 and cherries, lettuce and cream, 1,000.

(Remember that vitamin A from vegetables and fruits are carotenes, actually vitamin A precursors, and must be translated into vitamin A by the liver. This biochemical process is sometimes faulty in certain individuals, so values stated above for vegetables and fruits may not be completely realistic.)

Foods richest in vitamin E in International Units per less than four ounce portions are: wheat germ, 160; safflower nuts, 35 sunflower seeds, 31; whole wheat, 30; sesame oil, 26; walnuts, 22; corn oil and hazelnuts, 21; soy oil and peanut oil, 16; almonds, 15; olive oil, 14; cabbage, 7.8; almond oil, 7.5; brazil nuts and peanuts, 6.5; cod liver oil, 5.4; cashews and soy lecithin, 4.8; spinach, 2.9; asparagus, 2.5; broccoli, 2.0, butter, 1.9: parsley, 1.8; oats, barley and corn, 1.7; avocados and pecans, 1.5; salmon, 1.4; bee pollen, 1.3; rye, 1.2; and cheeses, eggs, leeks and coconut, 1.

John Valov's
Calf's Liver with Mustard Sauce

8 slices calf's liver	1 T. cider vinegar
3 T. raw certified Butter	½ t. dried tarragon
2 large onions, sliced and separated into rings	½ c. sour cream
1 c. poultry stock	1 t. french-style mustard
	¼ t. pepper

In heated skillet, melt 2 tablespoons butter. Add liver slices and saute quickly on both sides just until cooked through (do not overcook). Lift out liver, transfer to heated serving platter and keep warm. Add remaining butter to same skillet, along with onion rings. Saute, stirring until soft. Reduce heat, cover and cook until tender, about 5 minutes. Add stock, vinegar and tarragon. Cook over high heat until stock is reduced to about ½ cup. Blend in sour cream, mustard and pepper. Heat sauce through, but do not boil. Pour sauce over liver to serve. Serve with lightly steamed spinach, crowned with a patch of real butter. Makes 4 servings.

Organic Garden Salad

¾ c. carrot, grated	1 T. green pepper, finely chopped
½ c. celery, finely chopped	1 T. tamari (soy sauce)
2 T. cheddar cheese, shredded	2 T. peanuts, chopped
2 T. home-made mayonnaise (wheat base)	Vegetable seasoning

Mix all ingredients together. Add more mayonnaise if needed. Serves 4.

Wheatonnaise

1 c. spring water	¼ c. whole wheat flour
½ c. cashews, ground (optional)	

Whirl in blender. Boil 5 minutes, stirring constantly. Cool and return to blender.

CHAPTER 107

Water Retention (Edema)

Pinpointing the specific medical condition causing fluid retention, revealed by swelling — mainly in the hands, feet and near the eyes — is no simple matter.

It can be minor to major: an intake of too much salt or something as serious as congestive heart failure, in which heart pumping becomes inefficient or there is a fault with valves that control blood flow.

Edema can also result from adrenal exhaustion, allergic reactions, deficiency of certain nutrients — protein or vitamins B-1 or B-6 — injury to a part of the body; faulty kidney function; phlebitis — inflammation of the veins — pregnancy, premenstrual tension, or use of oral contraceptives.

Make No Mistake!

Some patients badger their doctors to prescribe "water pills" (diuretics), limiting him or her to dealing with symptoms, rather than trying to find and eliminate the underlying cause.

This could be a mistake for still another reason. Diuretics take away more than just the water: magnesium, potassium, and often more sodium than the body can spare, as well as precious members of the vitamin B family.

Loss of already deficient magnesium and potassium can contribute to high blood pressure. (See Section on High Blood Pressure). An extreme shortage of vitamin B-1 can increase the heart's demand for oxygen beyond the supply, and the heart's right side may become enlarged and injured.

Sodium And Adrenal Exhaustion

Sometimes too high an intake of salt causes the problem. And some research projects have shown that eating high amounts of refined carbohydrates — sugar and white flour products — encourages sodium retention.

At the other extreme, fluid accumulation could be brought on by heart disease or a blockage in the blood vessels, causing fluid to escape and pool in the tissues. The latter disorder demands the best possible medical attention.

The exact way that adrenal exhaustion brings on edema is not known. However, numerous studies show that proper stress management — see Section on Stress — reduction or positive adaptation, bedrest, and extra vitamin C and pantothenic acid can often restore adrenal function to normal.

Richest food sources of vitamin C per milligram in less than four ounce units are: rose hips, 3,000; acerola cherries, 1,100; guavas, 240; black currants, 200; parsley, 170; green peppers, 110; watercress, 80; chives, 70; strawberries, 57; persimmons, 52: spinach, 51; oranges, 50; cabbage, 47; grapefruit, 38; papaya, 37; elderberries and kumquats, 36; dandelion greens and lemons, 35; cantaloupe, 33; green onions, 32 and limes, 31; mangoes, 27; loganberries, 24; tangerines and tomatoes, 23; squash, 22; raspberries and romaine lettuce, 18; pineapple, 17; tangelos and royal jelly, 16; honeydew melon and quinces, 15; avocados and blueberries, 14; nectarines, 13; mulberries, 12 and cucumbers, 11.

Allergies, Fluid And Extra Poundage

Eating foods to which you are allergic is probably the most common cause of edema. Several of my friends have lost between 10 and 20 pounds — mainly fluid — by cutting out offending foods.

So how can you possibly manage that? By doing research with yourself, eating one food at a time and noting whether a negative reaction develops — eyes watering, generalized itching, sneezing, mucous congestion in nose or throat or a rash.

A second method is taking the Coca test to note racing of the pulse within minutes to hours after ingestion of a particular food. (Please see the Section on Allergies for how to take this test.) This is not foolproof, because sensitive or allergic reactions to foods are not always instantaneous. They can manifest as much as 15 hours after eating a food offender.

Favorite and much repeated foods are usually the culprits. Eliminating them often helps drain the accumulated fluid from the body.

Folksy Folk Medicine

Eliminating isn't the only way to go. Sometimes adding foods helps. Two of my neighbors called on me to show their swollen ankles.

It was near lunchtime, so I asked them to stay and prepared the soup and asparagus. They enjoyed the meal, saying they would prepare and eat the same thing for several days. To their delight, the edema went away. Now everybody in the neighborhood wants to live next door to me. (Cucumbers are on the list of vitamin C foods above, and asparagus is on the lists below for foods rich in folic acid and vitamin E.)

Missing Vitamins And Calcium

Already mentioned is that deficiency of vitamin B-1 can contribute to edema, as can insufficient intake of these vitamins: pantothenic acid, B-6, C and E, as well as protein and the mineral calcium. Providing more of these key nutrients can often draw off excessive body fluid and, in the process, correct certain causes of edema.

Clinical researchers tell me that when pregnant women do not have toxemia, edema can protect mother and fetus. Therefore, doctors closely supervise salt intake and use of diuretics.

Vitamin B-6 has been found to lessen or to eliminate symptoms of premenstrual tension and draw off accumulated body fluids.

Birth control pills sometimes bring on edema by interfering with the metabolism of vitamins B-6, folic acid and B-12. Aspirin and antibiotics sabotage vitamins and block their utilization, contributing to fluid accumulation.

Best Sources Of Deficient Vitamins

Foods Richest in Vitamin B-1 in milligrams per less than four ounce units are: soybeans, 1.10; sesame seeds, 0.98; brazil nuts, 0.96; bee pollen, 0.93; pecans, 0.86; alfalfa and peas, 0.80; millet, 0.73; beans, 0.68; buckwheat, and oats, 0.60; wheat, 0.57; hazelnuts, 0.46; rye, 0.43; sprouts, 0.40; lentils and corn, 0.37; brown rice, 0.34; walnuts, 0.33; egg yolk, 0.32 and chickpeas, 0.31.

Supplements and foods richest in pantothenic acid in milligrams per less than four ounce units are: royal jelly, 35; brewer's yeast, 11; torula yeast, 10; brown rice, 8.9; sunflower seeds, 5.5; soybeans, 5.2; corn, 5.0; lentils, 4.8; egg yolk, 4.2; peas, 3.6; alfalfa, 3.3; wheat, 3.2; peanuts, 2,8; rye, 2.6; eggs, 2.3; bee pollen and wheat germ, 2.2; bleu cheese, 1.8; cashews, 1.3; chickpeas, 1.2; avocado, 1.1; chicken, sardines, turkey and walnuts, 0.90.

Foods highest in Proteins are meats, fish, milk products, eggs, legumes and grains.

Supplements and foods with the highest content of vitamin B-6 per milligram for a less than four ounce serving are: brewer's yeast, 4.0; brown rice, 3.6; wheat, 2.9; royal jelly, 2.4; soybeans, 2.0; rye, 1.8; lentils, 1.7; sunflower seeds and hazelnuts, 1.1; alfalfa, 1.00; salmon, 0.98; wheat germ, 0.92; tuna, 0.90; bran, 0.85; walnuts, 0.73; peas and liver, 0.67; avocados, 0.60; beans, 0.57; cashews, peanuts, turkey, oats, chicken and beef, 0.40; halibut, 0.34; and lamb and banana, 0.32.

Foods Richest in Folic Acid in milligrams per less that four ounce units are: torula yeast, 3.0; brewer's yeast, 2.0; alfalfa, 0.80; soybeans, 0.69; endive, 0.47; chickpeas, 0.41; oats, 0.39; lentils, 0.34; beans and wheat germ, 0.31; liver, 0.29; split peas, 0.23; wheat, 0.22; barley, 0.21 and brown rice, 0.17 and asparagus, 0.12.

Foods with the highest amounts of vitamin B-12 in milligrams per less than four ounce portions are: liver, 0.086; sardines, 0.034; mackerel and herring, 0.0100; snapper, 0.0088; flounder, 0.0064; salmon, 0.0047; lamb, 0.0031; swiss cheese, 0.0021; eggs, 0.0020; haddock, 0.0017; muenster cheese, 0.0016 and swordfish and beef, 0.0015.

Foods Richest in Vitamin E in International Units for less than four ounce servings are: wheat germ, 160; safflower nuts, 35; sunflower seeds,

31; whole wheat, 30; sesame oil, 26; walnuts, 22; corn oil and hazelnuts, 21; soy oil and peanut oil, 16; almonds, 15; olive oil, 14; cabbage, 7.8; brazil nuts and peanuts, 6.5; cod liver oil, 5.4; cashews, 5.1; soy lecithin, 4.8; spinach, 2.9; asparagus, 2.5; broccoli, 2.0 and butter, 1.9.

Best food sources of calcium in milligrams per less than four ounce units are: sesame seeds, 1,200; kelp, 1,100; cheeses, 700; brewer's yeast, 420; sardines and carob, 350; molasses, 290; caviar, 280; soybeans and almonds, 230; torula yeast, 220; parsley, 200; brazil nuts, 190; watercress, salmon and chickpeas, 150; egg yolks, pistachios, beans, lentils and kale, 130; sunflower seeds and cow's milk, 120; buckwheat, 110; maple syrup, cream and chard, 100.

CHAPTER 108

Wrinkles

Although that first gray hair may come as a shock, you can quickly pluck it out. But what do you do about that first wrinkle? You take measures to feed your face properly. A lot of wrinkles arrive well ahead of schedule because poor nutrition invites them.

Glamorous Peggy Boyd, a Certified Nutritional Consultant who is the long-time owner and operator of Peggy's Health Center, a nutrition supermarket in Los Altos, California, looks young enough to be her own daughter. She says: "There's a growing awareness among women that beauty is an inside job. You are as beautiful as what you eat. Cosmetics will go only so far in covering nutritional sins."

Slow Sabotage Of The Skin

One of these sins is taking in too little of a particular nutrient, vitamin C, which assures integrity of connective tissue, a support and strengthener for the skin in much the same way as the chicken wire on the sides of a building underlies and strengthens plaster. If the support gives way, the skin becomes loose or wrinkled.[1]

Habituated smokers eventually develop dried up, lined and wrinkled skin, because smoking undermines the skin in two ways. Each cigarette burns up at least 25 mg of vitamin C. Smokers of twenty cigarettes a day use up 500 mg, putting themselves in a deficit situation, because vitamin C is not storeable. Their connective tissue literally caves in.[2]

The second act of sabotage by smoking is narrowing arteries and capillaries, limiting the oxygen and nutrients they can deliver to cells and the amount of wastes they can carry off.[3] If the fear of death from possible lung cancer isn't enough to make a smoker desist, the fear of looking old at an early age may do the job. (See the section on Smoking.)

A Hidden Skin-Destroyer

While smoking is a well-known ager of the skin, fluorides added to the municipal water supply are not. Studies disclose that fluoride levels as low as one part per million—the amount added to city water supplies—cause a breakdown of collagen, which makes up about thirty percent of the body. Disruption of this basic structural material—its synthesis and repair —results in skin wrinkling.[4]

This amount of fluoride, coupled with a poor diet, not only contributes to wrinkling but to speeding up of the entire aging process: weakening of bones, ligaments, muscles and tendons.[5]

A Turkish Tragedy

I received the greatest shock of my life when I visited Kizilcaoern, a village in Turkey, where the water supply has an even higher fluoride content —above five parts per million. I have never in my life seen so many prune faces. Women and men in their thirties looked as if they were in their seventies or eighties with deep wrinkles and flabby, hanging skin. Most of the natives in their thirties were so weak and decrepit they had to use walking canes to get around. One bent, hobbling woman with deep, crisscrossing facial wrinkles appeared to be in her late eighties and turned out to be twenty-two.

These people were pre-aged because of the water supply, about which they could do little. We can do something about ours. We can buy bottled, pure, mountain spring water as health and skin insurance or make sure our community's water supply is not fluoridated. If it is already fluoridated, we can circulate petitions to get rid of this chemical added to water to protect children's teeth. There are better ways to guard children's teeth from cavities—ways that won't harm all of us. See the section under the heading TEETH.

Skin wrinkling is caused not only by damage to underlying collagen, but also by a degree of calcium infiltrating the collagen. An extreme example of this condition is scleroderma, thickening and hardening of the skin and its becoming cemented to underlying structures, sometimes causing joints to become immovable.[6]

Little Known Facts About Skin

Any nutrition-oriented dermatologist can almost name the vitamins or minerals lacking by looking at the imperfect complexion of a patient. Deficient nutrition shows up first in the skin, because the body's God-given will to survive causes available nutrients to be rushed to the vital organs.

A not-so-amazing discovery by researchers at Texas Tech University is the fact that deterioration of the skin from poor nutrition is almost identifical to that from aging.[7] Several studies done some years ago indicate that many symptoms typical of old age—wrinkles, loss of skin elasticity, loss of teeth and brittle bones — are symptoms of scurvy, indicative of a serious deficiency of vitamin C.

So how can you enrich your usual diet with more vitamin C? By adding the following supplements and foods which, in a serving of less than four ounces, have these milligram ratings of vitamin C: rose hips, 3,000; acerola cherries, 1,100; guavas, 240; black currants, 200; parsley, 170; green peppers, 110, watercress, 80; chives and kiwi fruit, 70; strawberries, 57; spinach 51, oranges 50; cabbage, 47; grapefruit, 38; papaya, 37; elderberries and kumquats, 36, and fruits and vegetables ranging down to a rating of two milligrams.

Feeding Skin From Outside In

Ever since the first wrinkle spoiled someone's day, individuals or their beauty experts—the latter existed thousands of years ago in Egypt and elsewhere — have been trying to feed the skin from the outside: by applying lotions of all kinds. Then and in recent times, these preparations did little good for anybody but the sellers—for a very good reason.

Moisturizers have combined water and oil. Water was to add moisture, and oil was to hold it in place. However, once the solution was removed from the face, the moisture went with it, and the skin looked just as dry.

Then a better way was discovered: applying hyaluronic acid, a chemical that is natural to the body. The largest percentage of us is water, and what holds it in place is hyaluronic acid, a thick, transparent goo which is an important ingredient in a substance called mucopolysaccharides. The latter keep the skin young-looking, moist, pliable and smooth.

Hyaluronic acid binds well with the skin as well as with water, holding 1,000 times its own weight in water. (8) Now, that's moisturizing! I have experienced how well hyaluronic acid works in one skin-care formula. It is hard for me to believe the youthful glow it gives.

Feeding The Skin From Inside Out

Tell-tale signs make it quite easy for the nutrition-oriented dermatologist to recommend the right nutrition for the condition.

Observing an extra-sensitive skin and a reddish nose or cheeks ruddy from broken capillaries, he or she knows there is a nutritional shortage of bioflavonoids, vitamin C and, possibly, zinc.

Best sources of bioflavonoids are the inner rind and pulp of citrus fruits, tangerine juice—not orange or grapefruit juice—apricots, cherries, grapes, green peppers — especially the inner, white pulpy parts — tomatoes, papaya, broccoli, and cantaloupe—as well as buckwheat. (Per milligram ratings are not available.)

Foods with the highest zinc content in milligrams per less than four ounce serving are: herring, 110; wheat germ, 14; sesame seeds, 10; torula yeast, 9.9; blackstrap molasses, 8.3; maple syrup, 7.5; liver, 7.0; soybeans, 6.7; sunflower seeds, 6.6; egg yolk, 5,5; lamb, 5.4; chicken, 4.8; oats, 3.7; rye, 3.4; wheat, 3.2; corn, 3.1; coconut and beef, 3.0. When the nutrition-oriented physician observes many bumps or dryness, roughness or scales on the skin, he or she suspects a deficiency of vitamin A, most lavishly concentrated in the following supplements and foods, whose International Unit ratings per less than a four ounce serving follow: Cod liver oil, 200,000; sheep liver, 45,000; beef liver, 44,000; calf's liver, 22,000; dandelion greens, 14,000; carrots, 11,000; yams, 9,000; kale, 8,900; parsley and turnip greens, 8,500; spinach, 8,100; collards greens and chard, 6,500; watercress, 5,000; red peppers; 4,400 squash, 4,000;

egg yolk, 3,400; cantaloupe, 3,400; endive, 3,300; persimmons, 2,700; apricots, 2,700; broccoli, 2,500; pimentos, 2,300; swordfish, 2,100; whitefish, 2,000; romaine, 1,900; mangoes, 1,800; papayas, 1,700; nectarines and pumpkin, 1,600; peaches and cheeses, 1,300 (See Milk Intolerance); eggs, 1,200 and cherries and lettuce, 1,000.

Lines at right angles to one another or tiny wrinkles on the lower lip indicate vitamin B-2 deficiency. Later this lip develops a crinkly, crepe-paper look or appears to be chapped with small white flakes peeling from it.

In acute vitamin B-2 deficiency, cracks develop and persist at the corners of the mouth. Monkey lines may also form between the upper lip and the nose. When deficiencies endure for a long period, the upper lip may disappear entirely. Today's dermatologists find these conditions much more frequently since the cholesterol scare has driven people away from dairy products, reliable sources of vitamin B-2.

Some of the other major sources of vitamin B-2 in milligrams per less than four ounce servings are yeast supplements—torula, 16 and brewer's yeast, 4.2—and liver, 4.1; royal jelly, 1.9; alfalfa, 1.8; bee pollen, 1.7; almonds, 0.92; wheat germ, 0.68; mustard greens, 0.64; egg yolk 0.52; cheeses, 0.46; millet, 0.38; chicken, 0.36; soybeans and veal, 0.31 and eggs and sunflower seeds, 0.28.

Skin-marring ailments such as acne and eczema have often been traced to insufficient essential fatty acids (as well as zinc.) An experiment-established corrector of these ailments is the supplement evening primrose oil, which contains gamma-linoleic acid. (See the sections Acne and Eczema.)

Richest sources of essential fatty acids are cold-processed salad oils such as the following, listed with milligram concentrations per less than four ounces: safflower oil, 77,000; sunflower oil, 60,000; corn oil, 54,000, soy oil, 52,000; wheat germ oil, 44,000, sesame oil, 42,000 and these foods: sunflower seeds, 30,000, walnuts, 29,000; brazil nuts, 23,000; sesame seeds, 20,000; pecans, 114,000; peanuts, 12,000; almonds 11,000, and, among others, hazelnuts, 9,300.

Stress And Wrinkles

Dr. Hans Selye, who fathered the stress theory, found in rat experiments that in stressful situations, calcium is withdrawn from the bones, and when such conditions persist, many signs of premature aging develop — arthritis, wrinkles, cataracts and shriveled sex glands.[9]

Selye also discovered that large amounts of vitamin E prevented the wrinkles developed under stress. Other forms of stress can cause wrinkles, too: among them a negative attitude, reflected in habitual wrinkles-encouraging facial expressions; insufficient exercise to promote good blood circulation; harsh soaps, detergents and hair coloring and working daily under a baking sun.

Many seekers of a sun-bronzed skin live to regret it, because excessive sun-exposure rushes the appearance of old age: a parchment skin or premature wrinkles.

Reversing the damage of sun-caused wrinkles without a face peel is almost impossible. Yet a supplement of vitamin E has helped certain individuals to some degree.

Major sources of vitamin E in International Units per less than a four ounce serving are wheat germ, 160; safflower nuts, 35; sunflower seeds, 31; sesame oil, 26; walnuts, 22; corn oil and hazelnuts, 21; soy and peanut oils, 16; almonds, 15; olive oil, 14; and cabbage, 7.8.

Another Enemy Of Wrinkles

Alpha hydroxy acid (AHA), found in apples, grapes and other fruit, has been discovered by Temple University researchers to remove shallow wrinkles and rejuvenate the skin.

Supposedly, it removes dry skin, scaly patches, age (brown) spots, and acne, as well as wrinkles, states dermatologist Diana Bihova, M.D., of New York City, writer of the book Beauty From the Inside Out (Rawson Associates).

Bihova tells her formula for making a cream of the acids. Cook a cored and peeled apple in a little milk. Mash the apple in the milk. Cool the mixture. Then apply it once weekly and leave it on the face for 15 to 30 minutes.

A word of caution is issued by Bihova to try the mixture on a small spot of skin to assure that you are not sensitive to it. Even persons who can eat a particular fruit without reacting too much to it, sometimes are reactive when the mixture is applied to the skin. If there is any undue reaction, this should signal the end of the experiment.

A stinging sensation on the skin is common. Bihova says this is not a problem.

She states that the mixture costs little to make and really works!

Swiss Liver

2 lbs. calf's liver	3 T. onion, chopped
(seasoned with whole wheat flour)	3 T. parsley, chopped
2 T. wheat germ	3 T. kelp
3 T. butter	Pepper to taste
3 T. sesame oil	1 c. dairy sour cream

Cut liver into ½ inch slices, then into strips. Dust with flower and wheat germ. Heat butter and oil in skillet. When hot and bubbly, add onion, parsley and liver. Saute liver quickly turning strips to brown on all sides. Do not overcook. Strips should be pink in the center. Season with kelp and pepper. Add sour cream. Heat cream through, but do not let boil. Serve

Maureen's Waldorf Salad

10 fresh, ripe apricots	2 c. celery, sliced
3 large apples, cut into bite-size pieces	½ c. dark, seedless raisins
3 T. lemon juice	⅔ c. walnuts, chopped
¼ c. dairy sour cream (raw certified)	Crisp salad greens
¼ c. mayonnaise (home-made)	2 t. brewers yeast

Reserve 3 apricots for garnish. Cut remaining apricots into bite-size pieces. Sprinkle apricots and apples with lemon juice to prevent darkening. Blend sour cream and mayonnaise. Toss apricots, apples, celery and raisins with dressing. Chill several hours. At serving time, add walnuts to salad and toss. Spoon into lettuce lined salad bowl. Cut reserved apricots in half and arrange around edge of salad. Serves 8.

Alternative Doctors

(Please Note: This list of alternative doctors is offered as a service to show availability, rather than to recommend. It is beyond the scope of this book and the authors to check into individual practices, to evaluate, and rate them.

Physicians are listed, first, according to general geographic location, then, according to city and state. A brief writeup describes the type of practice pursued.)

Send $15.00 for a more complete list of alternative medicine doctors. Please Contact:
The National Health Federation
212 West Foothill Blvd.
Monrovia, California 91016
1-818-357-2181
1-800-643-4968

NORTHEAST

New York City

Atkins, Robert, M.D.
Atkins Centers for Complementary Medicine
400 E. 56th Street
New York, N.Y. 10022
PHONE: (212) 758-2110

Under direction of best-selling author Robert Atkins, M.D., ("Dr. Atkins' Health Revolution") the Atkins Center covers all aspects of medical care, ranging from obesity, hypoglycemia and Candida albicans to heart disease, cancer and multiple sclerosis.

MIDDLE ATLANTIC

Indiana, Pennsylvania

Sinha, Chandrika P., M.D.
1177 South 6th Street
Indiana, Pennsylvania 15701
PHONE: (412) 349-1414

Clinic offers Nutrition for disease prevention and allergy; Pain Control by nine different non-drug means, including hydrotherapy, biofeedback, and, among others, chiropractic; Acupuncture for pain, smoking, weight control, substance abuse and Preventive Health and Longevity through nutrition, exercise, smoke-cessation, weight control and stress management.

SOUTHEAST

North Miami Beach, Florida

Dayton, Martin, D.O., M.D.
Medical Center, Sunny Isles
18600 Collins Avenue
North Miami Beach, Florida 33160
PHONE: (305) 931-8484

Dr. Martin Dayton has two doctorates and three specialties: Family Practice, General Medicine, and Chelation Therapy and is a licensed Homeopathic Physician. His practice covers the spectrum from prevention to acute medical care—chronic states to degenerative conditions: Cancer, Osteoporosis, Hardening of the Arteries, Chronic Viral and Candida infections, Fatigue and Pain, using the range of holistic modalities.

North Miami Beach, Florida

Willner, Robert E., M.D.
16400 Northeast 19th Avenue
North Miami Beach, Florida 33162
PHONE: (305) 949-6331 or 1-800-562-5445

Robert E. Willner, M.D., serves as a national director of the American College of Advancement In Medicine. His General Practice specializes in Pain Reduction, Chelation Therapy for artery impairment, Weight Loss procedures and other preventive medical measures.

Landrum, South Carolina

Rozema, Theodore C., M.D.
Bio Genesis Medical Center
1000 E. Rutherford Road

Landrum, South Carolina 29356
PHONE: (803) 457-4141 and (800) 922-5821 (for South Carolina) and (800) 992-8350 (for the nation).

The Family Practice of Theodore C. Rozema, M.D. deals with the full range of diseases and disorders but specializes in Preventive Medicine with emphasis on Chelation Therapy and Nutrition.

MIDDLEWEST

Highland, Indiana

Streeter, Cal, D.O.
Highland Medical Plaza
9635 Saric Court
Highland, Indiana 46322
PHONE: (219) 924-2410

Dr. Cal Streeter's Family Practice emphasizes detoxification for strengthening the body and immune response, specializing in treatment of Allergies and Cardiovascular ailments. Among Dr. Streeter's preventive medicine modalities are Chelation Therapy and Osteopathic Manipulations.

SOUTH CENTRAL

Oklahoma City, Oklahoma

Farr, Charles H., M.D.
Genesis Medical Center
8524 South Western, Suite 107
Oklahoma City, Oklahoma 73139
PHONE: (405) 632-8868

Genesis Medical Center, under direction of Dr. Charles Farr, specializes in Nutritional, Preventive and Oxidative Medicine. Dr. Farr is a pioneer in intravenous use of hydrogen peroxide. Some of his publications are "The Intravenous Use of Hydrogen Peroxide" and "Oxidative Therapy," both by University Press of Oklahoma City.

Humble, Texas (Next to Houston Intercontinental Airport)

Trowbridge, John Parks, M.D.
The Center For Health Enhancement

9816 Memorial Boulevard, Suite 205
Humble, Texas 77338 (Next to Houston Intercontinental Airport)
PHONE: (713) 540-2329

John Parks Trowbridge, M.D., who directs the Center For Health Enhancement, is author of "The Yeast Syndrome," Vice President of the American College of Advancement in Medicine, a Board Certified Specialist in Chelation Therapy and Diplomate in Preventive Medicine for graduate studies in nutrition. The Center specializes exclusively in nutritional and rejuvenation medicine — laser surgery, chelation therapy and FACE 2, Non-surgical Facelifts.

NORTHWEST

Kent, Washington

Wright, Jonathan, M.D.
Tahoma Clinic
24030 132nd Avenue, S.E.
Kent, Washington 98042
PHONE: 1-(800) 825-8924

Family practice at Tahoma Clinic emphasizes Preventive Medicine, Nutritional Biochemistry and Allergy and is based on access to latest medical and nutritional journal publications: 22,000 articles reviewed in 12,000 hours of library research. Dr. Wright, a best-selling writer ("Book of Nutritional Therapy," Rodale Press, 1979, almost 500,000 copies sold), presents yearly seminars for physicians with associate Alan Gaby, M.D.: "Clinical Applications of Nutritional Biochemistry."

CALIFORNIA

Northern California
Albany, California

Gordon, Ross B., M.D.
405 Kains Avenue
Albany, California 94706
PHONE: (415) 526-3232

Dr. Ross Gordon's Nutrition-oriented Preventive Medicine practice accents Chelation Therapy to avoid cardiovascular complications and diverse methods of weight control and weight loss.

Los Altos, California

Cathcart, Robert F., M.D.

127 Second Street, Suite 3
Los Altos, CA 94022
PHONE: (415) 949-2822

Robert F. Cathcart, M.D., specializes in Allergy, Environmental and Orthomolecular Medicine, uses massive doses of vitamin C—intravenously, when necessary—in combination with other orthomolecular and clinical ecology therapies. A major part of his practice deals with chronic fatigue syndrome caused by Candida albicans, Epstein Barr Virus and other conditions. Another specialty is chelation therapy.

North Highland, California (Near Sacramento)

Gordon, Garry, M.D.

Preventive Medical Clinic
3325 Myrtle Avenue
North Highland, California 95660
PHONE: (916) 348-4000

Offering a full spectrum of medical services from prevention to surgery to spiritual therapy, Dr. Garry Gordon's Preventive Medical Clinic features Chelation Therapy and Orthomolecular Nutrition. Dr. Gordon has an extensive referral service in the event that his clinic is not equipped to handle cases regarded by orthodox medicine as hopeless.

San Francisco, California

Lynn, Paul, M.D.

San Francisco Preventive Medical Group
345 West Portal Avenue
San Francisco, California 94127
PHONE: (415) 566-1000

Treatment is offered for the full scope of degenerative diseases: poor circulation, arthritis, osteoporosis and, also, Candida albicans, allergies and chronic fatigue. Therapies offered are Chelation, Electroacupuncture, Pain Control, Acupuncture, Clinical Ecology and Homeopathy.

Southern California
Covina, California

Privitera, James J., M.D.
105 North Grand View
Covina, California 91723
PHONE: (818) 966-1618

Dr. James J. Privitera's Family practice—children and adults—accents allergies, metabolical medicine, nutrition and prevention.

Santa Monica, California

Susser, Murray, M.D.
Bios Medical Group
2730 Wilshire Boulevard, Suite 110
Santa Monica, California 90403
PHONE: (213) 453-4424

In association with John Lamont, M.D., Dr. Susser practices in the office mentioned above and also at Bios Medical Group, 909 Electric Avenue, Suite 212, Seal Beach, California 90740. PHONE: (213) 493-4526. Dr. Murray Susser, who hosts the popular daily radio program, "Questioning Medicine," (9:00 A.M. to 9:30 A.M., Mon. through Fri., KFOX, 93.5 FM, Redondo Beach), specializes in Allergies, Chelation Therapy, and Nutrition.

REFERENCES

Chapter 1   ACNE
[1] Maureen Salaman, "Effects of Zinc on Acne", Let's Live, September 1980, p. 17, 19, 20.

Chapter 2   ALCOHOLISM
[1] Psychology Today, January, 1986, 16.
[2] Ibid.
[3] Ibid.
[4] Register (Orange County, California, September 10, 1987).
[5] Ibid.
[6] Ibid.
[7] Ibid.
[8] Ibid.
[9] Ibid.
[10] Richard A. Passwater, Super-Nutrition (New York: The Dial Press, 1975), 16.
[11] J. Douglass et al, "Effects of Raw Food on Hypertension and Obesity," Southern Medical Journal, (1985) 78 (7): 841.
[12] Ibid.
[13] Melvyn R. Werbach, Nutritional Influences on Illness (Tarzana, California: Third Line Press, 1988): 11.
[14] Ibid.
[15] Ibid.
[16] Register et al, Journal of the American Dietetic Association (1972) 61:159-62.
[17] Ibid.
[18] Ibid.
[19] L.L. Rogers, R.B. Pelton and R.J. Williams, "Voluntary Alcohol Consumption by Rats Following Administration of Glutamine," Journal of Biological Chemistry (1956) 220 (1): 321-3.
[20] G. Edwards and J. Littleton, Editors, Pharmacogical Treatments for Alcoholism. (London, Croom Heim, 1984), 331-50.
[21] Personal communication.
[22] Melvyn R. Werbach, Nutritional Influences on Illness (Tarzana, California: Third Line Press, 1988): 11.

Chapter 3   ALLERGIES
[1] James Braly, Dr. Braly's Optimum Health Program (New York: Times Books, 1985), 230.
[2] Ibid, 47.
[3] Gary Null, The Complete Guide to Health and Nutrition (New York, NY: Dell Publishing Company, 1984), 298.
[4] Staff of Prevention Magazine, The Encyclopedia of Common Diseases, (Emmaus, PA: Rodale Press, Inc., 1976), 777.
[5] K. Folkers, et al, Hoppe-Seylers Zeitschrift Fur Physiolozersche Cheme, Vol. 365, March 1984, 405.

[6] I Kueva et al, The Microecology of the Gastrointestinal Tract and The Immunological Status Under Food Allergy, Nahrung, 28(6-7); 689-93, 1984.

Chapter 4 ALZHEIMER'S DISEASE
[1] Robert J. Johnson, "Aluminum: A Threat to Mental Health", Bestways (December, 1985): pp. 28-29.
[2] Allen C. Alfrey, et al, "The Dialysis Encephalopathy Syndrome: Possible Aluminum Intoxication," New England Journal of Medicine (January 22, 1976): 185-6.
[3] Journal of Orthomolecular Psychiatry, First Quarter, 1981, 54-60.
[4] Robert J. Johnson, "Aluminum: A Threat to Mental Health", Bestways (December, 1986), 28.
[5] Science News, Vol. 123, No. 16, April 18, 1981, p. 245.
[6] Ibid., Vol. 126, September 15, 1984, p. 167.
[7] Barbara Bassett, "Aluminum: Treat It With Care", Bestways (June, 1987), pp. 36-37.
[8] Dr. Stephen Davies and Dr. Alan Stewart, Nutritional Medicine (London: Pan Books, 1987), 389.
[9] Blair Justice, Who Gets Sick, (Houston: Peak Press, 1987), 11.
[10] Edna Zeavin, "Foods That Influence Behavior," Bestways, September, 1985, 11.
[11] Science News, Vol. 128, No. 2, July 13, 1985, 24.
[12] Ibid.
[13] Gary Null, The Complete Guide to Health and Nutrition (New York, NY: Dell Publishing Co., 1984), 210.
[14] Robert H. Garrison, Jr. and Elizabeth Somer, The Nutrition Desk Reference (New Canaan, CT: Keats Publishing, Inc., 1985), 106.

Chapter 5 ANEMIA
[1] Encyclopedia of Common Diseases (Emmaus, PA: Rodale Press, Inc., 1976), 44.
[2] Robert H. Garrison, Jr. and Elizabeth Somer, The Nutrition Desk Reference (New Canaan, CT: Keats Publishing, Inc., 1985), 67.
[3] Ibid, 67.
[4] Ibid, 67.
[5] Stephen E. Langer and James F. Scheer, Solved: The Riddle of Illness (New Canaan, CT: Keats Publishing, Inc., 1984), 34.
[6] Edited by Jeffrey Bland, Medical Application of Clinical Nutrition (New Canaan, CT: Keats Publishing, Inc., 1983), 262.
[7] Ibid.
[8] Ibid, 263.
[9] Ibid.

Chapter 6 ANOREXIA NERVOSA
[1] Carl C. Pfeiffer, Mental and Elemental Nutrients (New Canaan, CT: Keats Publishing, Inc., 1975), 69.
[2] Ibid, 69.
[3] Ibid.
[4] Ibid.
[5] R.L. Casper and J.M. Davis, "An Evaluation of Trace Metals, Vitamins and Taste Function in Anorexia Nervosa", American Journal of Clinical Nutrition, Vol. 33, 1980, 1801

Chapter 7 APPENDICITIS
[1] The Encyclopedia of Common Diseases, (Emmaus, PA: Rodale Press, Inc., 1976), 66.
[2] Ibid, 66.

Chapter 8 APPETITE, POOR
[1] Jeffrey Bland, Nutraerobics, (San Francisco: Harper and Row Publishers, 1983), 232.
[2] Robert H. Garrison, Jr. and Elizabeth Somer, The Nutrition Desk Reference (New Canaan, CT: Keats Publishing, Inc., 1985), 210.
[3] Ibid.

Chapter 9 ARTHRITIS
[1] Robert Bingham, Fight Back Against Arthritis, Desert Hot Springs, CA: Desert Arthritis Medical Clinic (Publisher), 139.
[2] Ibid, 124.
[3] Ibid, 138, 139.
[4] Tufts University, Diet and Nutrition Letter, Vol. 2, No. 10, December 1984, 1.
[5] Paula Blake, "Arthritis and your Diet", Bestways (April, 1987), 38.

[6] Ibid, 38.
[7] Ibid, 38.
[8] James Braly, M.D., Dr. Braly's Optimum Health Program (New York, NY: Times Books, 1985), 328.
[9] Ibid, 47.
[10] Ibid, 47.
[11] A.F. Morgan, J. Biological Chemistry, 195, 1952, 583.
[12] L.J. Eising, Journal of Bone Joint Surgery, 45a, 1963, 69.
[13] Adelle Davis, Let's Get Well (New York, NY: Harcourt, Brace, and World, 1965), 123.
[14] Ibid, 123.
[15] S. Morgales et al, Journal of Biological Chemistry, 1/24, 1963, 767 and S.R. Ames, Journal of Biological Chemistry, 169, 1947, 503 and R.W. Lamont-Havers, Borden's Review of Nutritional Research. 24, No. 1, 1963, 15.
[16] Encyclopedia of Common Diseases (Emmaus, PA: Rodale Press, Inc., 1976), 80-81.
[17] Ibid.
[18] Ibid, 74-76.
[19] Ibid, 81.

Chapter 10 ASTHMA
[1] Los Angeles Times, June 4, 1985, Part V, 1.
[2] Gary Null, The Complete Guide to Health and Nutrition, (New York, NY: Dell Publishing, Co., 1984), 194-95.
[3] Patrick Quillin, Healing Nutrients (Chicago: Contemporary Books, 1987), 182.
[4] Brian L.G. Morgan, Nutrition Prescription (New York, NY: Crown Publishers, Inc., 1987), 145.
[5] Jean Carper, The Food Pharmacy (New York, NY: Bantam Books, 1985), 218.
[6] Ibid, 165.
[7] Linus Pauling, How to Live Longer and Feel Better (New York, NY: W.H. Freeman and Co., 1986), 269-70.
[8] Ibid, 270.
[9] Ibid.
[10] Alan Gaby, B6: The Natural Healer (New Canaan, CT: Keats Publishing, Inc., 1987), 170-71.
[11] Janice McCall, Natural Healing Encyclopedia (Peachtree City, GA: FC & A, Inc., 1987), 21.

Chapter 11 ATHLETE'S FOOT

Chapter 12 BAD BREATH
[1] R.E. Hodges et al, American Journal of Clinical Nutrition, Vol. 11, 1962, 181, 187 and W.W. Hawkings et al, Science, Vol. 108, 1948, 2802.
[2] The Encyclopedia of Common Diseases (Emmaus, PA: Rodale Press, Inc., 1976), 163-64.
[3] Ibid, 165.

Chapter 13 BALDNESS
[1] H. Maynard et al, Journal of Nutrition, Vol. 64, 1958, 85.
[2] A.H. Poznankaia, Biochemistry, Vol. 23, 1958, 215
[3] T.D. Kinney et al, Journal of Experimental Medicine, Vol. 102, 1955, 151.
[4] R. Gufner, Archives of Dermatology and Syphilology, Vol. 64, 1951, 688.
[5] F. Kazz, Archives of Dermatology, Vol. 78, 1958, 740.
[6] The Encyclopedia of Common Diseases (Emmaus, PA: Rodale Press, Inc., 1976), 765.
[7] Ibid, 764.
[8] Gary Null, The Complete Guide to Health and Nutrition (New York, NY: Dell Publishing, Inc., 1984), 285.
[9] H.L. Newbold, Mega-Nutrients: A Prescription for Total Health (Los Angeles, CA: The Body Press, 1987), 336-37.

Chapter 14 BED-WETTING
[1] The Encyclopedia of Common Diseases (Emmaus, PA: Rodale Press, Inc., 1976), 171-72.

Chapter 15 BIRTH CONTROL
[1] Jeffrey Bland, Nutraerobics (San Francisco: Harper & Row, 1983), 237.

Chapter 16 BLADDER INFECTION (CYSTITIS)
[1] Rex Adams, Miracle Medicine Foods (Englewood Cliffs, NJ: Prentice-Hall, 1977), 90.

[2] Ibid., 91.

Chapter 17 BODY ODOR
[1] The Practical Encyclopedia of Natural Healing (Emmaus, PA: Rodale Press, Inc., 1983) 65-6.

Chapter 18 BREAST AILMENTS (FIBROCYSTIC DISORDERS)
[1] Alan Donald, "Benign Breast Disorders," Bestways, November, 1984, 53.
[2] Ibid.
[3] Ibid., 54

Chapter 19 BREAST FEEDING PROBLEMS
[1] "Infants Eat And Grow at Their Own Pace," Scientific Research News, United States Department of Agriculture, April, 1988, 1.
[2] Ibid, 2.
[3] The Practical Encyclopedia of Natural Healing (Emmaus, PA: Rodale Press, Inc., 1983), 107.
[4] John D. Kirschman with Lavon J. Dunne, Nutrition Almanac (New York, NY: McGraw-Hill Book Co., 1984), 210.
[5] "Breast Milk for Preemies is There for the Taking," Scientific Research News, United States Department of Agriculture (April, 1988), 1.
[6] Ibid, 2.
[7] Harvard Medical School Health Letter, Vol. 2, No. 6, March, 1986, 7.
[8] Ibid.
[9] Stephen Jaksha, Ventura, CA, Star Free Press, September 21, 1986, Section B, 14.

Chapter 20 BRUISES
[1] Adelle Davis, Let's Get Well (New York, NY: Harcourt, Brace and World, Inc., 1965), 30.
[2] The Practical Encyclopedia of Natural Healing (Emmaus, PA: Rodale Press, Inc., 1983), 76-77.
[3] Jeffrey Bland, Nutraerobics (San Francisco: Harper & Row Publishers, Inc., 1983), 44.
[4] Patrick Quillin, Healing Nutrients (Chicago: Contemporary Books, 1987), 200.

Chapter 21 BULIMIA
[1] "How to Beat Bulimia," News Story, Hilton Head Health Institute, Hilton Head Island, SC, by William R. Biggs/Gilmore Associates.

Chapter 22 BURNS
[1] Gary Null, The Complete Guide to Health and Nutrition (New York, NY: Dell Publishing, Inc., 1984), 301.
[2] Robert H. Garrison and Elizabeth Somer, The Nutrition Desk Reference (New Canaan, CT: Keats Publishing, Inc., 1985), 96.
[3] Gary Null, The Complete Guide to Health and Nutrition (New York, NY: Dell Publishing, Inc., 1984), 301.
[4] Richard A. Kunin, Mega-Nutrition (New York, NY: McGraw-Hill Book Co., 1981), 239.
[5] Patrick Quillin, Healing Nutrients (Chicago: Contemporary Books, 1987), 161.
[6] Ibid.
[7] Ibid.

Chapter 23 BURSITIS
[1] The Encyclopedia of Common Diseases (Emmaus, PA: Rodale Press, Inc., 1976), 105.
[2] Ibid.
[3] Ibid.

Chapter 24 CANCER
[1] Spotlight, August 1, 1988, 12-3.
[2] Science Digest, November, 1983, 92.

Chapter 25 CANCER (BLADDER)
[1] J.U. Schlegel, et al, "The Role of Ascorbic Acid in the Prevention of Bladder Tumor Formation," Journal of Urology, 1980, 103:155-159.
[2] Linus Pauling, How To Live Longer and Feel Better (New York: W.H. Freeman and Company, 1986) 225.

Chapter 26 CANCER (BREAST)
[1] Stephen E. Langer with James F. Scheer, Solved: The Riddle of Illness (New Canaan, CT: Keats Publishing, Inc., 1984), 121.

[2] Ibid.
[3] Ibid, 122.
[4] Ibid.
[5] Ibid.
[6] Patrick Quillin, Healing Nutrients (Chicago: Contemporary Books, 1987), 129
[7] Ibid.
[8] Ibid.
[9] Ibid.
[10] Richard A. Kunin, Mega-Nutrients (New York, NY: McGraw-Hill Books, 1981), 109-110
[11] The Practical Encyclopedia of Healing (Emmaus, PA: Rodale Press, Inc., 1983), 95.
[12] Joan Harder, "Defense Against Breast Cancer," Bestways, September 1986, 367.
[13] Ibid.
[14] Ibid.
[15] "Women Doing Poor Job of Breast Self-Examination," News Feature, University of Southern California News Source, November, 1988.

Chapter 27 CANCER (CERVIX AND VAGINA)
[1] Brian L.G. Morgan, Nutrition Prescription (New York: Crown Publishers, Inc., 1987): 60.
[2] Encyclopedia of Common Diseases (Emmaus, PA: Rodale Press, Inc., 1976): 300.
[3] Medical Hotline, Vol. 5, No. 1, January, 1984, 4.
[4] The Practical Encyclopedia of Natural Healing (Emmaus, PA: Rodale Press, Inc., 1983): 109.
[5] Ibid.
[6] Ibid.

Chapter 28 CANCER (COLON)
[1] Linus Pauling, How to Live Longer and Feel Better (New York, NY: W.H. Freeman & Co., 1986), 347.
[2] Richard Kunin, Mega-Nutrients (New York, NY: McGraw-Hill, 1981), 81.
[3] Gary Null, The Complete Guide to Health and Nutrition (New York, NY: Dell Publishing Co., Inc., 1984), 146-47.
[4] Jean Carper, The Food Pharmacy (New York, NY: Bantam Books, 1988), 57-58.
[5] Ibid.
[6] Jeffrey Bland, 1984-85 Yearbook of Nutritional Medicine (New Canaan, CT: 1985), 302.
[7] Ibid.

Chapter 29 CANCER (COLON, PRECURSOR), FAMILIAL POLYPOSIS
[1] J.J. DeCosse, et al, "Effect of Ascorbic on Rectal Polyps of Patients with Familial Polyposis," Surgery (1975) 78:608-12.

Chapter 30 CANCER (EYE)
[1] James F. Scheer, "Sunlight Linked With Eye Cancer," Bestways, June, 1986, 20.
[2] Ibid.
[3] Ibid.
[4] Ibid.
[5] Ibid.
[6] Ibid.

Chapter 31 CANCER (LUNG)
[1] The Practical Encyclopedia of Natural Healing (Emmaus, PA: Rodale Press, Inc., 1983): 98.
[2] Richard Kunin, Mega-Nutrition (New York, McGraw-Hill Book Company, 1981): 95.
[3] Jean Carper, Nutrition Pharmacy (New York, 1988): 73.
[4] Ibid.
[5] Ibid., 74
[6] Ibid., 75
[7] Ibid.
[8] Ibid.
[9] The Practical Encyclopedia of Natural Healing (Emmaus, PA: Rodale Press, Inc., 1983): 92.

Chapter 32 CANCER, PROSTATE (SEE PROSTATE PROBLEMS)

Chapter 33 CANCER (SKIN)
[1] James F. Scheer, "Skin Cancer Detection," Bestways, July 1983, 20.
[2] Ibid.
[3] Ibid.
[4] Ibid.
[5] Ibid.
[6] Ibid.
[7] The Complete Book of Vitamins (Emmaus, PA: Rodale Press, Inc., 1977); 567-68.
[8] Ibid.
[9] Science Digest, November, 1983, 92.

Chapter 34 CANDIDA ALBICANS
[1] Based on interviews with William Crook, M.D. and John Trowbridge, M.D.

Chapter 35 CATARACTS
[1] James F. Scheer, "Latest on Cataracts," Bestways, September, 1986, 20.
[2] Ibid.
[3] Ibid.

Chapter 36 CHOLESTEROL (20 NATURAL WAYS TO LOWER)
[1] Stephen Langer and James F. Scheer, Solved: The Riddle of Illness (New Canaan, CT: Keats Publishing, Inc., 1984): 96-97.
[2] Ibid., 95.
[3] Personal communication with Edward R. Pinckney, M.D.
[4] R. Sable-Amplis et al, "Further Studies on the Cholesterol-Lowering Effect of Apples on Humans: Biochemical Mechanisms Involved," Nutrition Research (1983) 3:325-328.
[5] Ibid.
[6] A. A. Qureshi, et al, "Suppression of Cholesterogenesis By Plant Constituents to NC-167." Lipids, November, 1985. 20 (11): 817-824.
[7] J.W. Anderson, et al, "Hypocholesteremic Effects of Oat Bran and Bean Intake For Hypercholesteremic Men," American Journal of Clinical Nutrition (December 1984) 40:1146-1155.
[8] J. Robertson, et al, "The Effect of Raw Carrot on Serum Lipids and Colon Function." American Journal of Clinical Nutrition (September, 1979) 32 (9): 1889-1892.
[9] K. Sambaiah, K. et al, "Hypocholesterolemic Effect of Red Pepper & Capsaicin," Indian Journal of Experimental Biology (August 1980) 18:898-899.
[10] Jean Carper, The Food Pharmacy (New York: Bantam Books, 1988), 186-187.
[11] M. Secur, "Effect of Garlic on Serum Lipids and Lipoproteins in Patients Suffering From Hyperlidemia." Diabetology Croatica (1980) 9:323.
[12] Personal communication.
[13] Jean Carper, The Food Pharmacy (New York: Bantam Books, 1988), 214-215.
[14] L.A. Simons, et al, Australian and New Zealand Journal of Medicine, Vol. 7, 262.
[15] J.W. Anderson, "Physiological and Metabolic Effects of Dietary Fiber," Federal Proceedings (November 1985) 44 (14): 2902-2906.
[16] S.M. Grundy, "Comparison of Monounsaturated Fatty Acids and Carbohydrates for Lowering Plasma Cholesterol." New England Journal of Medicine (March 20, 1986) 314 (12): 745-748.
[17] Jean Carper, The Food Pharmacy (New York: Bantam Books, 1988), 32.
[18] V. Usha, et al, "Effect of Dietary Fiber From Banana on Cholesterol Metabolism." Indian Journal of Experimental Biology (October 1984) 22:550-554.
[19] Y. Yamori et al, "Dietary Prevention of Stroke and its Mechanisms in Stroke-Prone Sontaneously Hypertensive Rats—Preventive Effect of Dietary Fibre and Palmitoleic Acid." Journal of Hypertension (Supplement) (October 1986) 4(3) S449-S452.
[20] C.R. Sirtori, et al, Studies on the Use of a Soybean Protein Diet for the Management of Human Hyperliproteinemias. Animal and Vegetable Proteins in Lipid Metabolism and Atherosclerosis. (New York: Alan R. Liss, Inc., 1983), 135-148.
[21] N. Iritani, et al, "Effect of Sopinach and Wakane on Cholesterol Turnover in the Rat." Atherosclerosis (1972) 15:87-92.
[22] Jean Carper, The Food Pharmacy (New York: Bantam Books, 1988), 312.
[23] Ibid., 317.
[24] Stephen Langer and James F. Scheer, Solved: The Riddle of Illness (New Canaan, CT: Keats Publishing, Inc., 1984), 111. 25. Ibid., 108.

Chapter 37 CIRCULATION BLOCKAGE (LEGS)
[1] A.M. Boyd and J. Marks, "Treatment of Intermittent Claudication," Angiology, Vol. 14, 1963, 198-208.

Chapter 38 CIRCULATION PROBLEMS
[1] Stephen Langer and James F. Scheer, Solved: The Riddle of Illness (New Canaan, CT: Keats Publishing, Inc., 1984), 109-110.
[2] Ibid, 110.
[3] Ibid.
[4] Ibid.
[5] Robert M. Downs with Alice Van Baak, "Improving Circulation," Bestways, July, 1986, 22.
[6] Ibid.
[7] Ibid.

Chapter 39 COLDS
[1] Linus Publishing, How to Live Longer and Feel Better (New York, NY: W.H. Freeman & Co., 1986), 26.
[2] Ibid., 26-27.
[3] Ibid., 27.
[4] Ibid.
[5] Ibid.
[6] Ibid., 146.
[7] Ibid.
[8] Ibid.
[9] Ibid., 157.
[10] Ibid.
[11] Ibid., 309.
[12] Ibid.
[13] Ibid.
[14] Ibid.
[15] Ibid., 309-310
[16] Ibid.
[17] Norman Ford, Eighteen Natural Ways to Beat the Common Cold (New Canaan, CT: Keats Publishing, Inc., 1987), 72.
[18] Ibid.
[19] Ibid., 72-3.
[20] Ibid., 73.
[21] Ibid.
[22] Ibid.
[23] Ibid., 83.
[24] Ibid., 88.
[25] Ibid., 86.

Chapter 40 COLON COMPLICATIONS (DIVERTICULAR DISEASES)
[1] Adelle Davis, Let's Get Well (New York, NY: Harcourt, Brace & World, 1965), 189.
[2] Patrick Quillin, Healing Nutrients, (Chicago, IL: Contemporary Books, 1987), 35.
[3] Gary Null, The Complete Guide to Health and Nutrition (New York, NY: Dell Publishing Co., Inc., 1984), 155.
[4] Mark Bricklin, The Practical Encyclopedia of Natural Healing (Emmaus, PA: Rodale Press, Inc., 1983), 153.
[5] Ibid.
[6] Ibid., 154.
[7] Ibid.

Chapter 41 CONSTIPATION
[1] American Journal of Gastroenterology, 77:599-603
[2] H. Andersson et al, Scandinavian Journal of Gastroenterology, 14:821-26, 1979.
[3] News Story, U.S. Department of Agriculture Human Nutrition research, March, 1986.
[4] Lancet General Advertiser, September 21, 1957

[5] M.I. Botez et al, "Neurologic Disorders Responsive to Folic Acid Therapy," Canadian Medical Association Journal 15:217. 1976.

Chapter 42   CRAMPS
[1] James F. Scheer, "Conquering Cramps for Good," Bestways, February, 1982, 95.
[2] Ibid, 96.
[3] Ibid.
[4] Ibid.
[5] Ibid.
[6] Ibid.
[7] Ibid.

Chapter 43   CRAVINGS (FOR FOOD)
[1] Edited by J.I. Rodale with Ruth Adams, The Health Finder (Emmaus, PA: Rodale Books, Inc., 1954), 80-83.

Chapter 44   DEPRESSION
[1] Stephen Langer and James F. Scheer, Solved: The Riddle of Illness (New Canaan, CT: Keats Publishing, Inc., 1984), 59.
[2] Richard Kunin, Mega-Nutrition (New York, NY: McGraw-Hill Book Co., 1980), 150.
[3] Ibid, 151.
[4] Ibid, 151-52.
[5] Ibid, 152.
[6] Ibid.
[7] Ibid.
[8] Ibid.
[9] Jeffrey Bland, Nutraerobics (San Francisco, CA: Harper-Row, 1983), 235.
[10] The Practical Encyclopedia of Natural Healing (Emmaus, PA: Rodale Press, Inc., 1983), 143.
[11] John D. Kirschman with Lavon J. Dunne, Nutrition Almanac (New York, NY: McGraw-Hill Book Co., 1984), 1180.
[12] Ibid.
[13] Stephen Langer and James F. Scheer, Solved: The Riddle of Illness (New Canaan, CT: Keats Publishing, Inc., 1984), 68.
[14] Ibid, 64-4.
[15] Ibid, 65.

Chapter 45   DIABETES
[1] Stephen Langer and James F. Scheer, Solved: The Riddle of Illness (New Canaan, CT: Keats Publishing, Inc., 1984), 76-77.
[2] Ibid, 77.
[3] Ibid.
[4] Ibid.
[5] Ibid, 77-8.
[6] Ibid, 78.
[7] Ibid.
[8] Ibid.
[9] Ibid.
[10] Ibid.
[11] Ibid.
[12] Ibid, 78-79.
[13] Ibid, 79.
[14] Ibid.
[15] Science News, Vol. 133, No. 4, January 22, 1988, 62.
[16] Jean Carper, The Food Pharmacy (New York, NY: Bantam Books, 1988), 133-34.
[17] Patrick Quillin, Healing Nutrients (Chicago, IL: Contemporary Books, 1987), 300.
[18] Gary Null, The Complete Guide to Health and Nutrition (New York, NY: Dell Publishing, Co., Inc., 1984), 123-24.
[19] Ibid, 124.
[20] Stephen Langer with James F. Scheer, How to Win at Weight Loss (Rochester, VT: Thorsons Publishers, Inc., 1987), 106-07.

Chapter 46 DIARRHEA
[1] James F. Scheer, "News & Commentary," Bestways, July, 1988, 20.

Chapter 47 EARS, RINGING, TINNITUS
[1] Jean-Pierre Taillens, Review Medicale de la Suisse Romande, 80/2: 65-78.
[2] The Encyclopedia of Common Diseases (Emmaus, PA: Rodale Press, Inc., 1976): 526-27.

Chapter 48 ECZEMA
[1] The Encyclopedia of Common Diseases (Emmaus, PA: Rodale Press, Inc., 1976), 1122.
[2] Stephen Langer with James F. Scheer, Solved: The Riddle of Illness (New Canaan, CT: Keats Publishing, Inc., 1984), 132.
[3] Ibid.
[4] Ibid. 133.
[5] Ibid.
[6] Ibid.
[7] Ibid.
[8] The Encyclopedia of Common Diseases (Emmaus, PA: Rodale Press, Inc., 1976), 1123.
[9] Ibid.

Chapter 49 EPSTEIN-BARR SYNDROME

Chapter 50 EYE (MACULAR DEGENERATION)
[1] Jeffrey Bland, Preventive Medicine Update (Audiotape), HealthComm, (August, 1988) Gig Harbor, Washington.
[2] Ibid.
[3] Ibid.
[4] Ibid.
[5] Edited by Jeffrey Bland, 1984-85 Yearbook of Nutritional Medicine (New Canaan, CT: Keats Publishing, Inc., 1985), 274.

Chapter 51 EYE PROBLEMS
[1] James F. Scheer, "New Slant on Night Blindness," Bestways, December, 1987, 16.
[2] Adelle Davis, Let's Get Well (New York, NY: Harcourt, Brace & World, 1965), 350.
[3] Ibid.
[4] Patrick Quillin, Healing Nutrients (Chicago, IL: Contemporary Books, 1987), 392.
[5] The Complete Book of Vitamins (Emmaus, PA: Rodale Press, Inc., 1977), 170.
[6] Adelle Davis, Let's Get Well (New York, NY: Harcourt, Brace & World, 1965), 354.
[7] Ibid, 353.
[8] Ibid.
[9] The Encyclopedia of Common Diseases (Emmaus, PA: Rodale Press, Inc., 1976), 682.

Chapter 52 FATIGUE
[1] Stephen Langer and James F. Scheer, How to Win at Weight Loss (Rochester, VT: Thorsons Publishers, Inc., 1987), 41.
[2] J.I. Rodale, Editor, The Health Finder (Emmaus, PA: Rodale Press, Inc., 1959), 81-82.
[3] Adelle Davis, Let's Get Well (New York, NY: Harcourt, Brace & World, 1965), 21.
[4] Ibid, 20.

Chapter 53 FROST-BITE
[1] J.M. LeBlanc, Canadian Journal of Biochemical Physiology, Vol. 32, 1954, 407.

Chapter 54 GALL BLADDER PROBLEMS
[1] H. Dam et al, Acta Physiology Scandinavia, Vol. 36, 1956, 329.
[2] F. Christenson et al, Acta Physiology, Scandinavia, Vol. 30, 1952, 256.

Chapter 55 GAS, INTESTINAL

Chapter 56 GLAUCOMA
[1] The Encyclopedia of Common Diseases (Emmaus, PA: Rodale Press, Inc., 1976), 661-663.
[2] Linus Pauling, How to Live Longer and Feel Better (New York, NY: W.H. Freeman and Co., 1987), 281.
[3] The Encyclopedia of Common Diseases (Emmaus, PA: Rodale Press, Inc., 1976), 663.

Chapter 57   GOUT
[1] J.I. Rodale, The Complete Book of Food and Nutrition (Emmaus, PA: Rodale Press, Inc., 1961), 188-89.
[2] Jean Carper, The Food Pharmacy (New York, NY: Bantam Books, (1988), 282.

Chapter 58   GUMS AND TOOTH SOCKET PROBLEMS
[1] Mark Bricklin, The Practical Encyclopedia of Natural Healing (Emmaus, PA: Rodale Press, Inc., 1983), 492.
[2] Ibid.
[3] Ibid.
[4] Ibid.
[5] Ibid.
[6] Ibid, 493.
[7] Ibid.
[8] Ibid.
[9] The Complete Book of Vitamins (Emmaus, PA: Rodale Press, Inc., 1977), 136.
[10] James F. Scheer, "Stress and Dental Ailments," Bestways, January, 1984, 16.
[11] Ibid.
[12] Ibid.
[13] Ibid.
[14] Ibid.
[15] News Feature, University of Southern California News Source, January, 1987.
[16] Ibid.
[17] Ibid.
[18] Ibid.
[19] Ibid.
[20] Ibid.

Chapter 59   HANDS PAINFUL, TINGLING (CARPAL TUNNEL SYNDROME)
[1] Jeffrey Bland, 1984-85 Yearbook of Nutritional Medicine (New Canaan, CT: Keats Publishing, Inc., 1985), 6.
[2] Jeffrey Bland, Nutraerobics (San Francisco: Harper & Row, 1983), 56.
[3] Jeffrey Bland, 1984-85 Yearbook of Nutritional Medicine (New Canaan, CT: Keats Publishing, Inc., 1985), 6.
[4] Jeffrey Bland, Medical Applications of Clinical Nutrition (New Canaan, CT: Keats Publishing, Inc., 1983), 56-57.
[5] Jeffrey Bland, Nutraerobics (San Francisco: Harper & Row, 1983), 56, 57.

Chapter 60   HEARING LOSS
[1] The Encyclopedia of Common Diseases (Emmaus, PA: Rodale Press, Inc., 1976), 516.
[2] Ibid, 517.
[3] Ibid, 506.
[4] Ibid.
[5] Ibid, 512.
[6] Science Digest, March, 1985, 28.
[7] The Encyclopedia of Common Diseases (Emmaus, PA: Rodale Press, Inc., 1976), 508.
[8] Ibid.
[9] Ibid.
[10] Patrick Quillin, Healing Nutrients (Chicago, IL: Contemporary Books, 1987), 393.
[11] Ibid.
[12] The Encyclopedia of Common Diseases (Emmaus, PA: Rodale Press, Inc., 1976), 507.
[13] The Complete Book of Vitamins (Emmaus, PA: Rodale Press, Inc., 1977), 128.
[14] The Encyclopedia of Common Diseases (Emmaus, PA: Rodale Press Inc., 1976), 507.
[15] Ibid.
[16] British Medical Journal, Vol. 283, July 25, 1981, 273-74.
[17] Ibid.
[18] Ibid.
[19] Ibid.

Chapter 61 HEART AILMENTS
[1] Patrick Quillin, Healing Nutrients (Chicago: Contemporary Books, 1987), 109.
[2] Stephen Langer and James F. Scheer, Solved: The Riddle of Illness (New Canaan, CT: Keats Publishing, Inc., 1984), 110.
[3] Stephen Langer and James F. Scheer, How to Win At weight Loss (Rochester, Vt.: Thorsons Publishers, 1987), 101.
[4] Ibid.
[5] Brian Leibovitz, Carnitine, The Vitamin B Phenomenon (New York, NY: Dell Publishing Co., Inc., 1984): 35.

Chapter 62 HEMORRHOIDS
[1] Edited by Jeffrey Bland, Medical Applications of Clinical Nutrition (New Canaan, CT: Keats Publishing, Inc., 1983), 279.
[2] Ibid.
[3] Ibid.
[4] The Encyclopedia of Common Diseases (Emmaus, PA: Rodale Press, Inc., 1976), 949.
[5] Ibid.
[6] Ibid.
[7] Ibid.
[8] Ibid.
[9] Ibid, 950.
[10] Ibid.
[11] R.E. Hodgen et al, American Journal of Clinical Nutrition, Vol. 11, No. 180, 1962, 187.
[12] Linus Pauling, How to Live Longer and Feel Better (New York, NY: W.H. Freeman & Co., 1986), 318.
[13] Ibid.

Chapter 63 HERPES SIMPLEX (INCLUDING GENITAL)
[1] Earl Mindell, Earl Mindell's Pill Bible (New York, NY: Paperbacker, 1988), 227.
[2] Ibid.
[3] Ibid.
[4] Conversation with Richard Kunin.
[5] Michael E. Rosembaum and Dominick Bosco, Super Fitness Beyond Vitamins (New York, NY: NAL Books, 1987), 64.
[6] Blair Justice, Who Get's Sick (Houston, TX.: Peak Press, 1987), 156.
[7] Ibid.
[8] Ibid.
[9] Emrika Padus, The Complete Guide to Your Emotions and Your Health (Emmaus, PA: Rodale Press, Inc., 1986), 584.

Chapter 64 HIATUS HERNIA
[1] Edited by Jeffrey Bland, Medical Applications of Clinical Nutrition (New Canaan, CT: Keats Publishing, Inc., 1983), 277.
[2] Ibid.
[3] Ibid.
[4] Robert W. Downs and Alice Van Baak, "When Heartburn Won't Go Away," Bestways, January, 1984, 38-42.
[5] Ibid.

Chapter 65 HICCUPS
[1] Mark Bricklin, The Practical Encyclopedia of Natural Healing (Emmaus, PA: Rodale Press, Inc., 1983), 287.

Chapter 66 HIGH BLOOD PRESSURE
[1] Robert H. Garrison and Elizabeth Somer, The Nutrition Desk Reference (New Canaan, CT: Keats Publishing, Inc., 1985), 159.
[2] Ibid.
[3] Ibid.
[4] Richard A. Kunin, Mega-Nutrition (New York: McGraw-Hill, 1980), 83.

[5] Elizabeth Barrett-Carmen and K.T. Khaw, American Journal of Clinical Nutrition, Vol. 39, 1984, 963-68.
[6] Ibid.
[7] O. Ophir et al, American Journal of Clinical Nutrition, Vol. 37, 1983, 755-762.
[8] The National and Nutrition Examination Survey, American Journal of Epidemiology, Vol. 120, 1984, 17-27.
[9] Science, 224 (4656) 1, 1984, 1392-98.
[10] J. Laragh and L.M. Resnick, Medical World News, March, 1985, 13-14.
[11] Nutrition Reviews, Vol. 42, 1984, 205-13: Nutrition Reviews, Vol. 42, 1984, 223-25.
[12] M.G. Sowers et al, "The Association of Intakes of Vitamin D and Calcium with Blood Pressure Among Women," American Journal of Clinical Nutrition, Vol. 42, 1985, 135-42.
[13] Ibid.
[14] B.M. Altura, B.T. Altura, "Magnesium Ions and Contraction of Vascular Smooth Muscles: Relationship to Some Vascular Diseases," Federal Proceedings, 40(12), 1981, 2672-9.
[15] Sciences, 223, 1984, 1315-17.
[16] Journal of the American College of Nutrition, 1, 1982, 317-322.
[17] Josef P. Krachovec, Keeping Young and Living Longer (Los Angeles: Sherbourne Press, Inc., 1972), 137-38.
[18] Mark Bricklin, The Practical Encyclopedia of Natural Healing (Emmaus, PA: Rodale Press, Inc., 1976), 58.
[19] Ibid, Revised Edition (1983), 59.

Chapter 67   HOARSENESS

[1] News Feature, "Handle Your Vocal Cords With Care," California State University, Carson, California, March 20, 1987.

Chapter 68   HYPERACTIVITY

[1] Carl C.Pfeiffer, Mental and Elemental Nutrients (New Canaan, CT: Keats Publishing, Inc., 1975): 412.
[2] Ibid., 413
[3] Ibid.
[4] Ibid.
[5] The Encyclopedia of Common Diseases (Emmaus, PA: Rodale Press, Inc., 1976): 64.
[6] Ibid.
[7] Carlton Fredericks, Carlton Fredericks' Nutrition Guide for the Prevention & Cure of Common Ailments and Diseases (New York: Simon & Schuster, 1982): 91-92.
[8] Ibid.
[9] James Braly, Dr. Braly's Optimum Health Program (New York: Times Books, 1985), 304.
[10] Richard Kunin, Mega-Nutrition (New York: McGraw-Hill, 1981), 143.
[11] Ibid., 144
[12] Carlton Fredericks, Carlton Fredericks' Nutrition Guide (New York: Simon & Schuster, 1982), 91.
[13] Alan Gaby, B-6, The Natural Healer (New Canaan, CT: Keats Publishing, Inc., 1984), 76.
[14] Stephen Langer and James F. Scheer, Solved: The Riddle of Illness (New Canaan, CT: Keats Publishing, Inc., 1984), 131, 132.
[15] Ibid., 132
[16] Ibid.
[17] Ibid.
[18] Matthew J. Venuti, "Behavioral Effects of Diet and Exercise on Seven Hyperactive and Emotionally Disturbed Children," Columbia Pacific University, August, 1983.

Chapter 69   IMMUNE SYSTEM PROBLEMS

[1] Robert H. Garrison, Jr. and Elizabeth Somer, The Nutrition Reference (New Canaan, CT: Keats Publishing, Inc., 1985), 277.
[2] Stephen Langer and James F. Scheer, How to Win at Weight Loss (Rochester, VT: Thorsons Publishers, Inc., 1987), 89.
[3] Ibid, 90.
[4] Ibid, 89.
[5] Ibid, 90.
[6] Science News, Vol 132, No. 3, July 18, 1987, 46.
[7] Ibid.

[8] Stephen Langer with James F. Scheer, How to Win at Weight Loss (Rochester, VT: Thorsons Publishers, Inc., 1987), 90.
[9] 1984-85 Yearbook of Nutritional Medicine (New Canaan, CT: Keats Publishing, Inc., 1985), 126.
[10] Stephen Langer with James F. Scheer, How To Win at Weight Loss (Rochester, VT: Thorsons Publishers, Inc., 1987), 91.
[11] Ibid.
[12] News Feature (AP), San Jose Mercury News, August 29, 1987, 2A.
[13] Ibid.
[14] Ibid.
[15] Blair Justice, Who Get's Sick (Houston: Peak Press, 1987), 158.
[16] James F. Scheer, "Positivism for Helping Cure Cancer," Bestways, July, 1986, 24.
[17] Blair Justice, Who Get's Sick (Houston: Peak Press, 1987), 232.

Chapter 70 IMPOTENCY
[1] "Diabetic Impotency: New Hope," (News Feature: Louis Lipson Interview) University of Southern California News Service, April, 1987.
[2] James F. Scheer, "Impotency: Not a Life Sentence," Bestways, May, 1986.
[3] Morton Walker and Joan Walker, Sexual Nutrition (New York: Coward-McCann, Inc., 1983), 225.
[4] Carl C. Pfeiffer, "Mental and Elemental Nutrients," (New Canaan, CT: Keats Publishing, Inc., 1975), 471.
[5] Personal Conversation with DeWayne Ashmead.
[6] Stephen Langer and James F. Scheer, How to Win at Weight Loss (Rochester, VT: Thorsons Publishers, Inc., 1987), 166.
[7] Personal Conversation with DeWayne Ashmead.
[8] Ibid.
[9] Carl C. Pfeiffer, Mental and Elemental Nutrients (New Canaan, CT: Keats Publishers, Inc., 1975), 282.
[10] Same as Number 1.

Chapter 71 INFERTILITY
[1] Patrick Quillin, Healing Nutrients (Chicago: Contemporary Books, 1987), 274.
[2] Mark Bricklin, The Practical Encyclopedia of Natural Healing (Emmaus, PA: Rodale Press, Inc., 1983), 303-4.
[3] Several clinical studies.
[4] Mark Bricklin, The Practical Encyclopedia of Natural Healing (Emmaus, PA: Rodale Press, Inc., 1983), 304.
[5] Ibid, 305.

Chapter 72 INTESTINAL (TOXICITY)
[1] British Journal of Nutrition, Vol. 52, No. 1, July, 1984, 97-105.
[2] Ibid.
[3] Ibid.

Chapter 73 ITCH (RECTAL)
[1] Mark Bricklin, The Practical Encyclopedia of Natural Healing (Emmaus, PA: Rodale Press, Inc., 1976): 303.

Chapter 74 JET LAG
[1] **Blair Justice, Who Get's Sick (Houston: Peak Press, 1987), 109.**

Chapter 75 LOW BLOOD PRESSURE
[1] A. Keys et al, "The Biology of Human Starvation," University of Minnesota Press, 1951; C.J. Tui, Clinical Nutrition, 11, 232, 1953 and J.A. Chazan et al, American Journal of Medicine, 34, 350, 1963.

Chapter 76 LOW BLOOD SUGAR (HYPOGLYCEMIA)
[1] Personal communication with Stephen Gyland, M.D.

Chapter 77 MEMORY LOSS
[1] The Complete Book of Vitamins (Emmaus, PA: Rodale Press, Inc., 1977), 162.
[2] Alan Donald, "How to Have and Keep a Better Memory," Bestways, July, 1987, 16.
[3] British Medical Journal, Vol. 5006, 1394-98.
[4] Blair Justice, Who Get's Sick (Houston: Peak Press, 1987), 110.
[5] Gary Null, The Complete Guide to Health and Nutrition (New York: Dell Publishing, Co., 1984), 423.

6 Stephen Langer with James F. Scheer, Solved: The Riddle of Illness (New Canaan, CT: Keats Publishing, Inc., 1984), 62-63.
7 Stephen Langer and James F. Scheer, How to Win at Weight Loss (Rochester, VT: Thorsons Publishers, Inc., 1987), 42.
8 Blair Justice, Who Get's Sick (Houston: Peak Press, 1987), 79-80.

Chapter 78 MENOPAUSE
1 C.J. Smith, "Non-Hormonal Control of Vasomotor Flushing in Menopause Patients," Chicago Medicine, March 7, 1964.
2 R. S. Finkler, "The Effect of Vitamin E on the Menopause", Journal of Clinical Endocrine Metabiology, Vol. 9, 1949, 89-94.
3 H. A. Gozen, "The Use of Vitamin E in Treatment of the Menopause", New York State Medical Journal, May 15, 1952, 1289-91.
4 N. R. Kavinsky, "Vitamin E and the Control of Climacteric Symptoms", Annals of Western Medicine and Surgery, Vol. 4, No. 1, 1950, 27-32.
5 The Complete Book of Vitamins (Emmaus, PA: Rodale Press, Inc., 1977), 483.
6 E.J. Christy, "Vitamin E in Menopause," American Journal of Obstetrics and Gynecology, Vol. 50, 1945, 84.
7 R. S. Finkler, "The Effect of Vitamin E on the Menopause", Journal of Clinical Endocrine Metabiology, Vol. 9, 1949, 89-94.

Chapter 79 MIGRAINES
1 Let's Live, March 1977, 110.
2 Ibid.
3 Ibid.
4 Eleonore Blaurock-Busch, "Holistic Help for Migraines", Bestways, July, 1984, 46.
5 Mark Bricklin, The Practical Encyclopedia of Natural Healing (Emmaus, PA: Rodale Press, Inc., 1983), 191.
6 Patrick Quillin, Healing Nutrients (Chicago: Contemporary Books, 1987), 233-34.
7 Mark Bricklin, The Practical Encyclopedia of Natural Healing (Emmaus, PA: Rodale Press, Inc., 1983), 192.
8 Harvard Medical School Health Letter, April, 1986, 6-7.
9 Mark Bricklin, The Practical Encyclopedia of Natural Healing (Emmaus, PA: Rodale Press, Inc., 1983), 192.
10 Ibid.

Chapter 80 MILK INTOLERANCE
1 Science News, Vol. 125, January 14, 1984, 26.

Chapter 81 MISCARRIAGE
1 Linus Pauling, How to Live Longer and Feel Better (New York: W. H. Freeman and Co., 1986), 358.
2 The Encyclopedia of Common Diseases (Emmaus, PA: Rodale Press Inc., 1976), 1026.
3 Edited by J.I. Rodale, The Health Finder (Emmaus, PA: Rodale Press, Inc., 1954), 918-919.
4 Ibid.
5 The Encyclopedia of Common Diseases (Emmaus, PA: Rodale Press, Inc., 1976), 1028-29.
6 Ibid, 1027, 28.

Chapter 82 MONONUCLEOSIS
1 This entire section is based on a TV Interview conducted with Robert Cathcart, M.D. in August, 1988.

Chapter 83 MOTION SICKNESS
1 Patrick Quillin, Healing Nutrients (Chicago: Contemporary Books, 1987), 394.
2 Personal Interview

Chapter 84 OSTEOMALACIA
1 Science News, June 4, 1983, 364.
2 Ibid.
3 Ibid.
4 Science News, June 4, 1983, 364.
5 Ibid.

Chapter 85 OSTEOPOROSIS

[1] Robert W. Downs with Alice Van Baak, "Calcium Balance: Tipping the Scales in Your Favor", Bestways, May, 1984, 18.
[2] Ibid.
[3] Ibid, 20.
[4] Robert W. Downs with Alice Van Baak, "Osteoporosis Update", Bestways, June, 1985, 10.
[5] Ibid.
[6] Los Angeles Times, June 25, 1986, Part II.
[7] Ibid.
[8] Ibid.
[9] Ibid.
[10] Robert W. Downs with Alice Van Baak, "Osteoporosis Update", Bestways, June, 1985, 10.
[11] Gary Null, The Complete Guide to Health and Nutrition (New York: Dell Publishing, Inc., 1984), 389.
[12] Mark Bricklin, The Practical Encyclopedia of Natural Healing Emmaus, PA: Rodale Press, Inc., 1983), 71.
[13] Ibid.
[14] F. Lengemann et al, Journal of Nutrition, Vol. 14, 1964, 98.
[15] Gary and Steve Null, Alcohol and Nutrition (New York: Pyramid, 1977), 59.
[16] Adelle Davis, Let's Get Well (New York: Harcourt, Brace and World, 1965), 170.
[17] John Kirschman with Lavon J. Dunne, Nutrition Almanac (New York: McGraw-Hill, 1984), 107.
[18] Gary Null, The Complete Guide to Health and Nutrition (New York: Dell Publishing, Inc., 1984), 388.
[19] Robert W. Downs with Alice Van Baak, "Calcium Balance", Bestways, May, 1984, 20.
[20] Ibid, 21.
[21] Mark Bricklin, The Practical Encyclopedia of Natural Healing (Emmaus, PA: Rodale Press, Inc., 1983), 70.
[22] James F. Scheer, "New Enemy of Osteoporosis," Bestways, March, 1988, 20.
[23] Science News, June 4, 1983, 367.

Chapter 86 OVERWEIGHT (HOW TO BE A GOOD LOSER)
[1] Journal of the Louisiana State Medical Society (1985): 137 (6): 35-8.
[2] Ibid.
[3] Ibid.
[4] Ibid.

Chapter 87 PREMENSTRUAL SYNDROME
[1] Los Angeles Times, August 16, 1984, Part VIII, 8.
[2] Ibid.
[3] Ibid.
[4] Ibid.
[5] Ibid.
[6] Ibid.
[7] Ibid.
[8] Ibid.
[9] Ibid.
[10] M.G. Brush, "Efamol in Treatment of the Premenstrual Syndrome", Report for St. Thomas Hospital Medical School, London.
[11] V.L. Pashby, "A Clinical Trial of Evening Primrose Oil (Efamol) in Mastalgia", presented at the British Surgical Research Society, Cardiff (Wales) meeting, July, 1981.
[12] Robert W. Downs with Alice Van Baak, "Natural Ways to Beat Premenstrual Tension", Bestways, December, 1983, 33.
[13] Ibid, 34.
[14] Ibid.

Chapter 88 PROSTATE PROBLEMS
[1] Sharon Faelten, The Complete Book of Minerals for Health (Emmaus, PA: Rodale Books, 1981), 427-28.
[2] Ibid, 429.
[3] Ibid.
[4] Ibid.
[5] Ibid.
[6] Jonathan Wright, Dr. Wright's Book of Nutritional Therapy (Emmaus, PA: Rodale Press, Inc., 1979), 283.

[7] James P. Hart and William L. Cooper, "Vitamin E in the Treatment of Prostate Hypertrophy", Lee Foundation for Nutritional Research, Milwaukee, WI, Report No. 1, November, 1941, 1-10.
[8] Jonathan Wright, Dr. Wright's Book of Nutritional Therapy (Emmaus, PA: Rodale Press Inc., 1979), 281.
[9] Sharon Faelten, The Complete Book of Minerals for Health (Emmaus, PA: Rodale Books, 1981), 428.
[10] Ibid.
[11] Ibid.

Chapter 89 PSORIASIS
[1] The Encyclopedia of Common Diseases (Emmaus, PA: Rodale Press, Inc., 1976), 443.
[2] Cutis (34:497).
[3] The Encyclopedia of Common Diseases (Emmaus, PA: Rodale Press, Inc., 1976), 443.
[4] News Feature, Royal Hallamshire Hospital, Sheffield, England, April, 1988.
[5] Ibid.
[6] News Story, University of California, March, 1988.
[7] P. Gross et al, "The Treatment of Psoriasis as a Disturbance of Lipid Metabolism", New York State Journal of Medicine, (1950) 50: 2683-86.

Chapter 90 SHINGLES (HERPES ZOSTER)
[1] A. K. Gupta, H. S. Mital, India Practitioners, July, 1967.
[2] Ibid.
[3] Fred Klenner, "The Treatment of Poliomyelitis and other Virus Diseases with Vitamin C," Southern Medicine and Surgery, Vol. 111, 1949, 209-14.
[4] Journal des Practiciens, Vol. 64, 1950, 586.
[5] K. Mikan, S. Ayers, "Post Herpes Zoster Neuralgia: Response to Vitamin E Therapy", Archives of Dermatology, December, 1973.
[6] T. Cochrane, "Post Herpes Neuralgia: Response to Vitamin E Therapy", Archives of Dermatology, Vol. 111, 1975, 396.
[7] Ibid.
[8] Ibid.

Chapter 91 SKIN IRRITATIONS

Chapter 92 SLEEPLESSNESS (INSOMNIA)
[1] Blair Justice, Who Gets Sick (Houston: Peak Press, 1987): 114.
[2] Journal of the American Medical Association, March 14, 1980.

Chapter 93 SMELL AND TASTE LOSS
[1] Popular Science, August, 1982, 8-9.
[2] Ibid.
[3] Ibid.
[4] Nature, Vol. 191, 1969, 1310.
[5] Ibid.
[6] Science News Letter, October 7, 1961.
[7] Popular Science, August, 1982, 8-9.
[8] Ibid.
[9] Stephen Davies, "Zinc and Special Senses," 1984-85 Yearbook of Nutritional Medicine (New Canaan, CT: Keats Publishing, Inc., 1985), 129.
[10] Jeffrey Bland, Nutraerobics (San Francisco: Harper & Row, 1983), 232.
[11] Biological Trace Elements Research, June/September, 1982.
[12] Ibid.

Chapter 94 SMOKING
[1] Karen Owens, "Beware of Second Hand Smoke", KA Owens & Associates, Public Relations, October, 1987.
[2] James F. Scheer, "Second Hand Smoke: Silent Saboteur", Bestways, November, 1987, 16.
[3] James F. Scheer, "Second Hand Smoke Can Be a Killer", Bestways, June, 1984, 18.
[4] Ibid.
[5] Ibid.
[6] Ibid.
[7] Journal of the American Medical Association, Vol. 254, October, 1985, 2271.

[8] Ibid.
[9] Orange County, California Register, August 10, 1983, Part A, 20.
[10] Ibid.
[11] Psychology Today, April, 1985, 14.
[12] Ibid.
[13] Ibid.
[14] Ibid.
[15] Harold J. Taub, "Better Protection for Smokers' Lungs", Let's LIVE, March, 1976, 8.
[16] Ibid, 10.
[17] Karen Owens, "Beware of Second Hand Smoke", KA Owens & Associates, Public Relations, October, 1987.
[18] Ibid.
[19] Harold J. Taub, "Better Protection for Smokers Lungs", Let's Live, March, 1976, 10.
[20] Ibid, 12.
[21] Personal Conversation.
[22] Ibid.

Chapter 95   SNORING

Chapter 96   STRESS
[1] Suzanne Kobasa, "Stressful Life Events, Personality, and Health", Journal of Personalty and Social Psychology, Vol. 27, No. 1, 1984, 1-11.
[2] Suzanne Kobasa, Salvadore Maddi, and S. Courington, "Personality and Constitution as Mediators in the Stress-Illness Relationship," Journal of Health and Social Behavior, 22, 368.
[3] Ibid.
[4] Ibid.
[5] S. C. Kobasa (1982 a), "Commitment and Coping in Stress Resistance Among Lawyers," Journal of Personality and Social Psychology, Vol 42., No. 1, 707-77.
[6] S. E. Locke et al, "Life Change Stress, Psychiatric Symptoms and Natural Killer Cells Activity," Psychosomatic Medicine, Vol. 46, No. 5, 441-453.

Chapter 97   STRETCH MARKS
[1] Carl C. Pfeiffer, Mental and Elemental Nutrients (New Canaan, CT: Keats Publishing, Inc., 1975), 231.
[2] Ibid.

Chapter 98   TEETH GRINDING (BRUXISM)

Chapter 99   THYROID FUNCTION, HIGH (HYPERTHYROIDISM)
[1] Isobel Jennings, Vitamins In Endocrine Metabolism (Springfield, Illinois: Charles C. Thomas, 1970), 99.
[2] Ibid., 31
[3] Ibid.
[4] Ibid.
[5] Ibid.
[6] Ibid.

Chapter 100   THYROID FUNCTION, LOW (HYPOTHYROIDISM)
[1] Stephen Langer and James F. Scheer, Solved: The Riddle of Illness (New Canaan, CT: Keats Publishing, Inc., 1984), 13.
[2] Ibid., 2-3.
[3] Personal communication
[4] Stephen Langer and James F. Scheer, Solved: The Riddle of Illness (New Canaan, CT: Keats Publishing, Inc., 1984), 27-32.
[5] Ibid., 27-28.
[6] Ibid., 28.
[7] Ibid.
[8] Ibid.
[9] Ibid., 28, 29.
[10] Ibid., 29.
[11] Ibid., 29, 30.
[12] Ibid., 30.
[13] Ibid., 25, 31, 32.

[14] Ibid.
[15] Ibid.

Chapter 101   TOOTH DECAY
[1] Letter from Cheryl Hirsch Associates (Public Relations), Sherman Oaks, CA, April 17, 1986.

Chapter 102   TOOTH, KNOCKED OUT
[1] "Coping With Knocked Out Teeth," News Story, University of Florida, July 2, 1982.

Chapter 103   ULCERS, STOMACH
[1] Catharyn Elwood, Feel Like a Million (New York: Pocket Books, 1968): 229-30.
[2] G. Cheney et al, "Anti-peptic Ulcer Dietary Factor, Vitamin 'U' in the Treatment of Peptic Ulcer", Journal of the American Dietetic Association, Vol. 26, 1950, 668-672.
[3] Ibid.
[4] Ralph Best et al, "The Anti-Ulcerogenic Activity of the Unripe Plantain Bananas", British Journal of Pharmacology, Vol.82, 1984, 107-116.
[5] Ibid.
[6] UCI Journal, University of California, Irvine, Summer, 1986, 2-3.
[7] Ibid.
[8] A. Rydning et al, "Prophylactic Effect of Dietary Fiber in Duodenal Ulcer Diseases, Lancet, Vol. 2, 1982, 736-39.

Chapter 104   VAGINITIS

Chapter 105   VITILIGO
[1] Paavo Airola, "Biological Medicine: Vitiligo," Let's LIVE, December, 1977, 49.
[2] Ibid., 50.
[3] Ibid.
[4] Ibid.
[5] Ibid.
[6] Personal communication.
[7] Paavo Airola, "Biological Medicine: Vitiligo," Let's LIVE, December, 1977, 50, 51.
[8] Ibid., 51.
[9] Carl C. Pfeiffer, Mental and Elemental Nutrients (New Canaan, CT: Keats Publishing, Inc., 1975): 183.

Chapter 106   WARTS
[1] Daniel Hyman, Modern Medicine, August 1, 1975, 22.
[2] Ibid.

Chapter 107   WATER RETENTION

Chapter 108   WRINKLES
[1] H.L. Newbold, Mega-Nutrients (Los Angeles: The Body Press, 1987): 347.
[2] Ibid., 346.
[3] Robert H. Garrison, Jr. and Elizabeth Somer, The Nutrition Desk Reference (New Canaan, CT: Keats Publishing, Inc., 1985): 159.
[4] John Yiamouyiannis, Fluoride: The Aging Factor (Delaware, Ohio: Health Action Press, 1983): 4.
[5] Ibid.
[6] Ibid., 41, 42.
   K.H. Neldner, Geriatrics, Vol. 39, February, 1984, 69.
[8] Rebecca James, "The Moisturizer of the Future," Bestways, September, 1987, 22-24.
[9] Hans Selye, "Calciphylaxis," University of Chicago Press, Chicago, Illinois, 1962.
[10] Adelle Davis, Let's Get Well (New York: Harcourt, Brace & World, 1965): 155.

INDEX

nutrition-oriented doctor required to guide recovery, 347
salt and water increase blood volume and pressure, 346
starvation diets, a major cause, 346
low blood sugar, 349-354
  causes:
  acute need for pantothenic acid, 347
  faulty use of carbohydrates, 349
  low thyroid function, 350
  cope with many small meals, 352
  symptoms, 351

M
memory loss, 355-358
  diminishing memory not always a symptom of Alzheimer's disease, 358
  lecithin improves memory of Alzheimer's disease patients, 356
  low blood sugar and low thyroid make brain sluggish, 357
  stress diminishes memory, 357
  undernutrition, most likely cause, 355
menopause (change of life), 359-362
  Carlton Fredericks' regimen to cope with syptoms, 360
  vitamin E reduces symptoms, 359
  vitamin E oil lubricates dried vaginal tissue, 361
methylxanthines, 99
migraines, 363-366
  feverfew, helps in coping, 365, 366
  symptoms, 363
  triggers for, 364
  estrogen and the Pill, 365
  foods, 364
  low blood sugar, 364
  refined sugar, 364
  sticky blood platelets, 364-365
milk intolerance, 367-369
  cause: inability to produce enzyme lactase to process milk sugar, 36
  solutions, 367
  yogurt, sometimes tolerated, 367
milk (skim)
  for lowering cholesterol, 167
miscarriage, 370-74
  are spontaneous abortions nature's way of rejecting a defective fetus?, 371
  bioflavonoids help prevent, shown by experiments, 371
  smoking women have 50% more miscarriages, 372
mononucleosis, 375-378
  Cathcart strategy, 375
  massive doses of vitamin C, 375, 376
motion sickness and morning sickness, 376-377
  gingerroot capsules win competition against Dramamine for motion sickness, 379
  scores with morning sickness as well, 379

N
near-sightedness, 240
night blindness, 238, 239
noise pollution, 282, 283

O
oat bran, 75, 193
olive oil
  for lowering cholesterol, 168

omega-3 oil, 404
onions
  for lowering cholesterol, 168
osteomalacia, 380-384
  40% of osteomalacia patients were found to be vitamin D deficient, 380, 381
  tennis players in the 55-65 age group had far more bone mass than non exercisers, 381
osteoporosis, 385-391
  best time to beat: teen years, 386, 387
  boron preserves bone calcium, 390
  calcium thieves, 388, 389
  exercise: bone-builder, 391
  higher calcium intake of teenage girls, the more retained, 387
overweight, 392, 393
  reverse system works with no calorie change: heaviest meal in morning, lightest at night, 392, 393

P

plantains, anti-ulcer treatment, 459
  for lowering cholesterol, 168
potato (red)
  for bruise healing, 410, 411
premenstrual syndrome (PMS), 392-397
  danger of over-dieting, 394
  evening primrose oil scores with PMS sufferers, 396
  junk foods must be junked, 395
prostate problems, 398-402
  enlargement makes cancer more likely, 399
  high fat refined food diet encourages cancer, 400
  pumpkin seeds folk remedy often reduces enlargement, 400
  risks of orthodox treatement, 398
  symptoms, 398
  zinc low in prostate patients, 399
psoriasis, 403-405
  causes: arachidonic acid, 403
  gluten, 403
  stress, 403
  lecithin helped patients recover, 404
  omega-3 oil gave relief, 404

R

Rankin method of managing bulimia, 112-114
rectal bleeding, 293-294
rectal itch, 340-343
retinitis pigmentosa, 234
rheumatoid arthritis, 55-63
Rinkel's diversified diet for allergy detection, 23

S

salivary gland cancer, 274
seaweed
  for lowering cholesterol, 168
second-hand smoke, 422, 424
serotonin, 413
shingles (herpes zoster), 406-408
  injected vitamin B-12 scored quick gains, 407
  injected vitamin C dried up rash, 407
  Jonathan Wright's do-it-yourself salve, 406
  orthodox measures limited, 406

522

MAUREEN KENNEDY SALAMAN
"A Speaker of Attraction"

Maureen Kennedy Salaman is a unique combination of talents and capabilities that have impacted the readers of her books, articles, plus her tapes, television, and live audiences around the world.

She is not only an award winning writer, but a speaker of extraordinary ability. Maureen has shared the wisdom, wit and insight of her health and motivational messages at over one thousand engagements in the last two decades and in over 300 cities around the country and around the world!

As a dynamic performer, she communicates a totally positive approach to health and problem solving, and helps listeners program their lives with strategies for healthy and successful living.

She is in touch with the wellness challenges confronting people everyday. Most importantly, she is able to share, through research and experience, what works and what doesn't, and why.

She has the unique ability to hold an audience's attention for an hour or an entire day by involving the group with the questions which they are the most concerned. She covers a wide variety of action oriented presentations, ranging from "Conquering Cravings" to "Correcting Hair Loss" to "Breaking the Bondage of Addiction."

Her special anointing is in communicating her totally positive approach to Christian audiences. The secular and business world respect her as a communicator of extraordinary ability.

To bring Maureen Salaman's life enhancing message to your church, or company, or to order her tapes or books, contact:

M.K.S., Inc.
1259 El Camino Real, Suite 1500
Menlo Park, CA 94025
Telephone: (415) 854-9355
FAX: (415) 854-9292